The Custom-Made Child?
WOMEN-CENTERED PERSPECTIVES

CONTEMPORARY ISSUES IN BIOMEDICINE, ETHICS, AND SOCIETY

Birth Control and Controlling Birth, edited by **Helen B. Holmes, Betty B. Hoskins,** and **Michael Gross**, 1980

The Custom-Made Child?, edited by **Helen B. Holmes, Betty B. Hoskins,** and **Michael Gross**, 1981

Medical Responsibility, edited by **Wade L. Robison** and **Michael Pritchard**, 1979

Contemporary Issues in Biomedical Ethics, edited by **John W. Davis, Barry Hoffmaster,** and **Sarah Shorten**, 1979

THE CUSTOM-MADE CHILD?

Women-Centered Perspectives

Edited by
Helen B. Holmes, Betty B. Hoskins, and
Michael Gross

The HUMANA Press Inc. · Clifton, New Jersey

The present work is one of two thoughtfully enhanced and carefully edited volumes that emerged from the conference on Ethical Issues in Human Reproduction Technology: Analysis by Women, held in June 1979 at Hampshire College in Amherst, Massachusetts.

ISBN: 0-89603-024-5 (hardcover); 089603-025-3 (paperback).

"This book was prepared with the support of NSF Grant #0SS 78 24508. However, any opinions, findings, conclusions, and/or recommendations herein are those of the authors and do not necessarily reflect the views of the NSF, The Federation of Organizations for Professional Women, or the Editors."

Library of Congress Cataloging in Publication Data

Main entry under title:

The Custom-made child.

(Contemporary issues in biomedicine, ethics, and society)

"The present work is one of two . . . volumes that emerged from the conference on ethical issues in human reproductive technology: analysis by women, held in June 1979 at Hampshire College in Amherst, Massachusetts."

Includes bibliographical references and index.

1. Obstetrics—Technological innovations—Congresses. 2. Diethylstilbestrol—Side effects—Congresses. 3. Prenatal diagnosis—Congresses. 4. Infants (Newborn)—Congresses. 5. Sex—Cause and determination—Congresses.

6. Feminism—Congresses. I. Holmes, Helen B. II. Hoskins, Betty B. III. Gross, Michael, 1948- IV. Series.

RG526.C87 174'.2 80-83824

ISBN 0-89603-024-5

ISBN 0-89603-025-3 (pbk.)

CONTENTS

The Neonate

Sex Preselection

Manipulative Reproductive Technologies

Preface

Women most fully experience the consequences of human reproductive technologies. Men who convene to evaluate such technologies discuss *"them"*: the women who must accept, avoid, or even resist these technologies; the women who consume technologies they did not devise; the women who are the objects of policies made by men. So often the input of women is neither sought nor listened to. The privileged insights and perspectives that women bring to the consideration of technologies in human reproduction are the subject of these volumes, which constitute the revised and edited record of a Workshop on "Ethical Issues in Human Reproduction Technology: Analysis by Women" (EIRTAW), held in June, 1979, at Hampshire College in Amherst, Massachusetts.

Some 80 members of the workshop, 90 percent of them women (from 24 states), represented diverse occupations and personal histories, different races and classes, varied political commitments. They included doctors, nurses, and scientists, lay midwives, consumer advocates, historians, and sociologists, lawyers, policy analysts, and ethicists. Each session, however, made plain that ethics is an everyday concern for women in general, as well as an academic profession for some.

The conference displayed the power of intense thought, motivated by passionate commitments—to other women, to free and rational inquiry, to the urgency of political action. The most carefully textured philosophical analyses were informed by felt experiences of pain and joy, anger and pleasure, frustration and satisfaction. The most impassioned calls for action were grounded in searching analysis. Yet across barriers, including age, class, race, status, training, sexuality, and politics, women talked together in mutual appreciation.

Early during the Workshop, members of each topic subgroup met together. These new colleagues, most of whom had never met each other in person, discussed the contents of each others' papers and planned together for the session that their subgroup would present. The Workshop was structured around eight sessions: contraception; Depo-Provera and sterilization abuse; diethylstilbestrol (DES); childbirth; prenatal diagnosis; neonatology; sex preselection; and such manipulative reproductive technologies as in vitro fertilization, egg fusion, and cell manipulation. A session on policy became devoted largely to balloting on specific resolutions. Each session here occupies a chapter that includes a brief summary overview of the topic in relation to the work of the panel, followed by the panel's technical, interpretive, and ethical papers. Each chapter concludes with panelists' formal responses to papers and the ensuing (edited) discussion.

Speakers and respondents were asked to direct their remarks toward the specific goals of the Workshop. These goals are:

1. To identify the ethical issues involved in setting priorities in research on human reproduction and in the application of such research.
2. To determine which values have heretofore been considered in resolution of conflicts.
3. To discover any alternative applicable social values that are now being offered by women.
4. To recommend new approaches for assessing values and determining policy.

As befitted a woman-planned, woman-oriented, and woman-conducted conference, the organization and format departed significantly from established practice. In the selection of participants, conventional academic qualifications weighed no more than deep concern, demonstrated interest, and previous personal experience. Each person had a place on the program and received the same honorarium. So that financial status would be less a factor in determining who could come, travel, board, and room were furnished to all. In the same spirit, participants provided for the conference directory a brief biography with suffficient personal background to acquaint participants with one another beyond their specific occupation or credentials.

The aim of many conferences and their ensuing proceedings is to reach closure and to arrive at a level of consistency and agreement. However the principles underlying both this Workshop and these volumes differ from such conventional practice. For decades men have been making decisions in the area of human reproduction technology: women have not been heard from. Hence, the purpose of the Workshop was not to resolve issues but, quite the contrary, to begin the discussion. It aimed to bring forth differences that heretofore had remained unexpressed and, in particular, to highlight the diversity of views that emerges from the varied experiences and situations of women. Therefore, in editing materials for publication, we guided ourselves primarily by the principle of remaining faithful to all contributors' intentions and, insofar as it allowed for a readable and coherent volume, to their exact language. For that very reason we considered but rejected the alternative possibility of a shorter, highly synthesized volume derivative from the multiplicity of views and approaches in the conference.

We intend that the completeness of this work will enhance its interest and usefulness. The technical papers have been written in such a way as to communicate expert information to the layperson, and we hope thereby to reach a wide audience, especially women and readers interested in women's studies. Yet these volumes will have particular interest as well for such professionals as providers of health care and social services, philosophers, and bioethicists. Beyond their immediate topical interest, these books become a critical historical document reflecting the development, at this time, of women's thought. Of most immediate practical importance, however, is that they make available to ethicists and policymakers women's views that hitherto have been ignored. Furthermore, this work establishes the urgency of incorporating many more women into all ethical and policy deliberations on issues of human reproduction.

Helen B. Holmes
Betty B. Hoskins
Michael Gross

Acknowledgments

The EIRTAW workshop climaxed four years of planning, starting with a small group of women who met for the first time at the Workshop on Medical Ethics at Manhattanville College, in June 1975 [sponsored by the Institute of Society, Ethics and the Life Sciences (The Hastings Center), Hastings-on-Hudson, NY]. I am grateful for the inspiration and impetus from those women. The Program in "Ethics and Values in Science and Technology" (EVIST) of the National Science Foundation (NSF) and the National Endowment for the Humanities co-funded the workshop. The Ford Foundation agreed to add supplemental funds as we sought to increase minority representation among the prospective participants. The NSF also funded editorial and clerical work toward the preparation of these volumes. The keen interest and encouragement of the EVIST Program Directors, first Dr. William Blanpied and, recently, Dr. Arthur Norberg, meant a great deal. Criticisms and suggestions by anonymous reviewers of the proposal contributed to the outcome of the project. Dr. Linda Atkinson and Ms. Jacki Ans of the Ford Foundation facilitated discussions with that organization.

Concrete assistance from officers of the Association for Women in Science—Dr. Judith Ramaley, Dr. Anne Briscoe, and Dr. Ellen Weaver—helped get the project rolling at its commencement. Later, our sponsor, the Federation of Organizations for Professional Women, gave indispensable aid: its officers, Dr. Naomi McAfee, Dr. Julia Lear, Ms. Ilene Wolcott, and Dr. Margaret Dunkle; and those who handled our finances so expertly, Ms. Louise Ott, Ms. Carolyn Feinglass, and Ms. Ruth Scott. Dr. Marie Cassidy, who served as the official representative of the Federation, handled critical paperwork in Washington, DC, which was crucial to the success of this project.

Useful suggestions in composing the grant proposal came from Dr. Malcolm Willison, Ms. Melissa Fountain, Dr. Mila Aroskar, and Dr. Judith Ramaley. From the Hastings Center Dr. Daniel Callahan, Ms. Margaret Steinfels, and Dr. Rosalind Petchesky gave useful advice during early planning stages. Dr. Robert Murray, Jr., Dr. Charles Lance, Dr. Joan Sieber, and Dr. Sally Kohlsted also helped in early shaping of the project. During the workshop, at its conclusion, and in a post-conference followup report, our evaluators—Dr. Ben Barker-Benfield, Dr. Claudia Card, and Dr. Maureen Flannery—offered keen insights and useful criticisms.

I am especially indebted to the dedication and creativity of Co-Director Dr. Janice Raymond, and the devotion and hard work of my interdisciplinary advisory planning and executive committee: Dr. Michael Gross (history of science), Dr. Betty Hoskins (biology and bioethics), Ms. Gerene Major (nursing), Ms. Norma Swenson (women's health and sociology), and Dr. Caroline Whitbeck (philosophy). Committee members, joined by Dr. Marie

Cassidy, organized the panels, playing a principal role in the selection, and at times the recruitment, of its members, and in the advance coordination of their presentations. In addition, the convener of each panel gathered the papers for this publication, undertook their initial editing, and contributed a summary overview.

The creation and execution of the Workshop and the preparation of these books would have been literally impossible without the dedicated labor and loyalty of Ms. Flora Johnson Josephs, Administrative Assistant. Her enthusiasm and spontaneous contributions went far beyond any reasonable expectations. Our Conference Assistants, Ms. Vivian Gabor and Ms. Julie Melrose, gave competent assistance during the Workshop, transcribed Workshop discussions, and typed early drafts of many manuscripts. Ms. Gale Storum's help with final manuscript preparation was indispensable. We are also grateful to the people at Humana Press for their kind assistance throughout the period of the book's accouchement.

Associate Editors, Dr. Michael Gross and Dr. Betty Hoskins, devoted long hours of painstaking, dedicated attention to each and every manuscript, with deep concern that each author's own ideas would come across clearly to our readers. Despite all this good advice, in a controversial, developing area such as this, errors, indiscretions, misinterpretations, and awkwardnesses invariably slip in. For them I take responsibility.

Finally, this project would have been totally impossible without the dedicated support and loyalty of my husband, Francis. Besides such customary husbandly duties as preparing meals, keeping the household running, and typing, he became a cheerful and competent volunteer whenever there was a deadline or job to do and no one to do it: providing office assistance before imminent deadlines, chauffering, advancing funds, proofreading, and reviewing of proposals and manuscripts. Whenever there were rejections, frustrations, disappointments, or cutting criticisms, his encouragement spurred me on and raised my spirits.

Helen B. Holmes

Reproductive Technologies

The Birth of a Women-Centered Analysis

Helen B. Holmes

Women have been the bearers of the next generation since human beings first existed. Yet today human reproduction hardly seems to be a natural process—a clutter of biomedical technology surrounds it. Drugs, devices, and instruments besiege us—to block or ease conception; to foster or terminate gestation; to monitor or hasten birth. And recently emerging uses of technology include the design of progeny to meet specifications, as well as the creation of embryos outside the human body.

Vast sums of money are spent in the development and marketing of such technologies. The public is expected to absorb these costs and to generate profits, but the public at large may not benefit. Sophisticated treatments may be available only to the rich, to the well-insured, or to the experimented-upon poor. Meanwhile even minimal medical care is unavailable to many ordinary people. Moreover, some do not know how to seek what is there, and others cannot afford what they find.

Women, although they are the principal consumers of reproductive technologies, have scarcely been involved in making the decisions about which technologies to develop and when and where to deploy them. The collective impact of the accounts of these technologies unveils a picture of inappropriate and distorted priorities, as will be seen in texts of the articles here printed. Our focus on the issues is entirely different from the usual one. Many questions that society considers to be major issues and dilemmas dissolve when the underlying patriarchal assumptions are brought to light, only to reveal entirely different sorts of questions.

The following synthesis is based on an analysis of some key ideas from the thoughtful papers and stimulating discussions presented in these books. I have tried to reflect accurately many of the valuable insights of our authors. However, I take full responsibility for my choice of the points to enlarge upon and, insofar as I have gone beyond their data, for my interpretations, my inferences, and my opinions. I shall begin with one example of the way in which women's perspectives evoke new questions. Next I shall enumerate existing values motivating the use of reproductive technologies and then shall present alternative values offered in the contributions to these volumes.

THE NEED FOR A NEW APPROACH

A contraceptive drug or device is developed to be powerful and effective. It is deemed essential that it be easy enough for use by poor women and women in developing nations who are judged to be the cause of overpopulation. It has a raft of side effects: documented immediate effects and suspected long-range effects, some inconvenient, some debilitating, some lethal. Currently society approaches the decision of whether to deploy this drug or device with a risk/benefit calculus such as this: the risk of death in childbirth for this population is greater than the risk of death from the contraceptive. Or, overall, the benefit to society from having fewer poor persons is greater than the benefit to society from avoiding morbidity among poor women.

We detected other motivations behind such an analysis. To us, mortality risks in childbirth and mortality risks from contraception do not belong in the same equation. They are not parts of the same dilemma.

In some cultures the risk of a woman's dying in childbirth is simply a necessary assumable risk. For her, the production of a child may well lead to her receipt of financial benefits from a man, to a rise in her social status, to support in her old age, and to the joy of having someone totally dependent on her for a few years.

In our analysis we approach the childbirth mortality problem in a variety of ways: on the one hand, through such policies as better prenatal care, health and nutrition education, training of midwives; on the other hand, through expanding opportunities for women by creating new ways for legitimating women's existence. *Our* ethical question would begin with individual respect: Which approaches are best for the women concerned? What do the women themselves want? Which methods would have the most input and leadership from the women at risk? Which choices would involve the least outside control from (male-dominated) political and business interests?

As for the question of risk from the contraceptive itself, in no way would we as women analysts condone the chance of death or disability in the service of contraception. Nor are women willing to accept what have been quoted as "inconveniences" (such as a disrupted menstrual cycle, loss of libido, a perforated uterus) as side effects of contraception. Furthermore, potential dangers to a fetus in case a woman happens to be pregnant when she receives the drug or device must not be risked. And a drug powerful enough to stop fertility should never be taken by a nursing mother.

Our values here are total—physical, mental, emotional—health and well-being, and concern for future generations.

Thus it is often clear that old questions are not valid questions to our participants, and that nonmeaningful values are being weighted heavily in the traditional methods of analysis. Now I shall point out those values that actually motivate current decision-making and then shall clarify our own set of values in order to define issues in new terms.

EXISTING VALUES

What are the desirable and worthwhile principles that heretofore have been considered in the resolution of ethical conflicts and in the setting of policy in reproductive technologies? Standard lists include: honesty, promise-keeping, truth-telling, justice, loyalty to patients, impartiality, obligations, and duties. I do not deny that these values *do* function in our health care system. Many individual physicians (hospital administrators, researchers, and others) *do* pattern their lives and orient their practices toward the above values. The warm and concerned physicians who are authors in this book serve as examples. And most other physicians believe in these values. However, I propose that, in most conflicts and dilemmas, the above values can be and often are overridden by other values such as the six to be described below. The overall impact of the American health care system on people's lives reveals these other motivations. Although policymakers may claim that decisions are made "in the best interests" of women, they do not *know* what is best; therefore they cannot be excused for failing to attempt to involve in their decision-making the input of the women at risk.

As we studied policies around each aspect of reproductive technology, the same underlying values were revealed over and over again. The actual principles used in making present-day decisions and choices were not those in the list above. Among the operative values, six salient ones turn out to be: technology, domination, objectification, exploitation, hierarchism, and profit.

Technology as Intrinsically Good

We discover that **technology serves as an end as well as a means.** All problems are expected to have technological solutions. Should a given device or machine fail to perform as expected, this is not taken as a refutation of the general aim of finding a technological solution. Simply, a better device must be produced. The "right" course of action is to develop a replacement, or a device to use with the first to correct its imperfections, or a new machine to monitor the first to tell whether its performance is satisfactory. Nontechnological solutions to problems are not sought: these are not intrinsically good. Furthermore, the emphasis is on finding solutions rather than on identifying causes.

Consider the electronic fetal monitor (EFM): Devised to monitor the fetal heart rate and display it on a screen, the EFM requires that the mother lie very still in a prone position with electrodes strapped to her abdomen. This position is unphysiologic for labor and delivery. The lack of movement of the mother and the pressure on the vena cava may adversely affect the baby's heart rate. As a result, women have been rushed for cesarean sections when their babies actually were not in distress; conversely some babies' real distress has gone undetected.

And so, a new technology was sought and found: internal monitoring. Rupture the amniotic sac, insert electrodes through the cervical os, and attach them to the baby's scalp. Result: still some false positives, some false negatives.

The next technology found was fetal scalp sampling. Through a cone inserted in the cervical os, a bit of blood is removed from the baby's scalp and tested for pH (acidity). The pH correlates with oxygen content, which, in turn correlates with fetal distress. Result: still some false positives, some false negatives. What will come next? Allowing the mother to sit up or move around does not fit the paradigm.

If technology is applied to the comfort and convenience of people (obviously I exclude military technologies), it may well make our lives fuller and richer, enhancing the inner quality of life, extending a productive life, reducing pain, and improving our relationships with each other. But we need to be vigilant critics about even the life-enhancing technologies. Often technology comes imperceptibly to control us and to turn us into slaves of our machines. And when do the negative aspects of any invention outweigh the positive? Negative aspects are seldom considered when the technology itself is assumed to be an intrinsic good.

This notion that technology is intrinsically good has several corollaries. Some of these are:

—A limited budget is better spent on a spectacular new machine than on public health measures.

—A hospital is better, the more machines and devices it has.

—A physician is better, the more technological solutions he uses.

—A patient is better cured, the more pills, the more injections, the more X-rays, the more tests, the more operations she has.

These latter two corollaries may well explain why the chemical diethylstilbestrol (DES) continued to be prescribed for threatened miscarriage long after some literature reported that it was less effective than a placebo; and why now DES is given to *terminate* pregnancy (the Morning-After Pill), with essentially no followup.

Efficiency is prized over working things out carefully and thoughtfully; speed, over a deliberative process. This translates to a preference for using machines instead of human beings to solve problems. Another consequence of short-circuiting deliberation is that only those problems with technological solutions are identified as real problems. Furthermore, experts are defined as those with technical competence.

Domination

A second current value is **domination,** by which I mean power over other human beings. It implies competition, putting out effort to be "better" than others. Physicians, hospitals, and pharmaceutical houses demonstrate that power over others is a primary value, as they compete for prestige or profit.

Only minimal health care information is made available to consumers and to health care workers low in the echelon, so that the physician remains indispensible. Consumer groups and women's health advocates have had to struggle to get patient package inserts for drugs and medications. Essentially each new drug requires another battle. When the medical system is finally forced to comply, the inserts they create are of little value. English fails to inform non-English readers; medicalese keeps most patients still ignorant; legalese protects physicians and pharmacists from malpractice suits. Language has been used to obfuscate.

Similarly, after the struggle to make informed consent forms mandatory before all surgery and experimental procedures, a victory seems to have been turned into a partial defeat. Those in power have learned how to use the forms to retain their power, by obtaining signatures when the patient is: in extreme pain or about to have an abortion; or intimidated by an atmosphere of authority; or under the guise of haste and urgency, without the legally required opportunity to get information.

The medical system also creates power for itself by defining nonmedical events as medical, i.e., with an emphasis on disease and cure. Birth control, pregnancy, and childbirth are three such areas. The plastic specula that many lay women in the women's health movement are using have been classified as prescription devices in some states, in order to make them no longer available without the hassle, cost, and subordination of a visit to a physician.

Another aspect of power is blind loyalty, meaning unthinking loyalty to the attitudes and individuals who constitute the network of the higher echelon in the health care system. Often this is unconscious because it flows out of shared values in a closed community. Or, it is manifested as a professional ethic of always speaking well of others in the same profession. It excludes those who differ in race, in class, in sex, in profession. Occasionally, it may slip over the line into cronyism and conspiracy, for instance, when FDA bureaucrats "summarize" a drug company's experimental data in such a way that negative results are not evident.

Objectification (Reification)

The professed value is "objectivity," "an attitude uninfluenced by personal prejudices and based on observable phenomena." But what is actually found is, "an attitude that turns persons into objects, that depersonalizes"; this is **objectification.**

Consider cost–benefit analysis. Should a certain drug be used? In the choice of what to count as costs and what to count as benefits, the personal is removed. Mortality is estimated for groups of people. The cost to the hospital is counted, but not the ultimate personal costs to individual patients. Suffering from side effects or pain during the procedure is rarely considered.

Also, the language used serves to depersonalize. The expression "target population" cancels out individual humans; "patient management" implies the nonexistence of a sentient brain; "target organ" focuses narrowly, blotting out the fact that the organ is part of a whole, living, feeling human being.

Women, who in fact are highly diverse, are lumped together as a class. The role for this class is wife/mother, a role that is assigned responsibility, but given no control. "The classic perception of woman as *Matter* becomes even more reified and objectified, because women are now biomedically manipulable."[1]

Exploitation of Nature

The earth is viewed as existing in order to be **exploited** by humankind. The consequence is a possessive, yet detached and callous, attitude toward the natural world: plants, animals, and minerals are here to serve us. As many resources as possible must be extracted; if we run out, we search for a technology that can extract even more, or that can extract something else. Furthermore, current practice seems to assume that nature is poorly designed or sick and needs to be controlled, that natural processes can and must be "improved" by technology (for example, that Similac is better than mothers' milk).

And short-term consequences may receive concern; long-term consequences tend not to be considered.

Hierarchism

Values, ideas, and persons seem to be viewed as occupying rungs on ladders, with some of them higher than others in a **rank-ordering.** When two values conflict, the one that outranks the other is chosen. When two human beings present their concerns, the person with the higher status is heard.

Invidious ways of ranking people are by their "normalcy" and by their culpability. Often, this means blaming a lower-status victim, for example, blaming rape victims and mothers of defective children for their own suffering.

Profit

This sixth value may underlie all of the others. Our health care system is a business run for **profit.** We see this in so many ways. Here I mention only five: unnecessary surgery, contraceptive development, attacks on lay health groups, patenting of techniques, and the short shrift given to preventive medicine and public health.

Surgeons are paid by the operation; surgeons have the highest income among physicians. From these two facts, even if we did not know of specific examples among our friends and relatives, we could conclude that there would be unnecessary surgery. Most pertinent to the subject matter of this book are the breast removals, the hysterectomies, the episiotomies, and the cesarean sections that may sometimes be unnecessary. Even if federal funds or private insurance pay the surgeon and the hospital, the patient pays physically in risk and discomfort, and financially in lost work time and convalescence expenses. And all of us will pay for her unnecessary surgery through higher taxes, higher insurance premiums, and general inflation. Surgeons and insurance companies grow richer while lower-level health workers and consumers grow poorer.

After World War I the pharmaceutical houses moved into the wide open field of contraceptive development; they foresaw, correctly, the huge profits possible. Nowadays, however, private industry in this country has essentially discontinued the development of new contraceptives: they cannot make enough profit because of the lengthy testing procedures currently required by the FDA. In the past, methods that seemed to have low profit possibilities, such as the cervical cap, did not get developed.

So that profits will keep coming, power and prestige must be maintained. Not only have those in control kept most lower status health workers semi-ignorant; they have also fought, sometimes viciously and violently, against lay health centers and workers, and against women's self-help procedures. Women who choose to have their babies at home have been accused of child abuse.[2]

Obvious examples of profit-orientation are the techniques for sex preselection recently developed by Ericsson and by Bovenkamp. Each has patented his invention and is selling it to clinics. The new in vitro fertilization clinic in Virginia is another example.

Public health physicians are the most poorly paid and have the least power and prestige. Public health programs get minimal support funding; is it coincidental that their goal is to help people take care of their own health, to prevent disease, and thus to keep people *out* of the medical system?

EMERGING WOMEN'S VALUES

Different indeed are the values offered in these books as the basis of moral action. Many of these women-centered values are described below.

Respect for the Individual

Each person has worth: first, simply because she is a human being, and second, because she is unique and different from every other human being. Her value priorities and her blend of values are unique, for they relate to her particular life experiences. In the selection of a contraceptive, her wish for a large, for a small, or for no family is a pertinent factor. In genetic counseling, her values should be the primary consideration.

Her physiology is also unique. Thus, before prescribing medicine for her, one should solicit information about her experiences with her own body and then proffer possibilities. A diversity of approaches should constantly be sought. "The best health care for a pregnant woman simply allows the discovery of her particular physical and emotional needs, and ensures a dignified, self-directed resolution to those desires, wishes and needs."[3]

The method of women-controlled (patient-controlled; consumer-controlled) research nicely illustrates individual respect. In this method, the same women design the experiments, participate as subjects, have full access to the records, and have input to modify or to withdraw from the experiment at any time. Clearly, this meets no definition of experiment that we learned as The Scientific Method. There is no blind-control group, no randomized design. Essentially, this type of experimental design serves to acknowledge that total objectivity is impossible. Such a design can be ethically—perhaps even scientifically—superior to current and past clinical experimental practices, which have had some widespread problems. For example, control groups may have been chosen to deny a treatment to some, or to enhance anticipated experimental results. Sometimes when data were disappointing, they were conveniently forgotten. Also, the ethical dilemma of how to give equity to both experimental and placebo groups often cannot be resolved.

Respect for the individual implies that individual differences are to be fostered, sought, and encouraged. Richness of the policy debate is to be expected from diversity. Ethical dilemmas are the better resolved, the wider the spectrum of inputs.

Respect for the individual further implies, of course, that we should not stereotype people according to class, race, sex, occupation, or educational attainment. This principle was, unfortunately, not uniformly followed by some of the Workshop participants. Thus, on occasion, a sort of reverse discrimination took place when speakers seem to have been condemned in advance because of their male sex, their white race, or their professional degrees. We have picked up pigeonholing and categorizing from our patriarchal society, and the habit is hard to break.

The Personal is Political

Every individual comes from a particular background, the influence of which she brings into every situation. This background stems from her personal experiences in life that modify the important effects of membership in a particular race, sex, and economic class. Therefore, for her policy proposals to be meaningful and valid, the listener must know from where she comes. This may not make the stance more true, but it increases its informational value. So, for good analysis, the analyst must bring all necessary factors out into the open. This also counters any tendency toward objectification and towards the blind application of any single ethic.

Let us take in vitro fertilization (IVF) as an example. Imagine how each of the following individuals could be of the same race and class, but could have her policy stance toward IVF shaped differently: an infertile woman whose marriage had broken up for this reason; a neonatologist who has worked with severely deformed infants; a developmental biologist who regularly in the daily course of her work discards mouse embryos. To take examples from the workshop, Judith Luce, as an advocate for birthing women, tells about the moment after the birth of her first child when she was scolded for trying to touch him.[4] Mary Ampola, defending the use of prenatal diagnosis, describes the joy and relief she felt after amniocentesis when she learned that her second child would not have Down's syndrome.[5] And Wendy Carlton,[6] before reporting on her sociological study of the training of medical students, lets us know that she was a rescued premature baby, and that, during her teen-age years, her eyesight was saved by high technology.

Facing up to one's biases and revealing them is quite in contrast to the practice of medical science. Researchers claim "objectivity," but seldom acknowledge their biases and interests.

Also, that which is usually condemned or treated as anecdotal or trivial is the personal, but the personal energy and passion that we commit to our work and to our lives may well be as important as or more important than the concrete results.

The Political is Ethical

Power is an ethical issue. Those in power define what is right and wrong and punish the deviant. Yet the demands made are contingent and idiosyncratic: fifteen years ago in a given hospital it may have been forbidden for a mother to touch her newborn right after delivery; today, it may be required.

As we in these books seek what is morally right, we automatically also perceive what ought to be done. Thus, an ethical discussion creates a political policy stance. For us, ethics is not negative (refrain from doing wrong), but positive (go out and see that what is right gets done).

Autonomy and Choice

Anyone who is affected by a policy or by a technology ought to have authentic choice of whether to submit to it and ought to be able to participate in controlling it. There was consensus about this value; this theme surfaced repeatedly in all sessions. This kind of autonomous control was proposed as a solution to the problems left with us by a patriarchal society, and as a means for preventing new problems from occurring.

At the personal, individual level, autonomy means that we may choose in an informed context whether, for example, to have home birth, to have the fetal monitor, to be sterilized, to have amniocentesis. Of course, we must have full access to pertinent information given by someone without a vested interest. Consent forms must be written clearly and presented well ahead of the moment for signature. It must not be made difficult for us to assert our choices. Also, since personal control is such an important value, user education for a self-help procedure would be ethically preferable to a high technology solution to a medical problem.

Autonomy extended to the group level means that policymaking groups working on the development or on the deployment of a technology should always effectively include persons on whom the technology has been used and/or include some who are at risk for its future use. For example, population planning for underdeveloped nations ought to involve the *poor women* of those nations. In fact, most of us believe that policymaking boards should include a *majority* of potential consumers. Some make the case that *all* members of these boards should be such consumers and that specialists and scientists should merely testify before these boards.

There was consensus that consumers at risk would be competent to cope with technical details and to make involved decisions. Determining an acceptable contraceptive, for example, is so complex an issue that it *requires* input from consumers. Judgment of the acceptability of risks is a social decision that can be made validly *only* by the consumer.

If we have autonomy to make and act on decisions about our reproductive lives, we shall be empowered. This is not power over others in a hierarchical sense. We wish to use power differently—to hold our own as strong equals, to pass it on to others who need it.

Wholeness of the Individual

No focus on a particular organ or on a particular disease should leave the entire body out of consideration. Wholeness of a person includes her psychological, physical, and emotional aspects. It takes into account her entire life span. A primary concern for *safety* stems from this value.

For example, the first priority in selecting a contraceptive is total well-being. Non-invasive techniques that leave the body intact are preferable. Depo-Provera with its numerous, diverse, and often irreversible side effects—psychological, emotional, as well as system-wide physical effects—clearly is unacceptable under this ethic.

And in childbirth, the choice of who should be present at birth obviously depends on considering the psychological, emotional, and physical wholeness of the mother-to-be and the baby.

Wholeness of the Community of Women/ Women-Centeredness

A sense of community leads us to strengthen our bonds with women everywhere. It leads us to be concerned about minority and disadvantaged women, and to avoid objectifying classifications about any of us. Actions that one takes for her own benefit should not serve to harm others.

Some of us believe that ending the isolation of women from one another will foster basic self-knowledge about our fertility. This knowledge, shared among women, may be far more liberating and empowering than any imposed contraceptive technologies. It may also be more effective—but effectiveness seems not to be an overriding value.

One of the ways in which our authors openly state their biases is in their clear and refreshing pro-woman stance. Some deplored the presence of even a few men; they yearned for the special exchanges that can take place in woman-only space. Woman-centeredness is a very positive, buoyant, conscious effort to bring us from the periphery of a man-centered world into a core together with each other. It is inspiriting and empowering. For it is essential that women have self-regard; it is valid for women to give ourselves first priority when we have been denied this for so long. The nurturing done by women, their calling-forth of persons, has kept our species in existence on the earth's surface in spite of the repeated scenarios of total destruction planned and partially executed by men. It is long past time for us to come together, for by doing so we may well save the human species.

Although we approach each issue with the question, "What is really in the best interests of women?" rather than with the question, "What is in the best interests of society?" correct answers to the first question will automatically answer the second.

Wholeness of the Human Community into the Future

We have a deep concern for the unborn, including those whom we shall never see, generations hence. We must not leave a legacy of disability. Taking an untested drug when one is pregnant or leaving radioactive wastes buried in salt deposits both conflict with this ethic.

We do believe that children must be chosen and cherished. Most of us would support the choice of a woman not to carry a particular fetus if she ascertains that she cannot parent well at a particular time in her life.

Many contributors note that they would avoid drugs, food additives, caffeine, alcohol, X-rays, and nicotine when pregnant or when nursing their babies. We seem to be fanatical about avoiding repetition of the DES and thalidomide tragedies.

Wholeness of the Ecosystem

We have a responsibility to the earth, a one-ness with nature. Our actions should disrupt as little as possible the other forms of life with which we share our planet. Furthermore, the inanimate parts of nature also should not be wantonly wasted.

This concern was especially deeply felt by the midwives, and eloquently expressed by Katsi Cook: "Feminists need to understand ... the suffering of our Mother Earth ... She's being raped for her natural resources ... The process that provides the ability for a human being to get to the moon requires a rip-off ... The reproduction of the four-leggeds—who is thinking about them? These plants outside—they are our medicine. And who's thinking about them?"[7]

Each part of nature has value. Each should be respected.

And note that I have come full circle, back to *respect*. Note the connectedness of values, without ranking them in priority. Thus we come to:

Connectedness and Nonhierarchism

Connectedness can be applied to persons and to our values. There exists a circle, not a rank-order.

Persons are connected one to another. This is egalitarianism but not the atomized view of everyone as separate; rather it is tempered by concern for and commitment to others as valued individuals. Is there ever a need to have hierarchies? Expertise cannot be compared or scaled because it comes in different forms—it is not institutionalized within certain professional or quasi-professional groups. Each of us is an expert in a different way—by study, by concern, by experience. A woman who has had a C-section and a surgeon who has done 100 sections both have expertise valuable to the policymaking process. A dilemma can be truly resolved only if all affected persons participate in determining the course of action.

Similarly, no one value in our circle is independent of any of the others. Each is influenced by and blends into the others. No one value automatically takes precedence over any one of the others. If two or more values seem to conflict over a given issue, then more ramifications need to be explored so that a real solution, an inclusive solution, is found.

THE PERSPECTIVE WIDENS

With these values as our frame of reference, we begin to see that issues in human reproduction technology encompass more and more elements of our lives. We cannot follow standard techniques of acknowledging that all social issues are related, and then ignore this relatedness in order to deal only with the bits and pieces. We strive to uncover all ramifications.

Take contraceptive choice and development as one example. Although most of us would favor offering any woman many options leading to an informed choice of contraceptive method, we were clearly biased toward nontraumatic, non-invasive methods with little chance of long-term side effects. Still, a safe, nontraumatic method of postcoital contraception is needed in case of failure of other techniques and in case of rape. However, most postcoital methods are risky and future technological solutions may well be also. Therefore, confronting the context of rape becomes an issue in contraceptive technology. Educating about rape, setting up rape crisis centers, caring for battered women, stopping pornography, and curbing violence in men are *all* issues in human reproduction technology.

Protection of the chosen fetus is another example. We see that potential person as a link to the future. We are concerned about possible harm to the fetus during pregnancy, especially during the first trimester when many women may not know that they are pregnant. We urge avoidance of X-rays with their known harm, and microwaves and ultrasound with less well documented ill effects. But there is an even more serious environmental insult: radioactivity. We are concerned about pregnant women who live near nuclear waste disposal areas, or whose houses are built on tailings, or whose husbands work in uranium mines. An increase in the number of nuclear power plants or in our stockpile of nuclear weapons leads to more waste disposal, more tailings, and more uranium miners. For some the question of nuclear power is seen in isolation as simply a matter of energy policy. But to us, these so-called "energy" issues become issues in human reproduction technology.

Furthermore, as we consider any particular technology for its effects on women, we also realize that the more technologies there are, the more the need for energy. Patriarchal society has assured us that the need for energy is at present a need for more nuclear power plants. Safety, the wholeness of individuals now and in subsequent generations, remains secondary to technology as an end in itself.

Another example is the dangerous contraceptive, Depo-Provera. We agreed that no woman should be given Depo-Provera, unless she gave truly informed consent. But we face our country's policy of not giving economic aid to underdeveloped countries unless they prove that they are tackling their "overpopulation," even if it be with an unsafe contraceptive. International economic policy thus has become an issue in human reproduction technology.

For a fourth example, consider the several biomedical technologies (some quite effective) that are now available to preselect the sex of a child before that child is born. Two stark realities hit us: the nearly universal preference that firstborns be sons, and the great

Diethylstilbestrol

An Interdisciplinary Analysis

Organized by
Helen B. Holmes
and
Anne J. Davis

Overview

Anne J. Davis

Diethylstilbestrol (DES), a synthetic estrogen, has been the focus of recent controversy because of the results of its use to prevent miscarriage in the 1940s, 50s, and 60s. Three groups were exposed by its use as an anti-abortifacient—mothers, daughters, and sons. Some of the daughters have developed a rare form of vaginal cancer and reproductive tract abnormalities[1]; some DES mothers have shown a higher incidence of breast cancer and reproductive tract cancer than normal[2]; and DES sons have shown a higher incidence than normal of genital abnormalities.[3] As early as 1953, the efficacy of DES was seriously questioned when two published studies showed that it was no more effective than a placebo in preventing miscarriage.[4,5] Yet it was used for almost another 20 years.

In this analysis of DES we have the advantages of hindsight. Our knowledge of DES and our experience, often tragic, with it permit us a greater understanding of this drug's long-term consequences. Additionally, we now have the long view of the social, political, and economic factors surrounding the development of DES. Our views have been influenced by the civil rights movement, the women's movement, and the concept of patients' and experimental subjects' rights, as well as the larger, and increasingly more public, concerns in bioethics. The importance of learning from, and acting on, this hindsight and knowledge cannot be underestimated. To paraphrase Santayana, if we do not know our history, we are doomed to repeat it.

The papers to follow examine numerous aspects of the DES controversy. One basic ethical principle, informed consent, lies at the heart of these issues. A discussion of informed consent is best understood within the larger context regarding the moral justification of conducting research with human subjects. One moral justification for conducting research with human subjects is the ethics of good consequences. Everyone, directly or indirectly, derives social benefits from research. After a sufficient number of animal trials, a drug or procedure must be tested under controlled conditions on humans so that the knowledge gained can be used for the larger social good. In addition, serious harm would develop from not conducting research on humans since scientific advances would be greatly hampered. Most of the curative and preventive measures we now take for granted and from which we benefit once involved research on human subjects. We can morally justify using humans in research by arguing from a utilitarian position of good consequences for the greatest number.

Using the principle of justice, we can develop a nonconsequential argument for moral justification of research, including nontherapeutic studies. We, as a society, benefit from the risks that others have taken in previous experiments; so is it just for us to reap these benefits without reciprocal action? On the other hand, should we employ agents that enhance the reproductive capacity of women if we know those agents may endanger future generations?

To justify morally the use of human subjects in research does not eliminate the myriad of ethical dilemmas that can and often do confront the researcher. Freedom of choice and coercion, the rights of the individual and the needs of society, the meaning of "the good," the problem of uncertainty in determining the risk–benefit ratio in research and experimental treatment are some of the more obvious ethical dimensions involved. The privacy of medical records may conflict with a later need to identify persons at risk.

The scientist and the clinician both have ethical obligations to provide disclosure of information that includes the proclamation of benefits, the warning of risks, and the discussion of quandaries in order to obtain a truly informed consent from a subject–patient. In the last analysis, only the integrity and ethics of such groups as drug companies, the health care professions, and researchers will safeguard the rights of the subject–patient–consumer. The history of and continuing situation with DES dramatically illustrate both the need for regulations and the possibility of violating them. They point to the important role that individuals and groups of concerned citizens interacting with the health care industry must assume. Let us do all we can *not* to repeat this history.

The DES Controversy

Discovery, Distribution, and Regulation

Susan E. Bell

"Nearly every disease, and certainly every experimental animal, has been the subject of a DES trial," according to a 1974 review of the medical literature.[1] Some of these include the following: to stop production of milk after childbirth for non-nursing women; to relieve breast tenderness; to control symptoms of menopause and menstrual disorders; to treat breast tumors and prostate cancer; to treat gonorrhea in young girls; to prevent miscarriage and other problems of pregnancy; and to induce miscarriages. It has been used to produce feminized poultry and to fatten cattle. People exposed to DES include those who have produced it in industrial plants, people who have taken it as a drug or ingested it in their food, and those whose mothers took it while pregnant. And DES is still being used: as the morning-after-pill; to treat cancer of the prostate; to stop production of milk; and to control symptoms of menopause. Currently some physician-researchers are experimenting with it for use in infertility.[2]

Although it is generally accepted that DES did not prevent miscarriage, and evidence in one study even showed that it increased abortions, neonatal deaths, and premature births when prescribed to prevent miscarriage,[3] there remain physicians who believe it effective as an antiabortifacient. Why do they persist in this belief? The answers lie in examining the period when a belief in DES as a treatment was first created: the scientific, medical, economic, and political climate between 1938, when it was first synthesized, and 1941, when it was first approved for marketing by the Food and Drug Administration (FDA).

This history reveals, first, the anticipation with which individuals and members of the medical profession greeted DES, and second, the creation of a market for DES. Laypeople, scientists, and physicians have always been fascinated with the life cycle—birth, pregnancy, aging, death—and with the ability to control this cycle through the use of surgery, drugs, magic, ritual, or other intervention. The medical profession was ready and waiting to use estrogens to intervene and to control "female problems" during the 1930s. How did this shape the introduction of DES into the armamentarium of the physician?

Before the FDA would approve the drug for marketing in 1941, tests had to be conducted on animals and humans. This form of research was used to create a market by ethical drug manufacturers.[4]

First, some history: (1) Synthesized in 1938, DES was the first inexpensive synthetic estrogen to be produced and used. (2) DES was not patented when it was first discovered. This led, in part, to its rapid widespread use. (3) DES was one of the first major drugs approved by the FDA for marketing under the 1938 Federal Food, Drug and Cosmetic Act (1938 Act). It was the first time the FDA officials thought that a proposed drug might not meet safety standards set by the 1938 Act. The process of approval was seen as precedent-setting by both the FDA and the drug industry for interpreting and enforcing these standards. (4) Because of the nature of corporate policy, the organization of the American Medical Association (AMA), and this FDA policy, cooperation among these three groups developed during the early research, production, and marketing of DES. Yet both the drug industry and the medical profession were apprehensive about the intrusion of "The State" into their internal affairs. (5) Practicing physicians used DES as a treatment before it was approved for use beyond clinical trials. (6) Synthesizing and using DES benefited government, business, and scientific and medical institutions.

During the 1920s and 30s, in many industrial nations, clinical and biomedical research was conducted on the nature of hormones in humans and other animals. Besides their possible role in aging, menstruation, and menopause, hormones were thought to account for women's temperaments—they "got cranky" around the time of menstruation, "got hysterical" around the time of menopause, and became nurturing when pregnant. If physicians understood how women's hormones worked, they could keep women young, beautiful, cheerful, and healthy.[5] Belief in the power of hormones and, particularly, in the power of estrogens, was only a part of the belief that by nature women are ruled by their hormones and are not only different from, but inferior to, men. This ideology, combined with research into estrogens, led to the medical profession's widespread use of estrogens on almost every imaginable female condition. Estrogen therapy was combined with other therapies, such as "castration" or "hysterectomy." In this case, medically prescribed estrogens replaced production of estrogen lost by the removal of women's reproductive organs. Physicians prescribed estrogens during menopause to relieve conditions they believed were caused by insufficient supplies of estrogens, such as headaches, depression, hot flashes, dry vaginas, and excessive bleeding. They also prescribed them to control general menstrual "disorders," such as irregular or painful menstrual periods. In the 1930s, natural estrogens were used in these therapies and as early as 1934, one scientist wrote:

> It is difficult to call to mind any subject upon which more rubbish has been written than the sex hormones. This is largely the result of the general public's desire for the maintenance of youth and all that it implies, together with the successful exploitation of this trait by commercial firms.[6]

Natural estrogens were expensive to use because they were costly to extract in pure form and were potent only when injected. Thus, a woman being treated with estrogens needing treatment each day or several times a week, had to return to her physician or clinic for the injections. The cost includes both production (extracting the substance) and use (physician's time and woman's time). The chemical structure of estrogen was sought in order to synthesize an analog with the same effects.[7] Basic research—estrogens and synthetic chemicals in general fascinated scientists[8]—was allied with applied research. Ethical drug firms sought an inexpensive synthetic estrogen, a "cheap key."

E. C. Dodds, a co-discoverer of DES, received funds from the British government.[9] Since Medical Research Council policy required that all discoveries be freely available to the world, DES could not be patented; instead, it was publicized freely and synthesized widely, partly by government sanction.[10] Results of a number of therapeutic trials conducted under the auspices of the Medical Research Council's Therapeutic Trials Committee were published in January, 1939, and presented at two conferences that year in England.[11] This provided further incentive to use the substance. By May, 1939, a member of the British Medical Research Council wrote to an American drug firm:

> Apart from the evidence that it is apt to cause nausea, we have heard nothing here to indicate any special toxicity, or any action other than those in which it reproduces the effect of a natural estrogen. So far as I know, the therapeutic trial carried out under the Therapeutic Trials Committee on stilbestrol itself has now been completed, and the trials at present in progress are concerned with another substance of the same series.[12]

American medical, scientific, and business communities responded with tremendous excitement. The pharmaceutical industry was beginning to boom; sulfa drugs had only recently begun to be marketed and used widely. The "miracle drug" context hastened implementation of new substances at the expense of more careful clinical testing.[13] In the medical community, cheapness and efficacy orally accounted for the great popularity of DES.[14] Clinicians substituted it immediately, trying different dosages, different treatment forms, and different methods of administration (injection, suppository, and tablet form).

How did the clinicians obtain DES samples? The New Drugs section of the 1938 Act exempted all drugs used for investigative purposes only. Under the exemption, clinicians could obtain drug samples for "research purposes," even though a drug had to be proven safe before it could be marketed.[15] Therefore, the drug trade, distributing free samples to physicians for "research purposes," created a market. The American government sanctioned this in regulations administered through the FDA, and the medical community, anxious to use the newest drugs to enhance their prestige, to impress their patients, and to control conditions formerly untreatable, spurred it on.

DES, used for research purposes beginning in 1939, received FDA approval for general (prescription) use in 1941.

In mid-1939, Merck and Company filed a New Drug Application (NDA) with the FDA to market DES for "ovarial troubles."[16] Others followed. Typically, a company would file an NDA, learn that proof of safety was insufficient, consequently withdraw the NDA, and sometimes resubmit it. A company could withdraw an application without prejudice to future applications. All of the drug companies confronted the same barrier: numerous published reports questioned the safety of DES, and none of the companies could provide sufficient evidence of safety.

Almost as soon as DES was synthesized and tested, evidence of its toxicity, as well as of its efficacy, was noted. Its effects ranged from nausea to cancer. The same year that DES was synthesized, breast cancer was reported in animals exposed to it.[17] From the beginning, the association between a synthetic estrogen and cancer was known. Time and time again, in correspondence between the FDA and drug company officials, as well as between them and the executive director of the American Drug Manufacturers Association (ADMA), the FDA questioned the safety of DES. For instance, in reply to Sharp and Dohme's original NDA for "Stilbinol" the acting chief of the FDA wrote:

> We fail to note in this application any report dealing with a sufficient number of cases where it is indicated that appropriate observations were made in order to determine what the actual effect of this preparation was insofar as toxicity was concerned . . .[18]

Other examples of this criticism are in the correspondence.[19]

The early evidence of toxicity contributed to a curious situation. The FDA required evidence of safety. Since this could be proved only by clinical research, drug manufacturers looked into the possibility of distributing DES for research purposes. Sometimes a firm initiated correspondence with clinicians, and sometimes it responded to requests from them. One hospital administrator wrote to Sharp and Dohme requesting DES. He had previously used DES supplied by Winthrop, but was unable to obtain more from this manufacturer. In his letter to Sharp and Dohme he noted that:

> ... We have used [Diethylstilbestrol] on a large number of patients and under so many different conditions and circumstances that I believe we have gotten some remarkably fine results...
>
> ... when our supply... gave out and we could not get any more, it was rather embarrassing to have a number of patients coming back for it...
>
> ... I am aware that this preparation has not yet been approved by the Federal Food and Drug Administration...[20]

In the process of gathering enough information about the safety of DES to satisfy the requirements of the FDA, the companies created a market for themselves.

By the end of 1940, the drug companies could anticipate that a hearing planned for January, 1941, with the FDA would lead to the denial of approval. Therefore, a group of representatives from some of the interested companies met together informally in December, 1940, and later informally with some FDA officials and agreed to withdraw their applications. In January, 1941, at subsequent meetings and in private correspondence, they decided to refile as a group.[21]

FDA officials had made it clear that only a group NDA for DES would be approved, since no one company had sufficient proof of safety to warrant approval of its individual NDA.[22] FDA also said that a decision made about one NDA would apply to all NDAs. On their side, drug company officials thought that they would gain more rapid approval if they joined together to amass evidence of safety. They would begin to recoup the money spent on research into DES safety as soon as they could market the drug.[23] Some FDA officials coached the manufacturers on how to pass the safety regulations; and evidence of dissension within the agency itself existed.[24]

On May 19, 1941, 12 drug companies[25] filed a joint Master Application with the FDA, having amassed almost 5000 clinical reports on DES-usage.[26] They subsequently filed individual applications with the rest of the evidence required to complete their individual applications. To 1941, this was the largest number of clinical studies submitted to the FDA on any drug.[27]

The FDA formally approved the New Drug Applications for DES on September 12, 1941, to market it for use by prescription only in treatment of menopause, senile vaginitis, gonorrheal vaginitis, and suppression of lactation.

The approval of DES marked a victory for more than one group. The ethical drug manufacturers were well on their way to establishing credibility with the FDA and also leadership in their burgeoning industry.[28]. FDA officials successfully negotiated, on an informal rather than a formal basis, a way to evaluate a potentially unsafe drug. Physicians were able to prescribe, in large quantities, a substance that would dramatically change women's hormone levels, enhancing their image as bestowers of health, beauty, and youth. Scientists would be enabled to carry out further laboratory tests on hormones with an increased supply and legitimated use of synthetic estrogen.

Drug manufacturers filed Supplements to their applications beginning in 1947 to use DES in pregnancy and received FDA approval the same year.

Women who took the drug were completely uninvolved in the decision-making process surrounding the DES controversy at that time. (They *were* participants in the general climate of interest in life cycles, and the wish to control their reproductive lives.) The case of DES provides a dramatic example of the way in which decisions have been made in business, professional, and government institutions about women's reproductive lives.

In a critical analysis of the status of DES today, we must take into account the different institutions and individuals shaping the policies and practices for present and future research, development, and use. Consider the focus on DES at this time in history: Why is the emphasis primarily on those exposed to it through its use as an antiabortifacient, and not on its use with nonlactating women or industrial workers? Why is the focus on its association with cancer?

In closing, I would like to suggest that we appraise the process of setting up and participating in such a meeting as this. It is crucial to examine the underlying economic, medical, scientific, and political climate in which the workshop came about. One of the stated goals here is to address the issue of women's participation in reproduction policies and in the development and use of reproductive technologies. I urge you not only to examine the particular topics that we are raising in this workshop, but also the process by which we arrived here, the processes by which we are participating in this conference, and the possible outcomes of our work.

Assessment of Risks from DES

An Analysis of Research on Those Exposed During Pregnancy or in Utero

Barbara C. Tilley

INTRODUCTION

This paper explores previous and current scientific studies on the effects of DES, and seeks to identify the resulting ethical issues. It describes the risks for women exposed to DES during pregnancy and the risks for their daughters and sons exposed *in utero.* Also, it discusses the recommendations of the HEW DES Task Force and the relationship of the DES experience to other research on women's health.

HISTORY OF THE DESAD PROJECT

As early as 1940 physicians began using DES and DES-type drugs as a treatment for threatened abortion. Peak use occurred from 1945 to 1955.[1] The early enthusiasm for DES to prevent miscarriage derived, in general, from uncontrolled studies.[2] Efficacy was not evaluated to the extent that current standards require. A simultaneous, randomized double-blind clinical trial at the University of Chicago, published in 1953, indicated that DES did not reduce pregnancy loss[3]. However, this study and other similar studies[2] had little immediate impact on clinical practice. Only after 1955, when other drugs became available for this purpose, did the use of DES decline. DES was seldom prescribed for pregnant women after 1970.[1]

In 1971 Herbst et al.[4] reported the association of vaginal adenocarcinoma (clear cell cancer) in young women with their exposure to DES *in utero.* Clear cell cancer or adenocarcinoma differs in cellular structure from the more common squamous cancer, a disease detected by Pap smears. Since 1970 numerous studies on DES-exposed daughters, sons, and the DES-exposed mothers themselves have been reported.[6–26]

In response to public and congressional pressure, the National Cancer Institute funded the DESAD (Diethylstilbestrol Adenosis) Project in 1974. Although originally designed to study *in utero*-exposed children, both daughters and sons, insufficient funds limited the study to daughters. The DESAD Project is a national cooperative study, underway at various sites (Baylor College of Medicine in Houston, Texas; Massachusetts General Hospital in Boston; Gundersen Clinic in La Crosse, Wisconsin; Mayo Clinic in Rochester, Minnesota; University of Southern California in Los Angeles). It is an observational study of the incidence, prevalence, and natural history of genital tract changes and cancer in DES-exposed daughters.[6] Women became Project participants in a variety of ways. "Record Reviews" are participants identified through the review of their mothers' prenatal records. The DESAD Project contacted these daughters and asked them to participate. "Walk-ins" are women who asked to be examined by the Project and "Physician Referrals" are women referred to the Project by their private physicians. The latter two groups obtained documentation of *in utero* DES exposure. Since the referred and self-selected women might have more health problems than those women invited to participate,[24] we analyzed these groups separately.

THE EXPOSED POPULATION

Estimates, based on marketing 1959–1965, indicate that from two to three million American women received DES during pregnancy resulting in exposure of between two and three million sons or daughters.[5] Additional information from the DESAD Project, which presents a varied and inconsistent pattern of DES usage among the participating centers, demonstrates that gross estimates may be quite misleading. For example, in the same geographic area some physicians prescribed DES prophylactically to all pregnant patients, others gave DES for particular medical reasons, and others would not prescribe DES at all. Even the medical reasons for prescribing DES were not consistent. Although the largest percentage of women received DES for pregnancy problems, some received it for headaches or nausea, and a few, for such reasons as nosebleed, backache, fatigue, ear trouble, tooth pulled, psoriasis, and severe sneezing. Among those physicians using DES no consistent pattern was found in the dose prescribed or the duration of the prescription.In the four geographic areas studied, the median total dose given during pregnancy ranged from 10,424 mg in the Boston area to 1625 mg in the Houston area. Median duration of exposure ranged from a high of 150 days (Boston area) to a low of 93 days (Houston area).[5,7,19]

Heinonen also found that, among the 12 hospitals participating in the Boston Collaborative Drug Study, two used no DES and, in the others, DES was used for 2.67% of pregnancies in Boston down to 0.05% in New York City and Providence, Rhode Island.[5]

Most daughters in the DESAD Project were 24 to 28 years of age in 1980, since the peak period of prescribing DES was in the 1950s.[1] Most DES-exposed mothers received DES during pregnancies before 1955. Since their average age then was 28 years they would be over 50 now. In the DESAD Project 98.6% of the women are white.[6] In the Heinonen hospital study,[5] which included hospitals in various parts of the United States, 73% of white women studied received DES as compared to 18% of the nonwhite women studied. Although many black women and other women of color were spared a risk incurred by millions of white women, this difference presents another ethical concern. Apparently, nonwhite women of the 1950s and 1960s in general did not receive what then was widely held to be an important therapeutic aid in carrying pregnancies to term.

DES-EXPOSED MOTHERS

New information on DES-exposed mothers who participated in the randomized trial at the University of Chicago[8] suggests the possibility of an increased risk of cancer of the reproductive organs in these women. Thirty-two cases of breast cancer were reported in 693 exposed women versus 21 cases in 668 unexposed control women. (The value of p obtained was 0.10, based on a one sided chi-square test. This implies that the difference in rates in the two groups is insignificant.) There were more ovarian cancers (4 vs 1), more cancer of the uterine cervix (7 vs 3), and fewer endometrial cancers (3 vs 5). The Chicago data also suggest that, if an increased risk does exist, pre-menopausal women (under age 50) will be most affected. This suggestion of increased risk in pre-menopausal women in the absence of excess risk in post-menopausal women is contrary to the usual experience in epidemiological studies of breast cancer, suggesting the need for further careful evaluation. However, most DES-exposed mothers, being already over age 50, are beyond the age when this particular excess risk is alleged to occur. Data from the Mayo Clinic, where doses of DES were generally lower than doses given at the University of Chicago, show no increase in breast cancer. Seven cases occurred and, based on current Olmstead County rates, 7.7 cases were expected.[9] (Early in 1980, NIH funded Dartmouth to coordinate a new breast cancer study of DES-exposed mothers and controls—unexposed mothers—identified by the DESAD Project.)

DES-EXPOSED SONS

The limited available information regarding DES-exposed sons comes mostly from a followup study of the sons of the women in the University of Chicago study.[10–13] Of 308 exposed sons examined, 97 had one or more genital abnormalities (including hypoplastic testes, undescended testicle, microphallus, and epididymal cysts) as compared to 23 out of 307 unexposed sons. (If this is a representative sample of exposed and unexposed, the probability that a difference this size or greater owes to chance is less than 5 out of 10,000. This is a highly significant risk.) Among the 39 exposed and 25 control sons willing to provide semen specimens for analysis, decreases in sperm count, average sperm density, average number of motile sperm per ejaculation, percent motile sperm and average motility grade of sperm were observed in the DES-exposed as compared to the controls. However, the numbers are small and the group is a self-selected subset. In addition, it is not known if this abnormal semen will result in decreased fertility since few of these men had yet tried to father children.

Another study, reported in California,[14] used questionnaires mailed to mothers of exposed and of unexposed sons. The letters to the mothers of DES-exposed sons included the information that their sons were exposed. As a result, 225 out of 306 (74%) mothers of exposed sons returned the questionnaire versus 111 of 231 (48%) mothers of unexposed sons. Although mothers of DES-exposed reported more genital abnormalities in their sons, the response bias makes it difficult to interpret these data.

To date there is no demonstrated association between testicular or prostate cancer and DES-exposure, although the increased incidence of testicular hypoplasia and undescended testicle could increase a DES-exposed son's risk of developing testicular cancer. However, testicular cancer is rare and so might not be detected in only 308 men. At this time no increase in cancer of the prostate has been reported. Since this cancer usually occurs in older men, it may be too soon to detect an increased risk for the DES-exposed sons.

To learn more about DES sons, NIH recently funded a study of DES-exposed males identified by the DESAD Project at the Mayo

Clinic. Since the Mayo Clinic used fairly low doses of DES, data on these sons should provide a valuable contrast with the higher dose group at the University of Chicago.

DES-EXPOSED DAUGHTERS

After the initial report on clear cell cancer in female adolescents,[15] Dr. A. L. Herbst and associates (1978) established the International Registry of Genital Tract Cancers in Young Women. As of 1978 the Registry had collected information on over 350 cases of clear cell cancer. Two-thirds of them have documented *in utero* exposure to non-steroidal estrogens, and the other third may have been exposed.[16] Exposure can be documented, but non-exposure cannot be. Questioning the mothers does not help: many women with documented DES-exposure did not remember taking any medication during pregnancy.[19] Registry data[16] show that reported disease was rare below age 14, peaked at age 19, and decreased thereafter. Detection before age 14 is unlikely unless the disease is advanced. Their estimate of risk for women through age 24 (0.14 to 1.4 per thousand) must be interpreted with care. A registry is dependent on voluntarily supplied information and so is subject to underreporting; hence the numerator may be too low. The true denominator is unknown.

A Mayo Clinic study[17] based on the population of children born in Olmstead County from 1948 to 1959, found no evidence of vaginal or cervical adenocarcinoma in the group of 803 DES daughters who were examined or contacted for information. (Of those identified as exposed, 99% were contacted.) Based on these data the 95% confidence limit for the risk was determined to be 4 per 1000 for women in the age group studied. However, not all of the women were actually examined since many provided information by mail or telephone only. Also, the Rochester community was a relatively low-dose area.

Currently, the DESAD Project has detected no cases of clear cell cancer in participants identified by prenatal record review. Those women having adenocarcinoma had been referred to the Project by physicians or had themselves requested entry.[7] Although adenocarcinoma continues to occur in rare instances, the DES-exposed daughters are not yet in the age group (50 years) when clear cell cancer might normally appear. So this risk can be assessed only as these women become older.

Although clear cell cancer to date is rare in these women, other changes in the vagina and cervix such as adenosis are not rare. (The term adenosis indicates the presence in the vagina of glandular tissue, similar to tissue lining the uterus.) For these changes some physicians originally recommended treatment, and a few physicians recommended extreme measures such as 5-FU cream or a vaginectomy. Although the changes appeared abnormal, little was known about their seriousness at the time that severe treatments were being recommended. As data began to show that the risks of cancer were low in these young women, treatment was no longer recommended for those without medical problems.

For the DESAD Project, examinations were performed using a colposcope, an instrument that magnifies the visual image of the vagina and cervix. Physicians in the DESAD Project observed adenosis and other changes, such as thick white epithelium. Biopsies of these areas often showed remnants of glandular tissue. Therefore, all epithelial findings in the vagina including adenosis were grouped as VEC, "vaginal epithelial changes." An early study based on self-referred women reported that over 90% of the DES-exposed women examined had adenosis.[18] In the DESAD Project the proportion of women with VEC differed drastically among the participant groups. The prenatal-record review group had 34% (the lowest and probably the most representative percentage) of women with VEC; the walk-ins, 59%; the physican referrals, 65%.[7]

As of early 1980, the DESAD Project had no documentation of a progression from typical adenosis to clear cell cancer. Some clear cell cancers have been reported to occur in the same area with adenosis,[4] but these were *simultaneous* findings.

A multivariate statistical analysis of the record review group showed that those daughters with VEC generally had mothers who were given higher doses of DES starting early in pregnancy and continuing for a longer duration than mothers of women without VEC. Also, the group of women with VEC was in general younger than the group without VEC.[7] This is consistent with a report by Antonioli that many DES-exposed women had changes which disappeared as they grew older.[23]

Following the reports regarding clear cell cancer, Stafl and Mattingly[18] reported that DES-exposed daughters were also at greater risk of cervical or vaginal squamous dysplasia, or of cancer. Dysplasia is *not* cancer, but is thought to be part of a continuum of changes that may become cancer. Depending on the degree of cellular change, dysplasia is called mild, moderate, severe, or carcinoma *in situ.* Dysplasia does not always become cancer and, if left untreated, may revert to normal. Both squamous dysplasia and cancer can be detected by a pap smear. Stafl's report was based on a highly self-selected walk-in and physician-referral population. Later information published by the DESAD Project showed clearly the bias in such groups. The rate of cervical dysplasia or cancer, per 1000 examined, in the prenatal-record review was 7; for walk-ins, 11; and for physician referrals, 12.4.[6,7] Since participants identified by prenatal record review more closely represent the general DES-exposed population, this suggests that there is little or no increased risk in the age group studied. However, although the rates in all groups are low, these young women are just entering the higher risk age groups where cervical cancer more commonly appears. Continued followup of these women is necessary.

In addition to epithelial changes, changes in the shape and structure of the vagina and cervix (coxcombs, collars, absent pars vaginalis, transverse vaginal septa, hypoplastic cervixes) have been observed. Again, of the DESAD Project participants enrolled as of December 1976, the self-selected and referred groups had more of these changes than the prenatal record review groups (302/1256 or 24% of record reviews, 337/787 or 43% of walk-ins, 364/711 or 51% of referrals).[7] Because of the presence of these structural changes, investigators at Baylor College of Medicine selected a group of women for hysterosalpingography, a radiographic examination of the uterus and fallopian tubes. Sixty-six DES-exposed women agreed to the procedure. Of these women, 44 had varying structural changes of the upper genital tract. Twenty-three of the 44 women had a T-shaped uterus with a horn-like extension off the upper end of the uterine cavity. These women had more structural changes than a comparison group of unexposed women who were examined and had the procedure at an infertility clinic. However, because both the exposed and unexposed women may have tended to be volunteers as a result of various previous medical problems, generalization cannot be made to the exposed population. A larger study is now about to be published.[25]

The presence of structural changes to the vagina and cervix suggests the possibility that problems with fertility or with pregnancy loss may also be associated with DES-exposure. The DESAD Project compared 618 exposed daughters to 618 unexposed matched and sibling controls. No difference in ability to become pregnant was detected. Of the group studied, 220 exposed women and 224 unexposed women had at least one pregnancy which did not end in an induced abortion. Thirty-eight percent of these DES-exposed women had unfavorable pregnancy outcomes (stillbirth, miscarriage, premature birth, or ectopic pregnancy) compared to 22% of the unexposed women. About half of those exposed women with unfavorable outcomes also had at least one full-term live baby. Over all pregnancies, 81% of exposed and 95% of unexposed had one or more full-term live baby.[21] DESAD is gathering further details about pregnancy history in order to determine more precisely the effects of DES-exposure on reproduction and to perhaps determine the biological mechanism. Other studies of pregnancy outcome by Kaufman[25] and Herbst[26] show similar results.

Studies of the menstrual histories of these women, conducted at the University of Chicago[12] and at Massachusetts General Hospital,[19] showed no difference in age at menarche. The Chicago study did show some increase in menstrual irregularities among the exposed, but the Massachusetts study did not. Further data are being collected in both studies.

No evidence indicates that the exposed daughters are at a higher risk of other diseases. The limited number of studies on the psychosocial effects of DES-exposure provides no conclusive results.

RECOMMENDATIONS OF THE DES TASK FORCE

In March, 1978, after public pressure, including pressure from DES Action, an organization representing the DES-exposed and their families, HEW formed a DES-study Task Force, which made recommendations for future research on the mothers, daughters, and sons.[27] Since little is presently known about the long range cancer risks for DES-exposed, and more needs to be learned about the fertility and pregnancy history of the daughters, the Task Force recommended that research in these and the other specified areas must be continued. However, it has no funds to allocate for such research. Also, the Task Force did not set up a mechanism to expedite grant or contract applications or to direct them to appropriate HEW agencies.

The Task Force also recommended educational programs for physicians and the public, and has recommended that those physicians prescribing DES notify those exposed. Physician education is essential since both the physical findings observed at an examination and the microscopic findings need careful interpretation. The appearance can suggest cancer when the findings are actually benign and the result can be needless surgery. Currently, Cancer Communications (HEW) is educating physicians by mailing pamphlets and reprints to their offices.[28] However, because physicians receive so much mail, DES information can easily be overlooked. In addition, Cancer Communications is preparing a detailed atlas on DES for physicians, complete with photographs of colposcopic and pathologic findings.

To educate the total DES-exposed population is also difficult, since many women are unaware of their exposure. Although all DES-exposed should be notified by the physician who prescribed DES, in the DESAD Project experience many medical records are incomplete and do not supply necessary drug information. Also, many physicians of the 1950s are dead or retired. Although some transferred their practices, others simply stored or destroyed their records. Even with complete records, in a mobile society, many mothers and their offspring cannot be found. In addition, the Task Force has no power to require physicians who gave DES to review their records and notify those exposed. Thus, the Task Force's recommendations will be difficult to implement.

CONCLUSIONS

DES mothers may be at higher risk of breast cancer than unexposed women, but this association has not been proven. DES sons have more genital abnormalities than unexposed young men, but the implications are unclear. Association of DES exposure *in utero* with clear cell cancer, and with vaginal and cervical structural and epithelial changes, has been demonstrated. However, no increased risk of squamous cancer has appeared in the age groups studied to date. Some daughters exposed to DES have greater difficulty carrying pregnancies to term.

Although the physiological problems related to DES may be unique, the problems relating to DES research are not. Studies of walk-ins and referral groups can be misleading; yet much of the available information on cervical (squamous) cancer comes from such studies. Long term prospective studies, following carefully identified populations over time, are expensive, and the limitations upon funds for women's health problems often force investigators into using easily accessible, walk-in populations.

Aside from funding, there are design issues. If all studies showing adverse or beneficial effects of therapy are accepted without considering their quality, DES history will repeat. Studies using mailed questionnaires, contrived control groups, or volunteers can be misleading or inconclusive. Women scientists and women's consumer groups must insist that the limited funds be spent on scientifically sound research. More women must become active in the review process, both prior to allocation of funds to study women and prior to publication of study results.

The DES story also vividly demonstrates problems with medical records. Twenty years from now it will be no easier to identify women given Valium during pregnancies in 1979 than it now is to identify the 1950s DES-exposed women. Some private physicians' medical records will still likely be illegible and incomplete. To date no uniform guidelines have been developed for recording medical information or for storage of records after a physician dies or retires.

To protect ourselves and our children we must begin to ask our physicians about the research behind recommended procedures or drugs. Has efficacy been clearly demonstrated? We should insist on knowing what drugs we receive during pregnancy and indeed what drugs we or our children are given for other reasons. We must actively participate in our own health care.

ACKNOWLEDGMENT

Prepared with support from the DESAD Project funded by the Division of Cancer Control and Rehabilitation of the National Cancer Institute, Contracts Cn-45092, CN-45122, CN-45124, and CN-45127.

The Legal Aspects of the DES Case

What Can Be Done

Fay A. Rozovsky

Few matters arising from medical technology are as complex as the medicolegal and ethical issues encountered in the DES controversy. One may well question who can initiate the DES lawsuits, who should be sued, and what legal theories should be utilized in any litigation. Indeed, one may question whether litigation is the answer. This paper examines briefly some of these issues and finally encourages an extensive legislative campaign at state and national levels.

In order for a person to bring a lawsuit, she must have "standing," that is, a sufficient stake in the outcome to show that she will pursue the matter to a conclusion. Moreover, she must have been a forseeable party at the time of the alleged tort or civil wrong.

To be sure, the DES children and their mothers have standing. The DES children, under modern trends in tort law, can be seen as victims of harm incurred as the result of medication prescribed and dispensed to their mothers during pregnancy. Yet, some may question whether the DES children are cognizable parties in any litigation based on negligence since, under negligence law, one must prove that the tortfeasor—or the one commiting the negligent act—owed a duty to the injured party. If, for example, one is suing the DES-dispensing obstetrician for negligence, he may defend by arguing that he did not owe a duty to the fetus, that his obligation of care ran only to the mother. Such an argument, I submit, would not hold up in court since an obstetrician is charged with caring for both the pregnant woman *and* her potential offspring.

The plaintiff—the person instituting the legal proceedings—must establish in a negligence action what was the appropriate standard of care or practice at the time of the alleged harm. Here, the DES cases meet a difficult threshold of proof. Up until the publication of the Dieckmann study in 1953,[1] a physician may argue, there was no evidence in the literature that even questioned the appropriateness of prescribing DES for "problem pregnancies." Yet a number of researchers in the 1940s seriously questioned the carcinogenic potential of DES.[2] However, in the years following the Dieckmann study it is arguable whether physicians were "on notice" about the therapeutic value of DES in problem pregnancies. Physicians may be expected to counter with the argument that it was an approved use for the drug, that there are certain inconsistencies within the design of the Dieckmann study that raise questions as to its scientific validity, and, most importantly, that if the FDA allowed the use of DES during pregnancy for certain specific purposes, the physician who dispensed it for these reasons was meeting the appropriate standard of care at the time.

In negligence theory, there is one famous line of departure from the argument that those who meet the appropriate standard of practice are absolved of liability. The exception grew out of the 1932 *T. J. Hooper* New York Federal Court case[3] in which a tugboat went down during a violent storm. All on board were lost. The surviving families brought a lawsuit against the tugline owners asserting negligence in that they breached their duty to their employees in not having on-board radio telephones. Had such equipment been on board, the plaintiffs argued, the captain and crew would have received warning of the impending storm and could have reached safe harbor. The owners defended, asserting that the standard practice in the industry was not to have such equipment installed on tugs. Indeed, they argued, it was a novelty to have such equipment on any ship. Mr. Justice Learned Hand rejected the defendant's contention, saying:[4]

> In most cases reasonable prudence is in fact common prudence, but strictly it is never its measure, a whole calling may have unduly lagged in the adoption of new and available devices. It never may set its own tests, however persuasive be its usages. *Courts must in the end say what is required, there are precautions so imperative that even their universal disregard will not excuse their omission.* (Emphasis added.)

Only on one occasion has the theory of the *T. J. Hooper* case been used as precedent in a reported medicolegal decision. It occurred in a 1974 case[5] out of Washington state in which a woman sued her opthalmologist for medical malpractice. The woman had been under the doctor's care for ten years for contact lens treatment. During the period the plaintiff complained sporadically that the lens did not fit well. In one of her last visits the defendant performed an additional test, an eye pressure test, and found that the woman had glaucoma. The disease had progressed to the point that the plaintiff had lost her peripheral vision. The defendant argued that he had met the standard of care expected of him as a physician specializing in opthalmology. The standard in the field was *not* to conduct an eye pressure test for anyone under the age of 40, absent any medical indications for doing so, since the incidence of glaucoma was 1 in 25,000 under age forty. The court rejected this defense citing the *T. J. Hooper* precedent as authority. The court also noted the ease with which the test could be performed and its relative inexpensiveness.

It is doubtful that the limited precedent of the *Hooper* and *Helling* type of case marks the ultimate step in judicial activism or judicial legislating in an attempt to reach a desirable outcome. Indeed, in the *Helling* case one may argue that it should have never gone to court at all, but should have been settled by the insurance carrier for the physician on the ground that the woman's case presented enough symptomatology to justify performing the eye pressure test.

Even if the DES cases can get beyond the standard of care argument, the plaintiffs must still prove that harm actually occurred and that the harm was causally linked to the defendant's departure from the standard of care or practice. Each of these elements of a negligence case presents some difficulties.

In the case of DES children, some would contend that the harm is ostensibly demonstrable. But is it? In the case of the DES daughters, adenosis or adenocarcinoma of the cervix may be easily discerned with colposcopy and Schiller stain. Low sperm mobility as well as benign and malignant testicular lesions may be demonstrated in the case of some of the DES sons. The University of Chicago followup of the original cohort in the Dieckmann study had evinced excess rates of breast cancer in the mothers exposed maternally to DES as compared to the rest of the population. But one must ask: what will the future hold for the DES-exposed populations? What new associations of disease and DES will be discovered as the exposed population becomes older? Will there be an effect on the offspring of the DES children? Will the DES children follow the bimodal or two-stage distribution of cancers characterized so sharply in the case of the children who survived the atomic attack at Hiroshima?

I raise this horrible prospect for an important legal reason, not simply to heighten one's empathy for the DES mothers and their offspring. It is an accepted principle in law that one should have but one opportunity to litigate a dispute. It is based on a belief that the one who must defend in these matters should not be subject to litigation on the issue indefinitely. A genuine dispute should be *resolved* once and for all, and the courts should not be forums for the airing and re-airing of the same case.

In the instance of the DES children and their mothers this legal theory would mean that once they litigated their cases for adenosis, low sperm mobility, and breast lesions they would be precluded from bringing lawsuits at a subsequent time for new diseases related to their DES exposure. If they decided to "wait," to avoid this legal principle, they may be out of the ballgame altogether, since the statute of limitations may have elapsed. A "Catch-22" situation indeed!

However, the most difficult task for the plaintiffs in the DES cases based on negligence will be establishing a causal relation between their DES exposure and the physical harm they attribute to the drug. Unlike other drug cases in which the harm incurred is an externally observable anomaly, or the onset of the injury is comparatively rapid, the DES "bomb" took nearly two decades—in most cases—to detonate. During that time span, the DES population was exposed to a variety of toxic agents, carcinogens, and other environmental influences. DES has been a dietary supplement for cattle, and, in the past, for poultry being prepared for slaughter. Could not the symptoms be attributed to consuming cattle and poultry containing residues of DES rather than to maternal ingestion of the medically indicated variety?

Proving medicolegally a causal link between DES exposure during the gestational cycle and the onset of benign and cancerous lesions nearly two decades later is not an easy task. Statistical associations such as those described by Herbst[6] may not be sufficient in a court of law. It remains to be seen how the plaintiffs will overcome this hurdle.

Even if the plaintiffs have sufficient evidence with which to go forward, whom will they sue? Will it be the doctors who dispensed the drug? Will it be the DES manufacturers? Or, will it be the FDA?

In the case of the dispensing physicians one can anticipate a defense that it was the standard of care at the time to prescribe DES, given the expectant mother's medical history. Recalling my earlier remarks regarding the *T. J. Hooper* and *Helling* cases, one would be hard put to convince a court of a breach of the appropriate standard of care. Moreover, the byproduct of the so-called "medical malpractice" crisis of the early to mid-1970s has been a reformulation of statutes of limitations in several states. These revised periods in which one may bring a medical malpractice lawsuit have been so shortened as to make it virtually impossible for the DES children and their mothers to sue the prescribing physician.

And what of the DES manufacturer? The basis for suits against the manufacturers of DES will be slightly different. It will be based on a products liability theory. Such an action includes the concept of negligence, but it also incorporates the theories of strict liability and breach of warranty. For present purposes, we may define "strict liability" as a situation in which one manufactures a product that is defective or which is unreasonably dangerous despite his or her taking due care in the manufacture of the product to avert such consequences. Liability will attach without proving fault if it can be shown that harm occurred to the consumer or purchaser as the result of the manufactured product. A "breach of warranty" action is premised on the theory that the manufacturer made an express or implied statement that the product is suitable or safe for the purpose for which it was produced. In such cases one would have to show that the product did not measure up to its warranty and that one was injured as a result.

The DES cases, however, may not reach the subtleties of these legal theories, for there are fundamental hurdles that must first be overcome. When DES was first marketed, it was not manufactured by one or two companies. Instead some ninety concerns produced the drug. With the onset of DES-related symptoms not demonstrable until some twenty years after mothers ingested it, many plaintiffs are and will be hard put to identify the pharmaceutical company that manufactured the DES prescribed for their mothers. The physicians who dispensed it may be retired or dead. The medical records may be destroyed. Without knowing the identity of the manufacturer, who can one name as the defendant?

A novel theory has been developed in response to this question. Called "enterprise liability," it is based on the concept that the plaintiff is not at fault for his or her inability to identify the manufacturer.[7] Indeed, this inability arises as a consequence of the collective defendants' conduct. This theory requires a showing that the product manufactured by each defendant was generically similar to the product in question as manufactured by all the others. Besides demonstrating that they were injured by the drug, the plaintiffs must show that the industry lacked or did not use adequate safeguards for the production of the drug.

The enterprise liability theory is currently being tested before the Michigan Supreme Court.[8] The plaintiff's brief[9] before the lower court suggested that at the time of its initial approval by the FDA, DES was to be dispensed for menopausal purposes only. Without further documentation of its safety, a group of pharmaceutical houses banded together in support of one application to extend the approved use of DES to include problem pregnancies. It is this assertion, along with the demonstrable injury to the DES children, that forms the basis for the enterprise liability argument.

Much rides on the plaintiff's case before the Michigan Supreme Court. If the court rejects the enterprise liability argument, it is not necessarily the end of the argument. However, other courts faced with the theory may likewise reject it, citing the court's holding in Michigan as authority in support of their determination.

This leaves then but one possible defendant: the United States Government, and, in particular, the Federal Food and Drug Administration. Thus far, DES cases in which the FDA has been named as a defendant have proven totally unsuccessful.

In order to sue the federal government, or an agency of the government, action must be filed under the Federal Torts Claim Act (28 U. S. C. §1346, 267-2680). Until the enactment of the Federal Torts Claim Act,the government enjoyed the shield of sovereign immunity and could only be sued if Congress passed a "private bill" allowing the government to be sued. With the enactment of this Act, the opportunity to sue the government was enlarged. If the harm to an individual arises from the negligence of a federal employee engaged in a ministerial act, the shield of sovereign immunity does not apply. Thus, in one Sabin oral polio case[10] in which a private citizen contracted polio, the government was held open to suit. The evidence indicated that persons in the Division of Biologics of the FDA had failed to test appropriately a batch of the vaccine. Through this negligence, a live polio vaccine was distributed from which the plaintiff developed the disease.

In at least two DES cases,[11] the action of the FDA in granting a new drug application (NDA) to DES and allowing the drug to be shipped in interstate commerce was deemed a *discretionary* act and not a ministerial function. Discretionary acts include the application of policy judgments, the balancing of risks versus benefits, one court noted.[12] Indeed, it went so far as to distinguish the DES situation from the live oral polio vaccine case described earlier. According to the court, at issue in the polio vaccine situation was the application of scientific criteria set forth in regulations. No policy formulation was involved.[13]

The holding in the two reported DES cases against the FDA under the Federal Tort Claims Act paints a dark picture regarding the government, the last of the possible three defendants in any lawsuits. Certainly, other courts *may* take a position opposite to that of the US District Courts in Orlando, Florida, and Houston, Texas. This is not likely, however.

What is most disturbing in the court's decision regarding the applicability of the Federal Torts Claims Act is the way in which it distinguished discretionary acts from ministerial functions. Were not scientific evaluations pursuant to regulations to be utilized in assessing the new drug application filed for DES? Is the court really trying to say that the approval of an NDA for DES was a "policy judgment?" By what right may the FDA make such a *policy* determination affecting the reproductive capacities of women? Were the lives of the DES children actually relegated to a "risk-benefit" analysis made by a bureaucrat? These inquiries are deserving of a response!

If one assumes that the prospect is quite dim for successful litigation on behalf of the DES children, what recourse is left? The answer, I submit, is legislation.

From their first day in law school, lawyers are instructed that there are essentially four sources of American law. In hierarchial order these are: constitutional law, legislation, administrative rules and regulations, and lastly, common law or judicial decisions.

I am not suggesting that a constitutional convention should be convened to frame an amendment for the DES mothers and their children. Court action, as described earlier, is essentially an unsatisfactory alternative. Administrators will cry out that they cannot do anything without enabling legislation. Therefore, it is to the legislature one must turn for relief.

In approaching a state representative, state senator, or a member of Congress, one must be ready to state what she wants, the specifics of the proposed legislation. More importantly, she must be able to say how much it will cost. In the case of DES what we need is *not* revenge or retribution for the wrong done to the mothers and their children. Rather, what is essential is legislation creating a life-long DES screening program for the exposed population. The program should also provide appropriate care and treatment of any anomalies linked to DES. Important, too, is a psychosocial component designed to assist the DES mothers and children and their loved ones in coping with their medical problems. The legislation should also include a provision that precludes an individual from being discriminated against, on the basis of her DES exposure, in employment, life insurance, and health insurance. Stiff penalties should be written into this law for anyone who violates the antidiscriminatory provision. Should a national health insurance program or a catastrophic health insurance plan be adopted, specific mention of health care coverage of the DES population should be incorporated in the law.

New York State has taken the first major step in the legislative arena.[14] Through the efforts of Fran Fishbane and DES Action, one now finds in New York advertisements regarding DES placed, according to law, on billboards, on all forms of public transportation, and on television and radio. The New York legislation created the nation's first mandated screening program, but it is not enough. More must be done in other states, and initiatives should be taken by

Congress to effect change nationally, particularly as to research on future DES-linked pathology.

I am not so naive as to think such legislative efforts will be wholly successful. Screening and followup care will cost money. We live in times of cost consciousness, particularly in the health care field. Yet, the DES mothers and their children cannot be so easily dismissed. Even if litigation is successful for a few, what of the thousands who will not benefit by such court action? No, the answer lies in legislation. The DES tragedy should be examined carefully. Let us as a nation learn from this mistake and do justice to those for whom the nightmare of diethylstilbestrol will last a lifetime to come!

DES and Drugs in Pregnancy

A Consumer Reaction

Robin Erhart

I feel my response to what I have learned about DES in these past few days is that of a typical consumer, and my lack of prior knowledge reflects the ignorance of the general public about the issue of DES. I believed that DES was a past issue. I thought that the risks had been recognized; that DES was no longer in use; that a very few, select women were treated with DES a long time ago to prevent threatened miscarriage; and that these few women and their daughters must surely by now be aware of the situation and be receiving proper care. The truth is obviously far more serious.

We are beginning to take the risks of DES seriously; its use during pregnancy is being curtailed. However, much is left to do. The very large number of DES victims need care and support. Many women, unaware that they have been exposed, need to be located, educated, and medically observed. DES is still in use and action must be taken to discourage this use.

As for the identification and care of women already exposed to DES, I agree with and wholeheartedly support the recommendations of the HEW DES Task Force to increase funding for more scientifically sound research into the effects of DES on mothers, sons, and daughters; and for establishment of identification and education programs. Physicians should be pressed to take seriously their responsibility for reviewing their records and informing exposed mothers. Articles and advertisements need to be circulated impressing upon the general public the extent of past DES usage, that two to three million women have been exposed, and that the situation demands action. DES-exposed women must be informed of the necessity for long-range medical observation. They should also be informed of responsible doctors or DES referral programs.

As Fay Rozovsky proposes, we must influence legislators to introduce and support legislation providing care of DES victims. I'm certain consumers would prefer that pharmaceutical companies and physicians assume at least some of the burden of responsibility.

Although Ms. Rozovsky suggests that it may be impossible to establish legal liability, I believe that an attempt to prove such liability might at least instill a greater sense of responsibility on the part of physicians and pharmaceutical companies.

As a consumer, I am amazed that, given our knowledge about the dangers of DES, it is still used at all. Current uses include, but are not limited to, the "morning-after" pill, lactation suppression, and beef-cattle production. Even setting aside the question of safety, the efficacy of DES as currently used for medical treatment is highly questionable. Consumer efforts toward a total ban on DES are essential.

Until such a ban is effected, the need for immediate consumer education regarding current uses of DES and identification of those drugs containing DES is urgent. For example, women should be informed when the medications given after childbirth to suppress their milk supply contain DES. They should understand that DES only temporarily delays the discomforts of engorgement and that there may be a risk involved in taking it. They should be informed of, and supported in, alternative methods of drying up their milk, such as decreasing nursing over a week's time. Women should be allowed to decide for themselves whether the effect of the medication offered is worth the risk. I find it difficult to understand the evidence cited earlier of women making the decision to expose themselves when they knew of the risks. Perhaps this would not have been the case if the education of these women had also included knowledge of alternatives and an awareness that common drug usage does not necessarily indicate FDA approval and that approval does not necessarily mean they are using a safe or effective drug.

We have learned that the assumed effectiveness of DES for "improving" normal pregnancies and for preventing miscarriage was based on faulty research. The effectiveness of DES for postcoital birth control is also based on faulty studies, as Belita Cowan testified in 1975. The unsubstantiated trust in DES must be shaken to insure that exposure of potentially pregnant women and their unborn children does not continue.

To fight DES use in meat production, our consumer dollar is our most effective weapon. Once educated, consumers could choose to purchase meat only from animals not treated with DES, if so labeled.

But, the DES issue has much broader implications. DES was not the first or only unproven drug indiscriminately prescribed to women, and even worse, to pregnant women. Women have for too long been guinea pigs for untested medications and medical technologies. Action in two directions could insure that DES history is not repeated. First, we need tighter controls on the use of unproven medications and technologies and, second, women need health care education.

Regarding the first, I find it outrageous that any drug approved by the FDA for certain, specific, and restricted uses can be used at doctors' discretion for whatever treatment they fancy in the name of "research and testing." The kind of indiscriminate DES "research and testing" that was carried out on pregnant women following its approval for "ovarial troubles" stands to be repeated unless stricter controls are imposed. As a consumer, I want doctors to be restricted to the use of drugs for approved indications only.

As for FDA approval, I would want this to be based on thorough and reliable testing for efficacy and safety. The necessary research should be absolutely scientifically sound. The frightening fact is that DES gained popularity and trust based on erroneous research results. And it is even more frightening that such research was carried out on *uninformed* women with *perfectly normal* pregnancies. Research controls should include thorough testing on animals before approval for further research is granted. It angers me that although DES was known to cause cancer in mice and genital abnormalities in their offspring before it was made available for use, no attention was paid to these facts. As with food additives, any drug found to induce cancer in research animals should be prohibited for use on humans, *especially* during pregnancy. Following proof of safety in animal testing, strictly controlled studies could be carried out on fully informed, consenting adults. Then, and only then, should research begin for use in pregnancy. And, this testing should be allowed only on those problem pregnancies that stand to benefit enough from the drug to outweigh any potential risk.

I find it incomprehensible that most of the research and testing of medications leading to FDA approval is done by the drug companies that produce them! Surely there is a more ethical way. Once a drug is approved, doctors should be required to give full information to pregnant women of (1) the reasons for prescribing, (2) the alternatives, (3) the alleged benefits, and (4) the potential risks of the medication.

Another need of equal, if not greater, importance is the education of the consumer. With education, we can become active in and critically questioning of our health care. We can then be the best guardians of our own health and that of our children. Women are instinctively concerned about the well-being of their offspring; consumer health-care programs need to be established to nurture and complement this concern.

For instance, we need a massive, nationwide effort to inform women of the potential risks of any and all drug use in pregnancy. "No drug has been proven safe in pregnancy" should be a motto that is repeated and repeated until it becomes second nature. Women should abandon the physician who casually assures, "It's perfectly safe; it won't harm your baby."

We need to be encouraged toward an awareness of the very delicate developmental state in which our unborn exist. A proper chemical environment is crucial to proper development. We need to recognize that any and all drugs, including alcohol, caffeine, and nicotine, have the potential to alter the unborn's chemical environment. Any chemical alteration might damage or destroy developing cells and, thereby, disrupt the normal pattern of development. The embryo is most vulnerable in the very first days and weeks—a time when a woman is often not even aware of her pregnancy. Therefore, we must take responsibility for ensuring the safety of our unborn from the very moment we expose ourselves to the possiblity of conception.

Some drug-induced, intrauterine damage, such as the effects of thalidomide, is startlingly obvious. Other damage, as in the case of DES, is hidden and not detected until much later. Another threat we need to understand is the harm that may be too subtle or variable to be proven statistically. A slight learning disability, an increased susceptibility to disease, allergies, whatever, may never be linked statistically to drug exposure. But the possibility needs to be considered.

If use of a drug is determined necessary for a pregnant woman, her physician should be required to provide her with complete and clear information to be added to her home health record. If we were all trained to keep our own records, such problems as those currently experienced in efforts to locate and verify DES victims because of the unavailability of physician records would be alleviated.

As a provider of prenatal health care, a lay midwife, I take seriously my responsibility for providing this type of information to the women I care for. But because I'm involved in alternative health care, this information is not readily available to me either. I need to be provided with information before I can inform others. The privilege of attending conferences such as this is not readily available to most of us.

In summary: we must work to insure that current DES victims are cared for, that unidentified DES-exposed women and children are informed, and that future DES use is banned. But, from DES let's also learn that strictly controlled, reliable research is imperative in proving drug efficacy and safety, learn that we cannot rely on our government or our medical societies to protect us, and learn that we must be provided with the knowledge that will enable us to participate fully in our own health care.

advantage that any firstborn has in society. Therefore, strengthening bonds among women so that we *like* our own sex, expanding opportunities for women, and supporting the ERA *all* become issues in human reproduction technology.

SOME UNRESOLVED DILEMMAS

Clearly emerging from the values delineated above and from our wider perspectives were general recommendations for improved ways of setting policies dealing with reproductive technologies, so that these policies could better serve the interests of consumers at risk. These general proposals surfaced repeatedly and, in their essentials, were unanimously endorsed at the Workshop. As explicitly formulated for the final session and as voted in the form of fourteen "general resolutions," they can be found in the Appendix of the present volume, *The Custom-Made Child?*.

We also agreed on many specific policy proposals. These recommendations and the level of agreement reached on each follow the general resolutions in that Appendix.

However, our method of analysis also revealed ethical problems, dilemmas, and disagreements. Some of these are presented below. In each, a conflict appears between two or more of our women-centered values. Here the dialogue has just begun. I propose that, in each case, it will be possible, with continuing input from affected consumers, to resolve these dilemmas without resorting to the sacrifice of one value in favor of another. For as one maximizes one value in the circle, one ought to try to maximize all. Sustained discussion may reveal an underlying harmony of values or a novel approach.

The Contraceptive Cafeteria

The concept of a "cafeteria of contraceptives" provoked one issue. Increasing the number of options in order to respect individual differences and give autonomy to individuals seems to conflict with the concern that some contraceptives may entail such risks to the whole body and/or to future generations that they ought never to be offered. In short, the conflict is between regulation and free choice. Perhaps we began to resolve this dilemma with one observation that so far the cafeteria has been male-supplied, and that its problems might vanish if the cafeteria were to be female-supplied. Suppose profit and objectification were replaced by our women-centered values in motivating the development of contraceptives?

DES Daughters

Another dilemma was how to determine policy toward our sisters who happen to be DES daughters. We want to identify them in order to help them, but we do not want to stigmatize them. Emotional scars in addition to physical scars are not needed. We want them to get good medical care, but not unnecessary surgery and frequent, painful physical examinations and tests. Do we turn them back into the system that created the problem? As we groped toward a solution, we wondered if lay women could learn to examine and counsel DES daughters, considering that the cytological changes in their vaginas are so difficult to interpret that only a few—if any—gynecologists are now competent to do so. Only when we determine to answer *all these questions at once* will new answers emerge.

Records and Registries

We raised questions about potential harmful sequelae from just about every procedure, drug, and technology we considered. For each of these procedures and drugs, what sorts of medical records should be kept and by whom? To whom should they be made available? National registries may allow us to uncover long-term effects many years from now. Future mothers-to-be may benefit from these data. But such registries may violate autonomy and respect for the individual. Keeping our own records to assume personal responsibility and/or allowing women-centered health groups to set up registries were two suggestions to start the dialog in reaching an equitable policy on this issue.

EFM When Needed

How can we provide the option of electronic fetal monitoring for the few women whose babies will truly benefit from it, without making it routine for all women? If we apply EFM only to "high risk" mothers, since socio-economic factors are involved, the labeling process becomes racist and classist. Labeling may also become a self-fulfilling prophecy. Can we shift the emphasis toward minimizing the factors that lead to high risk pregnancies in the first place, by ensuring adequate nutrition and whole-body medical attention?

In Vitro Fertilization

Is the development of in vitro fertilization in the best interests of women? On the one hand it appears to help our sisters who are infertile and wish to become biological mothers. But on the other hand it binds us more tightly to the male-controlled medical system and legitimates our assigned roles as child-bearers.

Reproductive Ability as a Measure of the Worth of a Woman

How can we reconcile our advocacy for drug-free, technology-free childbirth with our view that the worth of a woman ought not to be tied to her reproductive ability? I fear that we are going to demand that our sisters "perform" well during labor and childbirth. Will a woman feel guilty if she fails to have a drug-free delivery, chooses not to have her husband present, or leaves decision-making to others? If *choice* becomes the norm, how much personal responsibility *must* the mother take (for the well-being of the child), and how much *may* the mother delegate completely to professionals? Society currently blames the mother for a defective or stillborn child. My concern is that we women may do so also, as well as blaming her for an unjoyful or nonstoical childbirth performance.

This sparks a broader concern. We demonstrate quite well in this book that it will be better to remove the control of all aspects of human reproduction from the overwhelmingly male policymaking boards. But, we need to be careful that in so doing we do not just reconfirm the male typecasting of us as the sex partners of men, existing essentially to bear and rear their children. The women's movement has struggled long and hard to extend the roles of women. There is no easy solution to this dilemma. If women can acquire a larger share of control over (rather than simple assignment to) this formerly traditional female role, we shall then be able to guarantee, for the women who choose to reproduce, the freedom to add other dimensions to their lives and to guarantee that they do not sacrifice their physical, mental, and emotional health in order to reproduce.

A LOOK AHEAD

We have major suggestions to make about new approaches in determining policy for research directions and for application of research results in reproductive technologies. Clearly, old questions need to be reframed and old solutions need to be scrutinized for the actual values used in reaching decisions. To facilitate this rethinking there should be diversity in the membership of policymaking boards. A variety of viewpoints will make it more likely that the ramifications of a given policy be ascertained ahead of time.

Women ought to be included in every group where policy

decisions are being made in the areas treated in these books. All levels of policymaking should include women: preparing budgets; reviewing research proposals; carrying out research; applying research; disseminating information; advertising; composing consent forms; composing patient package inserts; designing clinical trials; evaluating clinical trials; setting up FDA policy; compensating victims; and so on.

Furthermore, involved lay persons should be included in all such groups. "Involved lay persons" means active lay health workers, consumer advocates, and consumers at risk. Such consumers include those who in the future may be subjected to a given technology, as well as those who have had it used on them—both the disappointed victims and the enthusiastic advocates of that procedure. These lay persons should serve such roles as: community representatives on medical school admission committees, members of hospital policy review boards, monitors of HEW regulations, composers of patient package inserts, keepers of voluntary registries of drugs and procedures.

It is evident that the new debate has just begun. We have started to clear away the underbrush in breaking a new trail. There are many points of view, many issues to be examined, and many unresolved dilemmas. These volumes are the record of the gropings of one group toward a new synthesis. I have faith that there will be more struggles together toward the just, equitable, and woman-affirming policies we envision.

DES: Ten Points of Controversy

Joan Hirsch Holtzman

INTRODUCTION

My brief ethical analysis of the DES case will not provide answers, but will be an effort to show more clearly why the case is controversial and what specific and broader issues seem to be at stake. I shall be concerned with those difficulties that arise in connection with:

1. Assessing the *roles* of the various moral agents involved with respect to the issue of responsibility and moral blame.
2. Evaluating the *rules* under which those moral agents were supposed to operate with respect to the issues of consistency and adequacy.
3. Proposing *remedies* to compensate victims and prevent or limit future harms, with respect to the issues of fairness and rationality.

In this discussion I shall call attention to ten points of controversy within the above three categories.

ROLES

Given what is now known about the actual and potential harms of DES, it is natural to question the behavior of those who played a role in the production and dissemination of this drug. Was it wrong to develop DES, to approve its use, to prescribe it to patients? Should the drug companies, the FDA, and the physicians involved be held responsible for the consequences of their actions?

If we take the issue of legal responsibility as the first point of controversy, it appears that these matters have already been decided, for we have been told why litigation has not, and probably will not, produce findings of negligence or liability. If, however, we are concerned with the issue of moral responsibility, the questions are still open. Here we might also ask whether the courts themselves, in making the decisions they have, should be added to the list of those who stand in need of higher moral review.

In making moral assessments, one must be prepared to do more than cast aspersions; one must be prepared to identify the criteria to be used in making judgments, to specify the kind and degree of responsibility involved, and to explain how blame or moral censure is to be distributed. Since it is not sufficient to judge behavior by its consequences, we may proceed by examining the antecedents of behavior: that is, by considering the reasons or intentions that informed the actions taken (or the deeds left undone). But this brings us to our second point of controversy—where the following sorts of questions arise:

—Were those who developed DES motivated primarily by a narrowly focused interest in synthetic estrogens? Was it profits and prestige they sought?

—Were those who approved the use of DES careless in establishing restrictions? Were they callous in disregarding the available evidence?

—Were those who prescribed DES ignorant but well-intentioned? Were they arrogant and unfeeling in their lack of concern for patients?

—Did any or all of the above (including judges who decided cases) have biased attitudes towards women that affected their handling of the situation? Were the motives and behavior typical, simply a manifestation of normal operating procedures?

What makes these questions so difficult to answer is not only that motives, beliefs, and attitudes are likely to differ from person to person, but that such mental states or dispositions are notoriously hard to ascertain. Those who own them may lie, dissemble, or fail to recognize fully what they are, and outsiders can only infer them from behavior. Moreover, in order to be fair, one must not neglect to extend queries about roles and responsibilities to include women.

The third point of controversy is whether women were active or passive participants in the quest for an effective anti-abortifacient. Did they want and encourage such developments, or were they, as often characterized, trusting and non-assertive? If the latter, how are we to interpret such descriptions? Are non-assertiveness and trustfulness moral weaknesses or do such traits exculpate women and make them immune from moral blame? On the other hand, if women did give encouragement and support, does this mean they should be chastised for their complicity or lauded for their attitude of responsible self-interest? And apart from the issue of self-interest, ought women not be expected to have had and to have expressed some concern about the effects DES might have on their offspring and future generations? Should only men have these concerns?

Finally, and with respect to all the above questions, we might ask whether the historical context should be considered a mitigating circumstance. Does it make a difference that DES was developed during a period of depression when special economic and social pressures were imposed? And was it not also a simpler time when less was known about carcinogens and the women's movement had yet to arrive on the scene? To what extent these considerations should be factored in is our fourth point of controversy.

RULES

Thus far I have noted problems in understanding and assessing the behavior of those who played a role in the DES case. I shall now show that there are problems in interpreting and complying with the rules that were supposed to govern that behavior. At issue here is not whether individuals were more or less at fault, but whether the rules themselves left something to be desired. I do not doubt that in some cases perfectly good rules were ignored or abrogated. But even for the most conscientious and scrupulous, there will be difficulties when rules are ambiguous, inconsistent, or totally absent.

To illustrate this fifth area of controversy, consider the rules or principles governing drug research that both scientists and the FDA were supposed to observe. Safety, if not efficacy, was a basic concern; procedures involving testing with animals were mandated. Left unanswered, however, were such questions as: How much can experiments on animals tell us about effects in humans? When exactly are clinical trials on humans warranted? At what dosage and for how many generations ought tests to be conducted?

Similar problems arise when we attend to that portion of the physicians' code which stipulates: "Do no harm." How is this rule to be interpreted when the patient is severely ill or at considerable risk? Would more harm be done by leaving the patient untreated or by using a possibly effective, though not firmly proven, medication? And what generally are the rules regulating the doctor-patient relationship? At present we are moving away from a paternalistic model and towards a contractual one. But at that time notions of informed consent and patients' rights were even vaguer than they are today. Can we say that patients were denied their rights then or that physicians were deficient in living up to their duties?

A sixth area of controversy exists because the values inherent in some rules conflict with the values inherent in others, or because the values espoused are ideals that in the real world cannot (at least as yet) be achieved. To illustrate, we know that in principle all drugs should be safe and efficacious. But we also know that in practice no drug is without risk or always effective. How then are we to weigh risks against benefits, or to decide what level of risk is appropriate to what level of benefit? And, should these decisions be uniform or should they vary according to the context?

Further conflicts are generated when we ask who should decide these matters. Should it be the government who acts in the interests of or to protect the welfare of those who might be harmed? Or should individuals be allowed to determine their own interests and welfare? At issue here are some very large questions that go well beyond the DES case: about personal freedom and autonomy, about whether or not people have a right to choose things that may not be good for them. To see how inconsistently we treat these issues in our country we need only think about the way the government deals with alcohol and cigarets on the one hand, and laetrile and marijuana on the other.

REMEDIES

Whether or not these fundamental conflicts can ever be resolved, the questions now are what principles (rules) and what principals (decision-makers) will determine public policies about DES.

Our seventh point of controversy begins with the question: Should DES be banned? At one level this is a dispute between those who favor removing DES from the market and those who do not. At a deeper level, however, there are disagreements about the reasons used to support each position.

For example, if it is proposed that DES be banned is it on the grounds that it is a particularly noxious substance or is there a broader moral imperative which says in effect, "Don't fool with Mother Nature"? On the other hand, if it is proposed that DES ought not to be banned, is it because like other drugs it has in addition to its known dangers, some legitimate medical or commercial use? Or because it would be wrong to interfere with individual liberty and free choice? What counts here is not only what we decide, but what principles we appeal to in deciding it.

The eighth controversy involves a different but equally important concern, namely: how to deal with the victims of DES. Since attempts to provide compensation through litigation have failed, there is a question about who, if anyone, should come to the aid of those who have been harmed? Should society at large (taxpayers) assume this burden as a humanitarian gesture? Is this a precedent we would be willing to follow in other cases? Will the benefits to the victims be commensurate with the costs?

Even if we answer "yes" to these last three questions there will still be problems in implementing our good intentions. For example, if we endorse a legislative program like the one proposed by Fay Rozovsky, might we not in our efforts to track down, examine and, where necessary, treat DES children, violate their privacy? And couldn't the development of information systems for this purpose be used in other contexts to the detriment of those we mean to help? Might DES children, for example, be denied health or life insurance? Here we have our ninth point of controversy, which pits those who want to correct past abuses against those who want to avoid committing new ones.

The last, but certainly not the least, question to be considered is: How can situations like DES be prevented from happening again? Some would say that this matter has already been addressed since there is now a Federal Commission on the Protection of Human Subjects, and most hospitals, universities and research centers have institutional review boards (IRBs). Others, however, take little comfort in these new developments, not only because their effectiveness remains to be seen, but also because there are serious disputes about how these boards are composed and operate, who is represented on them, and in what proportions.

Our tenth and final area of controversy, then, poses the following sorts of questions: Should decision-making bodies be composed of people with expert knowledge and laypersons in equal numbers? Ought those with a special stake in the outcome—patients, consumers, women, minorities—have their votes weighted? Is it possible or desirable to include disinterested or neutral parties?

These questions about participation in formally assembled groups have a particular poignancy for those of us who attended this conference for, from the very beginning, we challenged each other to justify our presence and the absence of others. But this, after all, is only one of many genuine and serious controversies we have to deal with. This effort to put them in perspective will, I hope, serve to mobilize rather than paralyze our best efforts.

DES Discussion

Moderated by Anne J. Davis

Susan Peterson: Susan Bell, could you ethically analyze that process you described, of companies in a sort of "mini-Watergate" with DES?

Susan Bell: A lot of shenanigans were going on—collaboration, cooperation, etc.—among drug manufacturers, government, and the medical profession. There was also a process of struggle among them. American capitalism was then emerging from a depression, and family structure and the work force were changing. DES is an example of the kind of tragedy that can happen when we do not ask wider questions such as: Why is research into estrogens going on? Why was the drug industry so excited about DES? How are drug manufacturers, the medical profession, and the FDA evaluating safety?

Ruth Hubbard: It seems to me that the stress on ethics confuses the analysis in terms of power and control. They are what we've been talking about. To turn questions of "who has power over whom" into ethical issues is to depoliticize them, whereas I think we need to politicize these issues even more. What Susan has been saying and we have been hearing all day is that ours is not a homogenized society. *We* are not exporting drugs. Upjohn is. *We* are not poisoning people. Certain people and certain drug companies with certain interests are.

Susan Bell: I would characterize my paper as being a political paper. There are ethical questions that I examine in my political analysis.

Judith Luce: Power is a basic ethical issue, and I don't believe that political issues and ethical issues should be separated because they aren't separate.

Anne Davis: I would like to know why people think politics and ethics don't belong in the same arena. Ethical decisions are made in a social and political context. Always, when an ethical decision is made, it is a political decision. Questions such as: Who makes it? On what criteria? Whom does it affect?

Janice Raymond: It might be more appropriate to call it metaethics and go beyond the dictates of patriarchal ethics to get into a whole new way of defining ethics. We should ask, "Just what does ethics mean?"

Yvonne Brackbill: But the other ethical issue, in addition to the power issue, is the fact that thousands of women received DES experimentally without informed consent. Some of the women in the suit against the University of Chicago Hospital did not know that they had been experimental subjects until the hospital sought informed consent to study their daughters.

Anne Davis: Informed consent has been and will continue to be a major theme.

Elizabeth Kutter: It's easy to say that in retrospect, but we're talking about the 1940s when we first experienced "miracle drugs," as with the antibiotics. The informed consent concept was developed from the Nuremberg Code, at that time. The emphasis at that time was on consent. It's only in the '60s that emphasis has been put on "informed."

Byllye Avery: I can see us together at some future date looking at the effects of Depo-Provera. Like DES, it fits in with the whole issue of tinkering with the body and whether or not we want to have babies.

Kathy Karpeles: Could the pregnancy difficulties of DES daughters have to do with the daughters' mothers having received DES for their problem pregnancies, rather than with DES exposure itself?

Barbara Tilley: Since not all mothers were given DES for problem pregnancies, we adjusted for that factor in our analysis. There was still a relationship.

Carol Korenbrot: Could you detect an increased rate of cervical cancer of 2 to 3 fold in 1275 women, or is cervical cancer too rare an event?

Barbara Tilley: Cervical cancer occurs more often in all women as they become older. Currently, DES-exposed women are not old enough for us to know the final answer. It is important that these women be followed over time. The DESAD Project is funded only until 1982, far short of the time needed to answer this question.

Barbara Menning: I do infertility counseling, and we see an alarming number of women with a so-called inadequate uterus—inadequate both for conception and for maintaining pregnancy. In sons, we see decreased fertility as demonstrated by semen analysis—very low sperm counts and very poor mobility. This is definitely going to be an issue affecting many people in the '80s.

Helen Rodriguez: Did the Harvard investigators instrumental in promoting DES keep better records than anyone else, so that they are now able to identify the patients? And did you retrieve these charts on the diagnosis of threatened abortion, or on the basis of DES usage?

Barbara Tilley: The Massachusetts group did keep complete records and these records were reviewed to identify all DES-exposed women. Whenever the DESAD Project reviewed a physician's or clinic's records, every prenatal record was read. No attempt was made to retrieve selectively.

Michael Gross: Why wasn't there written into the grant some kind of self-help—teaching the women to examine their own cervixes and vaginas to see any changes—especially where you want to have followup over a long period of time, and where it's really crucial that these women pay close attention to their own bodies?

Barbara Tilley: That wasn't done because initially we just didn't know what to tell women. A woman cannot always see or correctly interpret these generally benign changes. Even a physician not educated about DES can misinterpret the findings at an examination. Also, a DES examination includes iodine staining in addition to regular procedures.

Susan Bell: On the other hand, I doubt that when they were drawing up the grant, someone thought, "Let's have a self-help group." In fact, one of the screenings that is done with DES daughters is palpation, feeling the cervix and vagina. That's something, like the breast self-exam, that any woman can do, and that women in groups can do as an ongoing process.

Belita Cowan: At present, there's a precedent-setting DES case in New York City. The young woman with cancer had part of her vagina removed. Recently, the lawfirm called Barbara Seaman and me to ask if we would testify as expert witnesses at that trial. I want to report that the judge ruled that neither of us would be allowed to be witnesses because we're not MDs.

Fay Rozovsky: DES Action National got a similar call, Belita, and I was asked what we should do. Having heard what had happened to you and Barbara, I knew what the answer would be—we would not be categorized as expert witnesses. It's a very dark picture. In that case, I was told—I don't know how true it is—that the drug company brought in a number of male physicians to sit in the courtroom, and there was an attempt to get some women to fill the courtroom in response.

Margaret Kohn: Isn't one of the problems that will occur repeatedly in the reproductive area, how people trace their medical records, especially when the administration of a drug was so long ago and the patients usually don't know what they got?

Fay Rozovsky: The only saving grace, if there is one, is that many of the doctors took copious notes on DES patients because they had problem pregnancies. Their patients' hospital-based records may have reference to DES.

Margaret Kohn: What legislative approaches do you think would be good? States might pass laws that, at the death of the practitioner, the medical records would be preserved on microfilm.

Fay Rozovsky: That might not be a bad idea. The only

contradictory argument is the great concern about confidentiality and privacy. There are certain trade-offs that will have to be made. Something has got to be done.

Kathy Karpeles: What about the case where the physician is still alive and has records, but the mother is dead and the daughter knows she was DES-exposed?

Fay Rozovsky: Is there a judicial responsibility? There is one case I want to mention dealing with the question of how far the physician–patient relationship extends. An Illinois hospital and physician failed to warn a young woman that her blood had been sensitized by a transfusion with the wrong Rh factor. She later delivered a severely injured child as a result of the mishap. The court found that the defendants had a duty to the plaintiff to warn her of the blood mix-up.

Byllye Avery: One thing that should happen is a challenge to the practice of keeping our medical records from us. We need to have our medical record in the safe along with the will and the insurance papers. That's one of the most important documents we have. With this information we can talk intelligently about our past medical history.

Fay Rozovsky: That, Byllye, is one of the most important things, in particular with adopted children. They search for their biological parents, particularly for things like DES. The problem is not one that can be easily remedied. A number of considerations must be taken into account.

Emily Culpepper: So many other types of drugs were used supposedly to prevent abortion around the time of DES; I wonder if anybody could say what they were?

Barbara Tilley: Progestins were introduced later than DES and are still being used. Natural estrogens such as Premarin and androgen–estrogen combinations were also given.

Emily Culpepper: On your legislative suggestion, I liked what you said about attention to the ongoing well-being of the women and their children. But I was disturbed with the idea that women found out by opening their mail that perhaps they had been given DES. In trying to track down something like this, what's the attention to the emotional implications?

Fay Rozovsky: Very low, right now. I recently spoke to a DES adenocarcinoma daughter. She asked, "Why has everybody forgotten about me? It's the potentially cancerous group that they are taking care of. I'm no longer a threat. They took everything out of me, but nobody gave me any psychosocial support." The only group that has tried to offer support is DES Action—on a national level.

Janice Raymond: This question was actually provoked by your long-term screening idea, but I'd like to address it to all the panelists. I think there's something implicit in what each of you said that the remedy you might suggest for what happened to the DES daughters is some kind of screening. Do you really think that is the answer—to put DES daughters back into the hands of the system which created this problem?

Barbara Tilley: If I were a DES-exposed woman I would not randomly enter the medical system. Some DES-exposed women have had unnecessary procedures or treatments given by inexperienced or uninformed physicians. Given the current state of DES knowledge and research, I would seek out gynecologists and pathologists with experience in dealing with the problems of DES-exposed women and go to them for my health care.

Fay Rozovsky: We're going to have to work with the people who subjected us—if you will—to DES, but we have a measure of control and participation different from the mothers. For example, we've got to get support in Congress to get Senator Kennedy's committee and Representative Waxman's committee to fund the study. Where are we going to get the support? I would say, "Look to the drug companies." A lot of people here would say "No!" But drug companies are the best allies, because if they are not sued, they'll turn the money they would use on litigation over to a legislative effort and get the onus off themselves. So—politics do make strange bedfellows, as does medical care.

Prenatal Diagnosis

Organized by
Gerene D. Major

Overview

Gerene D. Major

With growing self identification and confidence, women are beginning to impact upon prevailing norms. In this conference we have had the opportunity to test prevailing ethical standards and theory by their "fit" to women's issues. The abstract rational method of systematic ethics fails to account for the particular contingencies of changing conditions in individual women's physical and social environments. In those questions in which women are central, as is inevitable with reproductive issues, male-generated ethical debates have principally addressed peripheral and subsidiary issues constructed from male self-interest.

For example, consider the allocation of funds to centralized perinatal centers in large cities such as Chicago, even as its neighborhood health centers close from lack of funding. Were both providers and consumers involved in each of these decisions? What is the benefit of the above decisions to women?

Those involved in the establishment of perinatal systems set ethical standards from which they develop policy, as they exercise power and control over daily operations and events. Are women involved at any level in these decisions? What structure and provision are made to ensure that the perinatal care resource is a woman-centered, woman-controlled environment in concept and implementation? The use of evolving technology is greatest in large medical centers located in major cities. What means have these medical centers provided for women-determined control and criteria of usage? Many are teaching hospitals. As women we want to know the values and concepts of the teaching staff on issues we identify: we want an accounting from those learning on us, treating us, and earning a lucrative livelihood through our needs.

We want to keep a close watch over the subtle, less visible, dynamics of initiating change and gaining control. We need to examine and monitor the socialization process of students in health careers, both in academic curricula and clinical learning environments. This is another way to assure responsible assessment and use of evolving technology, particularly when knowledge of the control and effects of technology lags behind its use.

The complexity of real conditions is beyond the scope of established prescriptive ethical principles, as becomes evident in the discussions of the papers of Ampola, Kenen, Locke, and Abramson. Ampola lays out the available techniques of amniocentesis, ultrasound, and prenatal detection of heritable diseases by tissue culture and enzymatic analysis. Kenen sets acceptance of those technologies within the US social context of the value and quality of offspring. Locke presents issues of counseling and decision-making in the medical professional–patient mode, outlining ethical principles and questions to be considered. Abramson illustrates the multiple interest-group inputs in the decision to fund, study, and treat a given prenatal anomaly. His chosen example of fetal alcohol syndrome is nongenetic; it demonstrates how blame is placed upon the mother for a defective child.

The time has thus come to assess the value of timeworn ethical principles. Our first priority is to establish a method of analysis and develop a systematic ethics congruent with our experience of ourselves as women in our environment. Peterson's paper summarizes some of those directions within feminist ethics. Our second priority is to effect the incorporation of this woman-centered ethical analysis into the existing systems of concepts and operations in science, philosophy, medicine, law, and so on. That strategy and impact will ultimately happen in all communities to the extent that we become its active agents and advocates.

A Look at Prenatal Diagnosis Within the Context of Changing Parental and Reproductive Norms

Regina H. Kenen

The *New York Times,* on April 10 and 26, 1979, headlined[1]: "Clues to Fetus Found in Mother's Blood" and "Prenatal Test Detects Hemophilia," an indication of advances in applied human genetics. Women have always had concerns about the health of the fetuses they were carrying, but superimposed on this normal preoccupation can be an additional realistic fear when there is any suspicion of severe genetic disease in the family.[2]

In an era where "quality" of one's offspring is often a paramount issue, the disjunction between diagnostic breakthrough and therapeutic strategy currently poses conflicts for many couples genetically at risk of bearing a child with a severe defect. Although the new techniques of amniocentesis, ultrasonography, and fetoscopy have by no means become household words, they have entered the working vocabulary of the mass media. As a result of this dissemination of information, couples contemplating parenthood are becoming more aware of the options, decisions, and responsibilities regarding childbearing that were previously relegated to God, chance, or luck. Increasingly, couples seeking genetic counseling are self-referred,[3] although the vast majority are still sent by physicians after the couple has first had a child with a genetic disease or where there is a history of genetic disease in the family. In order to understand better the choices that applied genetic technology offers potential parents, we need to look, at least briefly, at changes in the reproductive and parenting norms in American society.

When the United States was primarily an agrarian country, children were economic assets. Large families provided hands to milk cows, cook meals, plant and harvest crops, and maintain the farms.

Most families expected to lose one or two of their offspring in childbirth or childhood. Now small families are in vogue. Few women die in childbirth, and child care encompasses a much smaller proportion of their life span. More women, particularly the college educated, postpone marriage. In 1960, 40% of 18- to 24-year-old white females had never married. This increased to 49% by 1974.[4] A similar trend occurred among black women. Greater numbers of married women participate in the work force, egalitarian marriages are fostered, the divorce rate soars, and single parent families are becoming more common. Most couples say that they want two children, one of each sex. In recent years, the US birth rate has fallen slightly below zero population growth.[5] The cost of raising children has skyrocketed along with the general inflation rate. One economist estimates that the cost of raising a child today and sending him/her through four years of a public college is $64,000[6] (see Table 1).

Children in urban, industrial America are largely economic liabilities, desired generally for psychosocial reasons: e.g., nurturing needs, ego extensions, or carrying one's family name and tradition into the future. Becoming a parent has great social significance; for the male, parenthood is thought to be a sign of virility and potency, and for the female, of fecundity and the fulfillment of a role internalized from childhood:

> . . . as children have become less valuable they have become more valued. That is, as children have lost their economic value to the parents, under the impact of modernization, they have gained value in a qualitative sense.[7]

Characteristics such as intelligence, attractiveness, and athletic prowess are deemed desirable in children. But if any baseline is drawn between those children considered to be of high quality and those of lesser value, it is drawn on the basis of physical and mental normality. A couple bearing a child with a severe birth defect is sometimes said to have a promise unfulfilled. Olshansky[8] refers to the "chronic sorrow" felt by parents with severely retarded offspring; Fletcher[9] discusses the "cosmic guilt" associated with genetic disease; and Birenbaum[10] cites the "differentness" parents feel while raising children who, in all probability, will never become fully normal, functioning adults.

In fact, the "quality" issue points up one of the ethical questions involved in reproductive technology. By providing couples with the opportunity to have healthy, normal children, will we foster an unwanted latent effect, allowing society to renege on its rather recently acquired commitment to the rights of the handicapped? Recent political successes of the handicapped in acquiring equal access to society's resources plus the budding interest in adoption of

Table 1
Marital and Family Trends in the United States

1900	1979
Low divorce rate; most families stayed intact until the death of one partner	High divorce rate; serial monogamy and an increase in the number of one-parent families
Clear-cut differentiation of sex roles within marriage	Search for more egalitarian division of labor within marriage
Duty to procreate	Marriage and procreation only one option, though still by far the dominant one
Children primarily economic assets; secondarily psychosocial assets	Children economic liabilities; primarily of psychosocial value
More emphasis on quantity of children than on quality	More emphasis on quality of children than on quantity
Contraception less accepted, reliable, and available	Contraception and sterilization promoted, accepted, and reliable
Wives and mothers were home-makers; sometimes worked in small family businesses and on farms	Wives and mothers spend a large portion of their lives outside the home as members of the work force
Nuclear family or extended family most typical	Nuclear family or single parent family most typical
Family size was large	Younger couples state that they desire one or two children
Men gained full adult status in the occupational sphere before starting a family	More men and women assume full adult status in family roles before completing higher education and achieving full adult status in occupational roles

handicapped youngsters, including the mentally retarded,[11] may be a sign that this fear is premature.

Most "experts" in the field of marriage and family counseling agree that the decision to have a child should not be based primarily on traditional assumptions and obligations to procreate. Yet the traditional values, often promulgated by friends and relatives, still influence reproductive decisions to a large extent. Despite the increasing acceptability of childlessness, fewer than 5% of the population say unequivocally that they *never* want their own children.[12] Couples undergo invasive and often painful procedures to determine the cause of infertility and its correction,[13] and sociologists study voluntarily childless couples as examples of deviant behavior.[14]

Despite the historical precedents, more couples are now thinking about whether they want children instead of just automatically assuming that they will have them; some try to simulate the flavor of parenthood by caring for friends' and siblings' children. The decision to procreate is far reaching, affecting the life style of the couple for nearly a score of years. Moreover, raising one's own child remains one of the few areas of commitment that is still considered irrevocable. Society now accepts divorce and remarriage as solutions for marital difficulties and encourages efforts to seek more promising and satisfying work opportunities. But it is only the very rare married couple who place their child for adoption,[15] and opinion is nearly evenly divided on abortion for purely personal reasons. In a 1975 survey, 50% of the respondents approved of abortion when the couple couldn't afford another child, only 44% found abortion acceptable when the couple didn't want any more children, although 80% approved of abortion when a child would probably be born with a deformity.[16] Rossi suggests that parents are likely to withdraw psychologically from their unwanted offspring because they are not given the choice of having ex-children the way they are given the choice of having ex-spouses or ex-jobs. Or child abuse may result.

Social pressures, expectations of having one's own biological children, and the emphasis on the quality of those children are factors that may persuade some couples considering parenthood to seek the advice of a genetic counselor. Some couples seek reassurance; others seek information to help resolve the conflict between themselves when one partner wants a child and the other does not; and still others seek professional support for their decisions to have or not to have children.[17] The great majority seen by genetic counselors, however, are thought to be genetically at-risk. Even within this category, individuals do not have the same alternatives available to them. Some individuals face risks for defects that are not yet detectable antenatally. They can rely only on recurrence risk estimations in their reproductive decisions; they face options of childlessness, adoption, artificial insemination with donor sperm (AID), or playing "reproductive roulette." None of these options is optimal or entirely socially acceptable. In 1970, a national poll found that only 26% of those questioned said that they approved of AID.[18] Furthermore, adoption may not be a possibility if only healthy white babies are acceptable; very few of these infants are now offered for adoption.

Other prospective parents are more fortunate in that prenatal diagnosis and selective abortion are also options. More than 95% of women undergoing amniocentesis find out that their fetuses are not afflicted with the at-risk defect. However, a dilemma that Haas describes as a double approach-avoidance conflict faces clients receiving a positive prenatal diagnosis. On the one hand, there are the desire for a child and possible anti-abortion attitudes. On the other hand, there are the perceived positive reasons for preventing the birth of a defective child—alleviation of the potential suffering of the child and the physical, psychological, and economic burden to the family. The decision to abort is by far the most common,[19] but many factors can soften or heighten ambivalence surrounding the abortion decision. Mode of inheritance is a major factor. When the disease is one with a sporadic or nonrecurring, rather than with a dominant or recessive, inheritance pattern, psychological depression appears to be less severe because the couple can expect to fulfill the social norm of bearing a normal child in the future. Sex-linked disorders create a high degree of ambivalence because only the sex of the fetus can be determined in most cases, and not the disorder. This makes decisions even more painful and difficult, especially when the pressures are compounded by the short time horizon to make a decision.[2]

Conflict between the spouses, between the couple and their friends and family, between the couple and the medical staff, and between the couple and the religious community about the decision to abort a fetus found to suffer from a genetic defect all appear to aggravate the already high level of anxiety and guilt (see Table 2). Very little information is available, not only on the emotional consequence of undergoing prenatal diagnosis or selective abortion, but also about the effects of these procedures on future reproductive behavior, marital relationships, and familial stability.[2,19] The draft *Task Force Report: Predictors of Hereditary Disease or Congenital Defects* recommends that long-term, carefully designed studies be undertaken to assess adequately the effects of amniocentesis and the accompanying genetic counseling provided, and to understand further the interplay of forces involved in the decision-making process.

Little is known about the long-term safety and efficacy of new, controversial procedures in any field. Users of the new technology in applied human genetics have to take this uncertainty into account and weigh it against immediate benefits. Often, it takes years for long-term hazards to reveal themselves, and advances in prenatal diagnosis are relatively recent. For example, ultrasonography is deemed safe now, but responsible investigator-clinicians remain alert to the possibility of unforeseen, untoward outcomes in the future.[19]

Table 2
Factors Influencing Stress Associated with Being at Risk for Bearing a Child with a Severe Genetic Defect

Mode of Inheritance
Recessive
Dominant
Sex-linked
Sporadic
Maternal Age
Desire for Pregnancy
Parental Status
No prior children
Previous normal child
Previous child with defect
Future Options
Childlessness
Adoption
Artificial insemination with donor sperm
Pregnancy, monitored by prenatal diagnosis with selective abortion as an alternative if the diagnosis is positive
Taking the genetic risk
Degree of Support for Reproductive Choice Made
By spouse
By friends and family
By medical personnel
By religious personnel and tenets

One medical ethicist,[20] while observing ultrasound procedures, noted the emergence of a bonding effect between mother and fetus. This apparently occurred as a result of the pregnant woman's identification with the fetal body outlined on the screen. If this, in fact, does happen with some regularity, then ultrasonography may have the latent, negative effect of increasing the stress involved in deciding whether or not to abort a defective fetus. This would be a particularly distressing side effect because most women electing amniocentesis have a wanted pregnancy.

Couples today have reproductive alternatives not available to previous generations, but along with the benefits accruing from these advances come decisions and responsibilities not borne before. For example, Fletcher[21] hypothesizes that owing to the abortion issue there is an alteration in the formation of trust between parent and child when the couple decides to undergo prenatal diagnosis and consider selective abortion. It is a difficult task for parents to explain to existing children their willingness to abort a potential sibling, even if the fetus suffers from a serious genetic defect, without damaging these children's faith in their parents' unqualified love and support.

Unfortunately, rapid technological innovations and supporting social norms seldom develop simultaneously. Lags occur and controversies erupt. Until prenatal medicine offers therapeutic solutions rather than sub-optimal choices, such as selective abortion, the institutionalization of antenatal diagnosis is likely to be entangled in a web of conflicting social norms. Advocates of adversary positions can attempt to legitimate their value systems by forays into the political and legislative arena and by court challenges. In the end, however, the nature of the new norms will probably depend to a large extent on society's emphasis on the quality of children, the definition of that quality, and, most of all, on society's tolerance for "imperfection" in its members.

Prenatal Diagnosis

Mary G. Ampola

Inevitably with each pregnancy, prospective parents have fears concerning their child's normalcy, especially if they have previously had a defective baby with a genetic disease. For this reason ways have been sought to detect the presence of such diseases early in pregnancy, either to reassure the couple if the result of tests of heritable disease is negative or, if they desire, to prevent the birth of a defective baby. Amniocentesis, the withdrawing of amniotic fluid for study, was first used in the 1950s for sex determination. Since then, study of the amniotic fluid has proven extremely useful for many diagnostic and even for some therapeutic purposes.

Ultrasound should be carried out prior to amniocentesis. It is helpful for locating the placenta, estimating fetal age by head size, and detecting twins. The ultrasound waves are pulsed high-frequency, low-intensity waves that pass through tissues and display the reflected sound waves on an oscilloscope. It is desirable to locate the placenta in order to avoid it when the amniocentesis needle is inserted. This helps avoid contamination of the fluid with fetal or maternal blood, thus maintaining at an absolute minimum the risk of poor cell growth and inaccurate diagnosis.

Amniocentesis is an office procedure. Using sterile technique, a long fine needle is used to enter the uterus through the abdomen under local anesthesia. Once the needle is in place, a syringe is attached to remove between 5 and 20 cc of amniotic fluid, in which are suspended cells derived from the fetus. The procedure is done at approximately 16 weeks gestation because at that time there is a relatively large volume of amniotic fluid in comparison with fetal size and because the uterus has risen well out of the pelvis. In addition there is generally sufficient time for analysis of the amniotic fluid so that if positive results are obtained there is still time for a therapeutic abortion. Initially the major concerns about amniocentesis included the risk of infection, trauma to the placenta, puncture of the fetus, and increase in blood group sensitization, as in Rh incompatibility. For the most part, these complications have been avoidable and therefore are rare. The major concern recently has focused on the risk of inducing an abortion because of the procedure itself. Two large studies by HEW and the National Foundation–March of Dimes, involving about 1000 and 3000 pregnancies, respectively, found that there was no significant increase in spontaneous abortions in the amniocentesis group versus the control group. Both groups averaged about 3% fetal loss between 14 and 18 weeks gestation. However, there have been a few rare cases in which it appeared very likely that the amniocentesis directly caused an abortion shortly thereafter. The risk currently being quoted is less than 0.5% or 1 in 200 for spontaneous abortion. It seems quite clear that the use of ultrasound, a fine gauge needle, a single puncture, and an experienced obstetrician can keep this figure to an absolute minimum.

The two most important uses for the amniotic fluid have been the study of cultured cells for either (1) chromosomal or (2) enzymatic content. The reliability of these analyses is over 99%. We will discuss each in turn.

Chromosome abnormalities occur in one of 200 live births. The risk of abnormalities of chromosome number (too many or too few), increases with the age of the mother. The risk is particularly high if the mother is 35 years of age or above. Enough cells can be cultured for chromosomal analysis from amniocentesis fluid in two to three weeks on the average. At least 30 cells are counted to rule out the possibility of two cell types. A typical cell or two is photographed through the microscope and a chromosomal pattern cut out and studied using photographic prints.

The single most important reason for doing amniocentesis is to rule out Down's syndrome in older mothers. The risks of trisomic Down's syndrome (an extra chromosome in addition to pair 21) at maternal age 20 is approximately one in 2400, but between the ages of 35 and 40 the risk is one in 250. By the age of 45 the risk has risen to one in 40. The general recommendation at present is that women 35 and over be offered amniocentesis for this purpose, but in fact only 5% actually choose to have the test. In addition, couples who have previously had a trisomic Down's syndrome child have approximately double the risk for the general population of comparable age. Finally, there is a rare inherited form of Down's syndrome. For such a carrier, the risk in subsequent pregnancies is far higher than in any other Down's situation and clearly these individuals should be offered amniocentesis as well. In terms of cost effectiveness, it has been estimated recently that the cost of detecting one fetus with Down's syndrome, if all women 35 years of age and over were screened with amniocentesis, is approximately $10,000. On the other hand, the total cost of the special care which a Down's syndrome individual requires lifetime has been estimated to approach one-half million dollars.

A further use of chomosome studies is to assist families with X-linked genetic diseases, that is, diseases in which the gene is carried on one of the mother's X chromosomes. Only three of these diseases can be specifically diagnosed by enzyme analysis. Standard amniocentesis technique has not afforded diagnoses of any other X-linked diseases, including such disorders as Duchenne Muscular Dystrophy and Hemophilia A. Since only males are at risk to have these diseases, some parents elect to have chromosome studies done to determine the sex of the baby, and may elect to abort all male fetuses, particularly when the disease is a totally untreatable one.

The second major use for cells derived from amniocentesis is to detect one of about 75, but certainly not all, diseases of body chemistry. If an enzyme is absent, these patients accumulate substances that, in large amounts, become damaging to one or more tissues. In the usual clinical situation, the parents are entirely normal and do not know that they are carriers for the disorder. After one affected child, the usual recurrence risk, since most of the diseases are autosomal recessive, is one in four. Once a child has been born with the disease in question, couples at risk will often choose to have an amniotic tap with each subsequent pregnancy and have the option of therapeutic abortion if the fetus is shown to be affected.

In general one can do only one enzyme analysis per amniotic tap, since 3–6 weeks are required to grow enough cells in culture for the single assay. The diagnosis of diseases in this way depends on the fact that the amniotic fluid cells grown in culture reflect the genetic makeup of that fetus in terms of the enzyme in question. An example is Tay-Sachs disease, a fat storage disorder that occurs predominantly in Ashkenazi Jewish populations. The affected baby appears normal at birth, but by 6 months of age has begun to lag developmentally. Progressive neurological deterioration occurs, with loss of muscle function throughout the body. Swallowing difficulties require eventual tube feeding; loss of respiratory muscles causes repeated pneumonias. These children usually die within two to four years after a long and heartbreaking downhill course. Fortunately, in this disorder there is an effective carrier test that can be done very simply on a small blood sample in Ashkenazi Jewish couples who wish to avoid the birth of even a first affected child.

The liquid portion of the material obtained at amniocentesis can also offer valuable information. The major use at 16 weeks gestation is to measure alpha-fetoprotein, a substance normally present in only small amounts in amniotic fluid. This amount is dramatically increased in about 90% of women carrying babies with a defect of closure of the brain or spinal cord. The closure defects include anencephaly, spina bifida, and myelomeningocele. There are a few "false positives" known, but in general analysis for this chemical has been a very useful diagnostic test for "at risk" couples. The recurrence risk is 5% after one affected child and 10% after two.

The fluid has also been used in an attempt to culture various organisms such as viruses. However, in the case of German measles this has not been helpful. It was hoped that pregnant women exposed to German measles could be assessed more accurately of their risk by study of this fluid. It turned out that in some instances the virus was cultured from amniotic fluid but the fetus turned out to be unaffected. Conversely, failure to find the virus in the amniotic fluid did not preclude infected fetuses. Thus, culturing the fluid for organisms has not proved reliable.

There are certain basic requirements for effective and safe diagnostic amniocentesis at 16 weeks. These include an obstetrician who is experienced in the technique, the use of ultrasound before the tap, and laboratories that are skilled both in culturing and in analysis of the fluid. It should be mentioned that there is a shortage of these facilities at present. In addition, facilities should be available to provide a late, usually a saline, abortion if an affected fetus is found. Finally, the disease diagnosis should be confirmed in fetal tissues wherever possible.

Recently, newer techniques have been developed that allow sampling blood from the fetus. This is done under direct visualization using a fetoscope and a long needle, blood being taken from the large blood vessels on the fetal surface of the placenta. This technique is now being used in a few centers, primarily for very serious hemoglobin diseases such as sickle cell and beta-thalassemia. It holds tremendous promise for other disorders such as hemophilia A, as well as perhaps for many immune deficiency disorders. Further, chromosomal studies could conceivably be completed in 5 days instead of 2–4 weeks, and some enzyme defects might be detectable within 24 hours rather than in 3–5 weeks required when amniotic fluid cells are cultured.

Let us turn now to the uses of amniocentesis later in pregnancy. First, in instances of Rh incompatibility disease, antibody titers are followed in the mother's blood. If these levels rise above a certain critical point, amniocentesis is done at intervals. If the amniotic fluid bilirubin level, which reflects the amount of red blood cell breakdown taking place, rises excessively, the child may require premature delivery or even intrauterine treatment.

There are many instances in which early delivery of a child is highly desirable for the baby and/or mother, for example, in Rh disease, severe maternal diabetes, or toxemia of pregnancy. In this instance, it becomes important to know whether the baby is safer in the uterus or in the nursery. The limiting factor is usually the baby's lung maturity, because of the great risk in prematures of hyaline membrane disease. There is now a reliable means of assessing the lung maturity of the baby by measuring in the amniotic fluid the concentration of a substance called lecithin. This chemical reflects the ability of the lungs to remain expanded. If it is found to be present above a certain crucial concentration, the baby is considered to be safe for delivery.

Whereas all of the above techniques are diagnostic, within recent years it has become possible to begin to approach the whole area of prenatal treatment for diseases that begin to do damage *in utero*. I would like to cite three examples of such efforts. The first is that of Rh incompatibility. In 1961 amniocentesis was first used to assess the severity of Rh hemolytic disease. If a fetus, after amniocentesis, is judged to be at severe risk (bilirubin levels very high) and is too immature to be delivered prematurely, the only hope of saving the baby is to give an intrauterine transfusion of Rh negative red blood cells, which cannot be broken down by the antibody that has been destroying the baby's own cells. Under local anesthesia a needle is inserted through the uterus into the fetus's abdomen and a small plastic catheter threaded in. The needle is withdrawn and the new red cells transfused through the catheter into the fetus's abdomen, from which the cells are absorbed into the fetal circulation. The procedure can be repeated again later if necessary.

The second example involves the disease galactosemia. This disorder of sugar metabolism causes liver cirrhosis, cataracts, and growth failure in infants as well as mental retardation if they survive the first few months. The offending sugar that these children cannot handle is galactose, which is derived from milk. There is evidence that damage in these children can occur even before birth through the mother's milk intake. It is now recommended that mothers who have had a previous child with galactosemia remain on a milk-free diet throughout subsequent pregnancies. This has no adverse effect as long as the mother receives plenty of protein from other sources and takes supplemental calcium tablets regularly.

The final example that can be quoted is that of the disease methylmalonic acidemia. This involves an abnormality of body chemistry in which a certain acid (MMA) derived from protein accumulates because it cannot be cleared. In one form of the disease, large doses of vitamin B_{12} help clear the acid and prevent severe acidotic crises that are life-threatening to the children involved. I would like to describe briefly two siblings with methylmalonic acidemia, one of whom became the first patient to be effectively and specifically treated *in utero* for a genetic disease.

The first child in the family became severely ill at 2½ months of age with a profound acidosis that was unexplained. She died about two weeks later and urine sent to our laboratory after death was found to contain large amounts of methylmalonic acid. Genetic counseling was given to the couple, during which they were assessed to have a one in four risk for each subsequent child. They elected to take the risk and diagnostic amniocentesis was carried out in the second trimester. Fetal cells were assayed, revealing that this baby also was destined to have the disease. It was further established that the particular form in this family was likely to be responsive to vitamin B_{12}. It was known from previous experience that significant acid accumulations during the latter part of pregnancy occur in this disease. Accordingly, after extensive review of the animal literature with respect to vitamin B_{12}, the decision was made after full discussion with the couple to give the vitamin to the mother from 32 weeks gestation to term. We were able to demonstrate, by following the acid levels in the mother's urine, that the vitamin had reversed the trend to acid production by the fetus. Indeed, at birth at 41 weeks gestation, the baby was a lovely healthy child with very low acid levels in blood and urine. She has since been treated with vitamin B_{12} and a low protein diet and is now six years of age. There has only been one serious acidotic crisis in her lifetime, which responded well to treatment. She is a healthy and thoroughly delightful youngster with an IQ of 134.

Allow me to close on a positive note in terms of diagnostic amniocentesis. For over 97% of the women who undergo this procedure, amniocentesis serves the critical function of reassuring the parents that the baby will probably be normal. This is tremendously relieving, particularly if the anxiety level is high. I can personally attest to this fact, having undergone amniocentesis when I was pregnant with my second child at age 35 and very concerned about the possibility of Down's syndrome. It was wonderful to be told that I was carrying a chromosomally normal child. He is a normal, healthy, and joyful addition to our lives.

Antenatal Diagnosis

The Physician–Patient Relationship

Elaine Locke

At the risk of oversimplification, the ethical dilemmas for patients and physicians surrounding antenatal diagnostic procedures can be approached most effectively by observing two principles:

1. There are several levels of decision that can be addressed at different times based on the developing integration of medical information and other factors defining "burden" for the woman or family.
2. Information, the values brought forth in counseling, and decision-making are shared responsibilities with the contributions of the individual participants building upon one another.

In this paper I address information, counseling, and decision-making in the physician–patient relationship. The process is *not* a single transaction in which the physician imparts information and offers counseling, and the patient/family makes a decision.

The physician–patient relationship exists primarily for the purpose of determining and achieving what is best for the patient, and not for society or its broad ethical or social concerns.[1] Both patients and physicians, nonetheless, often do include such considerations. Although this paper does not propose to discuss *societal* rights and responsibilities in the light of scarce resources, value-related information outside the patient's needs may become involved,[2] blurring the boundaries of the discussion at times.

THREE DECISION LEVELS

For antenatal diagnosis there must be information, counseling, and decision-making on three levels. At the first level is the question: is the individual, family, or pregnancy at risk? At the second level, a decision must be made whether to submit to diagnostic procedures. And then the third level comes after a positive diagnosis: decisions must be made about further diagnostic approaches and about management options.

The primary decision, whether to broach the question of a special risk, is often made without any conscious consideration by either patient or physician. Both physician and prospective parents, unfortunately, tend to communicate—or fail to communicate—as if this first step were less important. The reason for this behavior is, of course, the natural assumption that all is well, which is indeed highly probable.[3] Screening of an unselected population is one way of initiating the process but, with very limited exceptions (such as testing for Rh factor), is completely impracticable.[4] A medical and family history, the most basic tool, often lacks both relevant information and the kind of followup that suggests diagnostic studies.[5]

However, level two is reached only if someone has made the very important decision that there may be a risk. At this second level of decision-making, information must be provided about the potential for diagnosis of the at-risk condition, and about the nature and the probable degree of impairment. Options available after a positive diagnosis are a necessary part of the information given after such a diagnosis, but knowing such options beforehand also helps some individuals with the level two decision-making. A woman, often in concert with her mate or another family member, with this information, decides whether to submit to diagnostic procedures.

At the third level of decision-making, information is needed on the reliability of the diagnosis, and the impact of the diagnosis on the outcome of pregnancy. After preliminary study, further procedures may yield more information, and the options must be reconsidered. Finally, the patient and family face decisions about management options in relation to their situation and values.

SHARED RESPONSIBILITIES

In discussing the content of information and the levels of decision-making, the question of "By whom?" is often left open. The initial decision level is probably the best at which to raise the question. In certain cultures, the sufferer expects the practitioner's cure to begin with a magical discovery of what is wrong, virtually unaided by whatever could be told of symptoms, onset, and course of the discomfort.

Although we may smile, some vestige of this behavior persists even in our scientifically sophisticated society. It is the doctor's job to take a thorough history and interpret and apply it in light of physical findings—but not until the patient presents for care. It is a rare patient/couple that brings relevant information to the physician before a first pregnancy, asking what are their chances of conceiving and bearing a healthy child. Both physicians and patients in the past have accepted the fact that genetic studies usually *follow* rather than *seek to prevent* an initial pregnancy with poor outcome.[6] Given the state of the art, this will continue to be the norm for most populations and most conditions. But it is incumbent upon both physicians and prospective parents, with the rapid expansion and dissemination of knowledge in this area, to accept the full measure of responsibility inherent in the information they have.

In the past, patients often abdicated their total right to decisions regarding their medical care, on the basis of the physician's knowledge.[7] Although the patient has now taken some share of this responsibility back, it will never shift completely to the patient because the physician's scientific knowledge makes some residuum of responsibility the physician's at all times. In fact, the fiduciary relationship of physician to patient is predicated on the responsibility arising out of the physician's professional knowledge.[8]

Undeniably, some physicians resist patient-initiated exchange of information and particularly patient participation in medical care decisions. Just as undeniably, some patients resist taking responsibility for their own health, preferring to trust the doctor if they get sick, and to follow whatever advice is forthcoming. Although both men and women may be found at both ends of the responsibility spectrum as patients, changing self-awareness on the part of many women in recent years has highlighted the potential conflict between the women who are the most knowledgeable and the most eager to assume responsibility, and the physicians who are the most resistant to such participation. Although the conflict is probably not as frequently obvious in antenatal diagnosis as in some other areas of women's health care, the underlying principles in the relationship are just as important.

On the other hand, as Judy Luce said, if you tell a woman she is at high risk, she may well fulfill the prophesy. This is an important ethical issue in prenatal diagnosis. There will be physicians who raise the question of the need for a prenatal diagnostic procedure too often; and there will be some who don't raise it often enough. The former will be accused of pushing technology; the latter, of withholding information a woman has a right to know. Skilled people—not technologically skilled, but humanly skilled—physicians, counselors, and women—are needed to know when to raise the question in order to avoid bad judgment in both extremes.

It may be helpful to state four general ethical principles applying to the physician-patient relationship:

1. The right of the individual freely to seek or to refuse health care is to be protected.
2. The physician has the responsibility of assuring, insofar as is possible, that the patient is properly counseled concerning the need for medical care, its risks and benefits, and the alternatives available.
3. Physicians who assist patients in exercising the right to seek or refuse care must always conduct themselves primarily with the patient's good in mind, recognizing that the patient's personal values are to be respected as vital to that good.
4. While fostering the ability of patients to exercise this right, physicians must ever retain responsible control over their own decisions and actions so as not to become merely the agents of patients or others, especially in matters involving medical judgment and personal conscience.

These principles highlight a term that has been slighted so far in this overview, namely, counseling. Let me say I am talking about physicians as counselors, not because they are the only or necessarily the best counselors, but because when a patient encounters a physician, communication does take place. It is especially important because it is often the first counseling, and also, because of the potential for role inequality negating the value of counseling. Counseling is not simply a presentation of information, data, probabilities, and technical capabilities to the patient/family. Neither is it the physician's decision or advice, thinly disguised as counseling. It is the process of adding to the medical information what is important to the participants in terms of values, long-range considerations, and alternative ways of thinking about the impact of decisions.[9] As counselor, the physician (or whoever serves in that role) and the patient must seek to make the patient's values as relevant to the decision process as is the information sought in a history or a diagnostic study.

Hardly anyone would dispute that the decision-making in principle is ultimately reserved to the patient/family. But in practice, a physician's decision may subtly preempt the patient's latitude of, or capacity for, decision at any of the decision levels noted. The patient who is not made aware that something in her history could place her at risk (whatever her own definition of risk may be), has been preempted.[10] The woman who has been told: "We recommend all patients over 35 go for amniocentesis because of the increased incidence of chromosomal abnormality," may have been preempted, even though her consent has been sought and all appropriate medical and genetic information is given to her. She may *not* have been encouraged to consider whether the information to be derived is helpful and desirable to her as an individual. Similarly, she may feel that the results of a diagnostic procedure foreclose further consideration and virtually dictate management from that point on. This attitude will prevent her true engagement in making a decision on management; unfortunately, it is also likely, even before that point, to impair her capacity to make a decision about diagnostic studies. As stated earlier, the awareness of outcome options may be helpful in making a decision about having diagnostic studies; however, an implied commitment to a future decision can impair decision-making in the present regarding the diagnostic procedure. The patient/family cannot possibly enter into a future state of mind that may be created by the results of a diagnostic procedure. This does not argue withholding or delaying a discussion of options, but emphasizes the importance of keeping those options open.[11]

SPECIFIC QUESTIONS

The principles of separating decisions when possible, and of sharing information responsibly, are helpful in considering the following questions:

1. In a situation such as prenatal diagnosis, which is characterized by a sharing of information, values, and decision-making, how should these responsibilities be allocated among the patient, the physician, and others?
2. What is the responsibility of a woman/couple to inform themselves of the outcome risks in childbearing before undertaking a pregnancy?
3. Who should decide, and on what basis, whether information about the risks of poor pregnancy outcome, or the risks of diagnostic procedures, diagnostic findings, and options related to the findings, is material to those involved in decisions regarding medical care and care of the expected child?
4. Should a physician/counselor simply recommend a diagnostic procedure to a woman at risk (subject to her right to refuse), or inquire first whether the information to be sought is deemed important by the woman, or desired by her?

Several correlative questions that spring from the roles and relationships involved may, however, require a more elaborate theoretical frame of reference than has been outlined here:

5. When, if ever, is screening appropriate without explanation of the purpose and meaning of alternative findings?

   This may occur in screening to narrow the population at risk in order to increase the diagnostic yield from more definitive diagnostic procedures that may be more invasive or costly.[12] But, obviously, only extremely low-risk, low-cost screening could ever be considered as a routine not requiring knowledgeable participation by the patient.[13]

6. Is the patient's simple right to know, or the physician's traditional practice of pursuing a differential diagnosis, sufficient reason ethically for performing all prenatal diagnostic procedures available?

   Other participants have discussed triviality as a criterion, and what constitutes "burden" to a woman/family. But this question may arise even when circumstances are not trivial and when costs are comparable to benefits, although benefits are not necessarily realized by acting on the information developed through the diagnostic procedures.

7. Must diagnostic procedures be justified by the difference they make in management and behavior?[14]

   Although it is not a perfect analogy, refusing antenatal diagnostic studies to a couple who indicate that abortion is out of the question is a little like refusing an infertility workup to a couple that does not wish to consider adoption.

8. If it is ethically appropriate for decisions regarding allocation of scarce resources to be made apart from the context of the individual patient–physician relationship, who should make such decisions, and on what basis?[15] Is this a more immediate question for antenatal diagnosis than for any other medical service?
9. Need physicians and patients concern themselves with the effect individually and collectively of decisions for selective abortion on attitudes toward normalcy or the "abnormal" individual? How will such individuals and society in general respond to the knowledge that they could (or should?) have been selectively aborted as defective fetuses?

> This would seem to be a question for society in general to resolve, and one that should not interfere in the decision of prospective parents about their fetus, were it not for the fact that parents and physicians often are making decisions in emotional and physical proximity to a child with comparable abnormalities who is already born to and sometimes living in the family.[16]

The exploration of ethical and behavioral principles, through both research and public discussion, needs to keep pace with the advances in antenatal diagnosis. In this context, elimination of risk isn't everything, even if it could be achieved. Certainly this is a particularly valid caution in relation to antenatal diagnosis.

Policy Decisions in Prenatal Diagnosis

The Example of Fetal Alcoholism Syndrome

Fredric D. Abramson

I would like to comment on a number of issues related to prenatal diagnosis, and then discuss decision-making for policy in the area, using the specific example of the Fetal Alcohol Syndrome.

Concerning the norms and values affecting family size and spacing, a breakdown of statistical averages by ethnicity, religion, race, socioeconomic status, geographic factors, and so on reveals a wide diversity of appropriate values. But to what extent can the present society either support divergent values or force conformity? The answer bears on the choice of what technology to use or not to use.

Operationally, genetic counseling means advising a woman whether the problem that concerns her is hereditary. Concern about a pregnancy may not be associated with a proven abnormality, but usually arises after the birth of a child who has a malformation. If we want to extend genetic counseling to the population at large, we (and by "we" I mean all of us, all of our society) have to realize that counseling starts with a concern by the patient—by the woman—that her reproduction, her pregnancy, may terminate in a harmful outcome. I first realized that while attending a prenatal clinic when my daughter was being carried. With every visit, when a woman was asked, "What do you want—a boy or a girl?," inevitably I heard the answer, "I don't care, as long as it's healthy." To me, this translates to the observation that, in fact, women are aware of a significant risk of an unhealthy offspring. The chance of stillbirth may be only 2%, but to that must be added the 3 to 7% collateral risk of congenital malformation.

Yet there is a propensity to take risks. For instance, as a counselor, I have found women who have accepted a one in four chance of having a normal offspring, so great was their desire to have a child. On the other hand, others, when told their chances of having an abnormality were one in ten, declined at the time to seek a pregnancy. However, many of these people changed their values and their perception of the risk as their life situation changed. It was never constant. For a counselor, this poses a critical ethical question: Whose values are to be used? Mine? Yours? Or are there universal values that apply in this situation?

I believe we must maintain a frame of mind that continues to challenge and revalidate information that we have previously received.

In the early days of penicillin use, people died as a result of adverse reactions to impurities in the drug generated by its production process. I would have been reluctant to advocate at that time that the use and development of penicillin cease because people did die. Deaths associated with penicillin led researchers to explore and explain why these deaths happened, and how to eliminate them.

We tend to embed information in our value systems and our operating policies. For example, until the 1950s, it was understood that humans had 48 chromosomes. In the late 50s, that number was corrected to 46. Even in the late 1960s, *Scientific American* carried an article that said there were 48 human chromosomes. This was approximately a decade after it became common public knowledge that 46 was the human chromosome number. So we must be alert to situations where commonly accepted "facts" are refuted. And each one of us is responsible for evaluating and validating any information that comes to us.

The following comments highlight some aspects of decision-making that bear on ethics, using Fetal Alcohol Syndrome as an example. Fetal Alcohol Syndrome (FAS) was described in the early 1970s in association with alcoholic mothers, and is easily identified on examination. The events regarding FAS after the initial observations exemplify some of the biases that we all bring to examining certain kinds of questions.

We begin with a phenomenologic observation. That is: we observe a child with something physically and mentally wrong (in common medical parlance, that's FLK, funny looking kid.) And we observe, in association with that child, that the mother drinks. These observations stimulate quasi-research—*ad hoc* explanations that lead others to describe a case where the mother drank, or to ask whether the mother drank, and whether her child has mental retardation. With either anecdotal or carefully designed research, we end up with an interpretation: in this case, that alcohol causes a syndrome in children born to drinking women. But that's only the beginning of the story.

The interpretation of findings in relation to a phenomenon is seriously constrained by the social and professional mores and values that we all have. What is it that a person chooses to see, and does he or she have an investment in seeing something that may or may not be there? I do not believe that research is value-free. An example of an operative social norm here is that drinking is evil, and therefore it is appropriate to find that drinking does do something to a pregnancy.

Now we come to the area of policy. First, the findings and interpretations begin to reach the policymakers, who, for instance, may be at HEW, or in Congress, or defining medical curricula. Decision-makers begin by looking at what happens in other policy areas regarding other problems. In the case of FAS, one of the dilemmas for policymakers is: are they dealing with something like rubella, in which case there's compelling cause for alarm and immediate action; or is it something more like swine flu, where a massive public action tended to have rather adverse effects on some of the people who proposed the action, as well as on some people who received the vaccine?

Now, part of this internal examination means that the person evaluates his or her own propensity to take risks. For instance, is the person willing to take the risk of being found wrong in a public policy statement? That has career values tied to it; it has public censure tied to it. In addition, making a policy statement has to do with priorities. It must be important enough in competition with other things that are being brought to the policymaker's attention.

Finally, in the case of, say, an HEW-level response, what is the program visibility? If its visibility would help a career, then visibility is desirable. If, however, it is high-risk, relative invisibility is useful. So the visibility is weighed against the risk to the individual decision-maker.

Out of that process comes some kind of action, or inaction, as the case may be. But the process does not end there, because external forces act on this decision-maker. Out of our social and professional values and standards, the public begins to lobby. We citizens begin to take actions and to assert our values and judgments to the policymaker.

In the case of FAS, there are three examples of such value lobbies: DISCUS (the Distilled Spirits Council of the United States), a manufacturers' group; women's groups; and sections of HEW such as Family Planning. The FDA proposals to label every bottle of alcohol with a warning that drinking the contents may be harmful to pregnancy were countered by the DISCUS argument—from their interests and values—that such labeling is ineffective because nobody reads the label anyway, so it will not stop drinking. Rather than argue about the validity of their assertion, notice simply that it stems from their value system and interests.

Two questions raised in developing new programs are: How important is FAS? How much money should be given to the problem? Everyone said, "It's very important." And policymakers recommended that the money be taken out of the women's programs—for women's alcoholism—and put into FAS. The women's groups said, "Wait a minute. It's not a women's problem. It's a fetal problem." This sounds like a semantic argument. But what they were really saying was, "There's very little money dedicated to the treatment of the woman alcoholic." And to siphon off that money to a problem of the fetus when there are three million pregnancies and 40 million women was a misapplication of the funding priorities. They said, "Let somebody else fund it, like NICHHD [National Institute of Child Health and Human Development]."

A third example is the response of other HEW programs, because it is in their interest, perhaps, either to deny or to accept it. Family Planning said they were willing at least to provide information to pregnant women, many of whom are teenagers in the federally sponsored programs, about the dangers of drinking alcohol. And there are other examples like that.

In summary, then, there are three sectors of attention. One deals with "research" and "science"—with what we see, and how it is interpreted. The second sector—which overlaps with the interpretation phenomenon—has to do with who makes decisions about what affects us. Finally, external forces take into account the social and professional mores that we have, which powerfully color the interpretation of what we choose to see, and the amount of energy we choose to devote to the issue.

I wish now to explore further some of the value issues. For example, we hold as self-evident that prenatal care is good for the fetus, but perhaps we want to reexamine that value. We assert that drugs and other things will hurt the fetus. We know that pregnancy is mysterious and not understood. Yet our society holds the mother accountable for the outcome of the pregnancy.

The most insidious aspect of the FAS phenomenon is that we end up saying that women who drink two ounces of alcohol a day are endangering the health of the fetus. This is, in fact, buying into a value that says a woman is so fully responsible for her activities during pregnancy that if something goes wrong, it is entirely her fault. I have seen this occur in couple relationships where the husband blames the woman. Women have been blamed for riding horses during pregnancy, for promiscuity, for smoking pot, or taking aspirin, or taking LSD, or whatever. If there is a bad outcome, society wants to find someone to blame, so the woman is blamed. So a litany of possible failures is run down until a "yes" answer is obtained. I personally find that society has to reexamine this blaming behavior carefully and ask, if it is a value worth keeping—or is it worth challenging, and asking for more information?

The Politics of Prenatal Diagnosis

A Feminist Ethical Analysis

Susan Rae Peterson

THE PRACTICAL VALUE OF ETHICS FOR MEDICINE

Ethical decisions are presented to every one of us every day. It is my belief that most people not only reason morally often, but also do this with subtlety, with scrutiny, and at times, with great courage. The problem is that we rarely take time to articulate clearly and precisely the competing values or principles that account for our moral decisions. In the field of medicine, moral reasoning (ethics) takes on a new significance, because sometimes it may be a matter of life or death. For feminists in ethics, it is not only such extreme emergencies that merit close ethical analysis, however; more routine practices are also considered to be legitimate ethical topics, since a primary ethical principle is that, in general, suffering is wrong and ought to be alleviated.

Moreover, until very recently, medical practitioners (from midwives to neurosurgeons) have not found it expedient to study and become familiar with such things as values and moral language or reasoning. But there are two things to note here: first, it is extremely difficult to be a medical practitioner without this background and vocabulary, especially in something like prenatal counseling; and secondly, the alternative is a heartless (i.e., morally wrong) retreat to technical language and medical jargon.

No matter how bad it is for someone to be evil or cruel, it is even worse to deny that ethics is relevant. Many physicians today treat moral problems as merely technical ones, and this may be the biggest obstacle to medical reform—the denial by some practitioners that there *is* a moral dimension to their decisions. When the Nazis committed genocide and human experimentation for biological purification and scientific knowledge, we thought them monsters (or subhuman) not only because they were evil, but because they failed to see a moral dimension, and nowhere offered a possible moral justification (even during the Nuremberg trials).

Therefore the immediate benefit to medicine of ethics is a more precise language that specifically names values, such as honesty, integrity, fairness, health, promise-keeping, loyalty, duties, obligations, justice, equity, impartiality, equality, etc. The words themselves are not new or strange, so I am not advocating the substitution of a new jargon for the old. Rather, since many of these words are part of our overall vocabulary, I am advocating that we use *them* to reflect and communicate the depth and subtlety of our current moral thinking.

Accordingly, using words such as "acceptable" or "appropriate" in ethical contexts, as do many contributors to these volumes, is in my opinion only evasive or irresponsible. It is evasive if "appropriate" (in "It is appropriate to use Electronic Fetal Monitoring here") simply *means* "morally justified" and it is irresponsible for medical practitioners to think that something like EFM needs no moral justification. Feminists want to bring values out into the open and avoid a false "objectivity" that they correctly suspect to be a sham anyway.

In addition to *value clarification,* two other practical benefits are *question making* and *fallacy finding.* To find the right answers, we must ask the right questions. Some questions are loaded ("Did you stop beating your child?") while others are fruitless ("What is the purpose of life?"). In prenatal diagnosis, a primary question would be, "Is the practice of prenatal diagnosis morally good, given the absence (in general) of prenatal therapy?" In other words, since abortions are potentially harmful and therefore at first glance (*prima facie*) wrong, and since abortion is the only alternative when there is a sufficiently negative diagnosis, is it not wrong to institute this new practice?[1] We can begin to answer this by looking at both values and facts, facts such as the overall safety of modern abortions, etc., and values, such as the qualitative value of children mentioned in Kenen's paper. Also, we reason morally when we reply that possible benefits, such as fewer suffering humans and fewer burdened families, may outweigh these moral costs. It would be fallacious to say that because prenatal diagnosis benefits some, we should provide it for all, or to say that because it harms some, it should be prohibited. To provide it for all, the benefits would have to be clear and probable. To prohibit it for all, the harm would have to be qualitatively great and apply to large numbers of people.

Logical fallacies are dangerous, and so it is useful to be able to recognize them, e.g., the fallacy of common practice: "But everyone else is doing it." As with other moral and political battles—the two are difficult to distinguish most of the time—it helps to criticize the opponent by stating not only a moral charge, but also charges of inconsistency.[2]

A major criticism women have of medical practice today is that it is a business run by businessmen for profit, rather than a public service run for moral purposes such as relieving suffering, improving public health, and protecting individual patients. Thus feminists are "ethicizing" medicine, as it were, exposing the fallacy of present motivations.

VALUE-LADENNESS IN GENETIC COUNSELING

To counsel someone is to advise them, both with information and with action-guiding principles or judgments. It is common for medical practitioners to distinguish directive counseling (with guidance) from non-directive counseling (with only information). I think this distinction is misconceived. First of all, on a practical and psychological level, it is very difficult, if not impossible, to avoid making value judgments anyway, and to reveal these in tone or body language if not in words (e.g., saying, "You have a 50–50 chance of having a deformed baby" instead of, "You have a 50–50 chance of having a healthy baby").

Secondly, and more seriously, it is logically impossible to avoid making value judgments in *presenting information,* since we must present only information we believe worth imparting according to some value judgment. One may also wonder why anyone would ask a medical practitioner for counseling if advice or moral guidance is *not* what is wanted. Probably the only thing morally repugnant about so-called "Directive Counseling" is the fear some have of being coerced in their decision-making. But, in fact there is no such thing as "pure information" anyway, since human beings decide according to their desires and needs what to call informative, or a fact.[3]

I suspect that by Non-Directive Counseling practitioners really mean counseling in which no sentence of the following sort occurs: "You ought to do such-and-such." One nurse taking my Medical Ethics course told me she substitutes for this another kind of sentence: "In your place I would do thus and so," thus avoiding a direct recommendation. Morally, however, there is no difference in the two sentences, since in both cases a recommendation was actually made. However, psychologically there may be a benefit which has moral worth, since patients may feel less influenced in the latter method and more autonomous. Pehaps this psychological comfort goes some way toward morally justifying "Non-Directive" Counseling, but I concur with Elaine Locke in thinking that the best counseling *focuses* on values, namely, a combination of medical values with the patient's own values of lifestyle, quality of life, family preferences, and so on.

In prenatal diagnosis, value-ladenness shows up as well in concepts such as "normalcy" and "perfection," neither of which is a neutral or objective term. Since these are inevitably value concepts, feminists will want to insure that the meaning of any such concept complies with feminist values, and not with masculinist ones, as now seems to be the case[4].

UTILITARIANISM AND COST-BENEFIT ANALYSIS

Usually medical practitioners feel comfortable with ethics so long as it is utilitarianism (i.e., everyone ought to do that which maximizes the quantified happiness of the greatest number of people), since they frequently use quantification to make decisions. This is morally right insofar as we simply *must* do such weighing in practical decisions presented in all areas of life. If someone asks how we can decide about life or death in terms of cost and benefit, the answer simply is, "Easy, we do it all the time." One example would be our nation's high valuation of the automobile even in the face of a high probability of substantial traffic fatality rates.

On the other hand, feminists feel that it is simply morally misguided to reduce qualitative matters (such as conception, pregnancy, and childbirth) to quantities—it simply should not be done, or if it is done, it leads to no good. Rather, it would seem from this conference that feminist critics of medical practice tend to be deontologists (i.e., in contrast to utilitarians), who hold the theory that everyone ought to do what by its very nature is right, regardless of consequences. This, however, is a naive polarization, since each of us does reason on the basis of future consequences at times, for example, when our fetus seems to be having problems. Also *prima facie* wrong actions can be justified (such as killing in self-defense). Uncertainty simply is a fact of life, whether in medicine or not; although we may not like it, we must decide anyway.

THE ETHICS OF RIGHTS

Ethical language is varied. Talk about rights presupposes certain ideological frameworks, specifically contractarian philosophies such as Thomas Hobbes' and John Locke's. The ethics of rights is masculinist and patriarchal in several ways, only some of which shall I mention here. First, society is viewed as a collection of atomic particles (individuals) in which each individual's utility (happiness) is viewed as "mutually disinterested" from another's. Many women philosophers (and some men) find this picture of society much too abstract and unreal, for it does not account for communities or love relationships, such as are found in the family, where one person's happiness or lack of it directly affects another's.

Secondly, the moral model for this egoistic competitive creature is the promise or contract; something is justified if a contract was made by willing partners or moral agents.[5] (Human nature in this model is such that everyone tends to maximize his or her own self-interest.) There are limits to this contract model, also—too many to mention here. But our concerns here call for a comment on informed consent.

A rights ethic includes the basic theories that justify or rationalize bourgeois capitalist democracy. Many benefits resulted from the implementation of this theory, such as mass mandatory education, but certain inherent problems remain. John Stuart Mill (in *On Liberty*) pointed to the "tyranny of the majority" when he asserted individual rights over and against popular opinion or legislative rule of law. If one is totally manipulated by mass media, for instance, when and how can one obtain "information" adequate enough to consent? And even were that information adequate (since it can never be complete), does consent by one individual justify any action consented to by another party? It clearly does not, since it is not legally or morally allowable for someone to contract into slavery to another person.[6] Many women clearly consent to remaining with husbands who beat them. Does this consent justify the beating? I think not. Therefore, the limitations of the contractarian model of ethical justification are clear. Thus, the problem of informed consent (though it is significant insofar as no information or misinformation is given to women where no consent is possible), is a masculinist problem and not one that will get a feminist critique of medicine very far.

Moreover, rights are not absolute. Even worse, they do not help most moral discussions. Many heated discussions grow even more heated or more deadlocked over issues of rights than over any other issues. Even though I may have a right to some object, and you may have a right not to be deprived of it, it is still not clear that I have an obligation, duty, or anything else to give it to you. For example, our right to freedom of speech does not extend so far as to be able to slander and libel people. Some difficult rights questions in prenatal diagnosis are: "Does a mother with a known genetically transmittable disease have a right to avoid having a genetically defective child through prenatal diagnosis and abortion?," "Does such a mother have a right to have the child anyway, even though this will perpetuate a genetic disorder that causes suffering? " and even, "Does a child born with a significant genetic disorder have a right to procreate?" But even if we answer "yes" to all the above questions, there would be another rights question, "Does the public have a right to be protected from the consequences of an increase in genetically disabled persons?" which would present us with a new problem. So rights reasoning is not as productive in moral reasoning as one might think.

FROM RIGHTS TO RESPONSIBILITIES

Some ethicists have gone from a negative moral theory to more positive ones.[7] By this I mean to say that they have gone from theories emphasizing those things that cannot be taken from someone (a property theory at heart, and therefore capitalist and masculinist and patriarchal) to theories that emphasize positive values, such as helping, cooperating, and doing things because of love and friendship. These types of ethical theories are more appropriate for medical situations, I think, except in cases where total strangers deal with one another, such as in hospitals. A patient in a hospital must have her rights clearly set out and established at the outset. But, where a trust relationship exists with a particular physician, the rights relationship is out of place. Feminists are encouraging the de-emphasis of rights relationships. The vulnerability or helplessness of a patient does not give reason for a stronger assertion of rights; rather, the responsibility on the part of the practitioner to do his or her best is increased. Humans simply come related to one another, and thus duties are much more fundamental than rights. Feminists in medical ethics are operating in an ethics of duty.

VALUES IN MEDICAL AND PROFESSIONAL ETHICS

One source of tension in medical ethics exists between making decisions that are best overall for society in general and making decisions that are best in particular for the patient involved. In prenatal diagnosis this is most obvious. The new powers and controls we have over our reproduction signal changes in our own self-conception and in our relationship to nature. When prenatal therapy becomes normal, this will be even more problematic.

Feminism has seemed to find its strength in particular situations. Women have been found, in studies done by people like Kohlberg,[8] to make decisions in moral situations precisely on the basis of the characteristics of individuals involved, leaving overall societal concerns aside. However, such overall concerns cannot be left out entirely. Although it may be masculinist to assume that the most abstract and universal ethical principles are the best, it is not obvious that the most concrete and particular ethical decisions are the best either.

One new value in medical ethics is "demedicalization," which I translate loosely as "demasculinization." The medical technology involved in reproduction as well as in medical research institutions, etc., does seem to be masculinist. Therefore we can say that one central issue women have with reproduction technology is the "demasculinization" of the medical profession in America.

Professionalism embodies values that morally are highly objectionable, not only to feminists. Central to the notion of professionalism is an elitism, either through a supposed monopoly on knowledge, or through a monopoly of the services available through the particular profession in question. The positive value usually associated with professionalism is a dedication to the public interest. Such commitment is usually found in codes of medical ethics (although perhaps not always in the practice of medicine). Some feminists are quite justified in perceiving professionalism as a disvalue; laypersons in the medical field therefore see the moral path as lying outside of professionalism.

Although justified, the reluctance to work with medical professionals seems to me, however, to be misguided. First of all, true reform must involve medical professionals. Secondly, there are many medical improvements being made in private practice and in institutions. Some reform pioneers who have contributed to this book can say better than I how difficult such pushing from within can be. The primary feminist value in professional ethics seems to me to be *non-exclusiveness* either of professionals or of nonprofessionals. Besides, there are conceptions of a profession other than masculinist ones that we can use: we just need to strengthen and refine them.

VALUES IN FEMINIST ETHICS

One major moral problem involved with prenatal diagnosis and other medical technologies dealing with reproduction is a tendency toward "depersonalization" of women, childbirth, and children because of these technologies. A feminist value then would be a general *humanism,* which values *humane treatment* combined with a respect for persons' *self-determination.* Other feminist values would be *cooperation, kindness,* and *individualization.* We would do well here to try to come up with a more complete list of feminist values which we would then be able to use in reform and criticism.

There are five ways to be a feminist in general and therefore in medicine.[9] **Conservative feminism** asserts that there are real differences between men and women that are not merely products of socialization; these differences accurately reflect our natural condition and therefore ought not to be changed. **Liberal feminism** says that women have been oppressed owing to the lack of fair treatment given to them by the political and legal systems in bourgeois democracy, and that legal reform is therefore the source of women's freedom from oppression. Most pro-choice people in abortion and most women involved in this conference would seem to be liberal feminists. **Marxist feminists** think that the primary source of women's oppression is the class division and the exploitation of the majority of people by those who own the means of production. Individual men who are not the ruling class are not the oppressors of women. The source of women's freedom from oppression is therefore a revolution that abolishes private property and gives public ownership to the means of production.[10] **Radical feminism** sees that places where such revolutions have taken place have not abolished women's oppression, and therefore asserts that women's oppression is a result of a fundamental biological dichotomy in childbearing abilities. Therefore, the source of freedom is a freedom from our biology through the new technologies being developed now.[11] **Feminist socialism** tries to assert that women have been oppressed *both* through patriarchy (male control and domination of primary social institutions) and through capitalism, and therefore fights on two fronts. It would seem to me that this latter position is the most comprehensive.

THE OWNERSHIP OF BODIES AND CHILDREN AS PROPERTY

Women critics of medicalization and the medical profession seem to assume that women's mistreatment by the profession is wrong because it is the women's *own* bodies that are involved. However, it seems to me (and to Sarah Ann Ketchum[12]) that it is entirely misconceived to think of bodies as things we own. This is in fact a carryover from other masculinist ethical theories such as contractarianism and utilitarianism, which say that if someone owns something, then they have a right to do with it as they please. Now property rights are one thing, but to extend property rights to one's body (John Locke) seems inappropriate morally. I do not own my body; I am my body.

On the other hand, although my body is not a reproducing mechanism that *I* own it is also most certainly not owned by anyone else either, especially a man or some men. The moral difference, however, between being sexually and reproductively coerced by individual husbands on one side or male domination of the medical profession on the other is insignificant to me. Morally, the oppression is equally wrong. The latter group (medical profession) has a more oppressive function to those who think it is better to be hurt or oppressed by the ones you love. I am not one of those.

The moral crunch comes when feminists want to argue against the ownership of the female body in general by men, but who also want to argue that *they themselves* own it. One cannot have it both ways. If women own their bodies, children become *products* that can be bought and sold. We must reconceive of ourselves and our children in some other manner.

WOMEN'S RESPONSIBILITY IN REPRODUCTION AND THE FEMINIST DILEMMA

It is both a curse and a blessing that only women bear children. It is historically and economically a source of women's oppression. Yet the overwhelming significance of species survival through reproduction has guaranteed women a source of great potential power, power in the sense of ability rather than control.[13] It may even be that the awesome ability women have to produce human beings was the cause or source of patriarchy itself, if men out of fear or jealousy sought to control the powerful spirits women seemed to have.

But if women perceive of themselves as owning their bodies, nonwomen can then *steal* or *appropriate* them, either through burglary (marriage), robbery (rape), or theft (dating), if men do not bother to purchase them honestly but illegally (prostitution). No one can steal what is not owned in the first place.

So on the one hand some some see freedom from reproduction by medical technology as oppression, while others are reluctant to give up the only value women clearly have in a patriarchal society, i.e., as reproducing machines. Men *need* us now, for species survival, for "legitimate" heirs, for labor connected to reproduction, such as childrearing, education, and housework, and to supply the capitalist labor market.

But if and when they do not need us for this, I believe they would eliminate us. Misogyny (i.e., woman-hating) cannot be underestimated in a society with a high rape rate, with medical experimentation on women, and with the exportation of Depo-Provera and DES, such as has been reported here.

Therefore, one primary and fundamental moral and political decision needs to be made by women in medicine soon, namely whether or not to welcome technology that may free women from their bondage to biology. In making this decision, let us not forget that it is still disadvantaged women over the world who most need the benefits of technology and the freedom it can bring.

Prenatal Diagnosis Discussion

Moderated by Gerene D. Major

Michael Gross: I think we should expand the range of concerns here. For instance, an attempt is being made in Germany to measure and adjust "therapeutically" prenatal levels of sex hormones like testosterone. It is assumed, questionably, that the level of sex hormones at some critical period determines sexual identity. An explicit aim of this research on hormone-dependent sexual differentiation of the brain is to find a way to diagnose homosexuality *in utero.* Whether it succeeds or not, we should consider the implications and underlying values. These attempts are clearly linked to the general approach of all prenatal therapies, to "normalize" the child. Moreover, their aim is to reinforce sex differences by eliminating the "problem" of homosexuality—behavior that violates stereotyped sex roles. In short, this form of prenatal diagnosis most clearly seeks to reinforce sex role stereotypes. In fact, popularized accounts of ongoing research on brain differentiation already serve that aim by asserting a biological basis for a host of supposed sex differences.

Judith Luce: Katsi mentioned last night, about meeting in the longhouse, that everything that was done would take into consideration what the effect was going to be on their children's children's children's children—seven times. When I was little, every Saturday I went to the shoe store and took X-rays of my feet. I used to look at my toes wiggling in my shoes, and most of my friends did. There were supposedly no long-term effects of X-rays that anyone knew about.

I'm concerned that there's a bias that comes with working within any narrow discipline. When Mary Jane Gray said, "We think that there are no long-term effects . . . ," what she is really saying is, "We *hope* there are no long-term effects." There's really a bias towards accepting technology, whereas there's a bias on my part for *not* accepting it.

Renée Jenkins: Sonograms are done so often. I work with young teenagers who have no idea when their last menstrual period occurred, and almost every one of those young women end up with at least two sonograms to try to detect the fetal age. Is there some sort of registry? What kind of continual records are kept on mothers who get sonograms? Maybe there should be a sample national group over a period of, say, ten years, so that in some sort of systematic way you can go back and look at the early and the long-term effects.

Mary Jane Gray: We have *not* done research in this country involving large prospective studies of various problems. For years, we didn't study hormones and menopause, because that would have involved a prospective study of large groups, and the government has rarely funded such studies—often they still don't. You're going to have to depend on women knowing that they have had sonograms—and possibly on people someday going back and reviewing records and tracing these.

Joyce Lashof: There was discussion about a year ago, before I left HEW, of trying to set up a prospective long-term study on pregnant women. A special task force is probably still looking at the problems involved, the cost, the size of the sample required. I think it's badly needed.

I'm very familiar with the literature about X-rays during pregnancy and with how the data were gathered that eventually determined that there was an increase in leukemia. Dr. Alice Stuart developed a long-term study on childhood cancer. She obtained death certificates of all children who died of cancer in England from 1950 on, and then went back and got each birth certificate and took the next birth certificate—in order—in the birth certificate file. The mothers of the children born at the exact same time—the mother of the normal child and the mother of the child who had died under the age of ten of leukemia or any other cancer—were interviewed. From the data, she was able to determine that the one factor which correlated with an increase in leukemia was the performance of X-ray pelvimetry during the first trimester of pregnancy. So far, there are no data that X-ray pelvimetry performed after the first trimester has a detectable risk. That doesn't mean it doesn't have some risk. I'm convinced that there is no threshold in low-dose radiation. But in terms of detectable amount of risk, it has not been proven beyond the first trimester. That kind of study in cancer continues, and Dr. Stuart has a registry now of all childhood cancer deaths from 1950 on, and continues to look for other things. It's a lifetime's work, and it takes a dedicated epidemiologist to do it—and yet to *my knowledge* she's only turned up X-ray as a correlate.

Ruth Hubbard: I want to make it clear that we aren't just "anti-technology freaks." If one thinks about what ultrasound is—a form of mechanical disturbance—it stands to reason that it could cause changes either in the placenta or in the embryo. I would be more surprised if there are no effects than if there are. I go on the assumption that there must be some; the question is their extent. Coming at it from that direction, I worry about what the women are told to caution them about possible ill effects.

Mary Jane Gray: These kinds of studies, I think, are done better in countries like England and Sweden, where record-keeping is better than it is in this country. It's very hard to take the teenagers Renée is talking about and even follow where they're going to be.

Yvonne Brackbill: A national registry is quite different from a study. The question that was raised originally, to which nobody really responded, was what to do if we find out in the future that the risks are far greater than we anticipate at present. I'm adding to that question and saying: Don't you physicians who are using that technique feel that you have some obligation to press for the establishment of a national registry?

Mary Jane Gray: I know of no way we can set up a national registry, but I think—as an individual obstetrician—maybe we can, through the bureaucracy, get something like this that can function. If this is done prospectively, you've got to register everybody who gets a particular procedure. I know this is a crucial issue because of the DES crisis.

Yvonne Brackbill: It isn't necessary to set up a new agency. There is already a structure within the World Health Organization for national registries for adverse drug reactions. The United States has been a token member for some time now, although we've never really contributed.

Fredric Abramson: The existence of computers has promoted and enabled the construction of very large data banks about people. Two issues are being raised concerning this. One is invasion of privacy, with the ability to track us through a myriad of life experiences and to aggregate information. There is a very powerful sense in this country that absolutely opposes the incorporation of information about us into data files—no matter how noble the purpose.

The other aspect is that health registries are being formulated using that computer technology. Tufts New England is developing a birth defects computer-base that has the intention of providing malformation case entry by physicians all over the country. It is hoped that the pooled information will facilitate better diagnostic techniques, and better understanding of the outcomes of children with disorders. The American Red Cross maintains a national registry of all rare blood donors that come in to the Red Cross. Fifty percent of the blood in the

United States is handled by the American National Red Cross. They also attempt, and get cooperation from other participating blood banks, to locate rare donors.

Carol Korenbrot: You must recognize that in order to use this information technology ethically, you have to face the pragmatic problems of following these people: investing money and time, and invading people's privacy to follow them for life.

Barbara Andolsen: Yvonne, you are asserting a physician obligation to set up this registry. Fred and Carol are making another ethical point: "Is it a violation of my rights as an individual to have mandatory reporting?" Or, if this registry contains only names of women who gave consent for release of this information to a data bank, then the population will still be self-selected.

Maureen Flannery: As a physician I support Yvonne's idea of a registry very strongly. I suggest that we, as a group, ask ACOG and American College of Radiology, together, to set up a registry for ultrasound studies. Sonograms are being done now, and there may be no records of them in ten years unless we do something about it. Ultrasound may turn out to be like DES. One of the spookiest things, to me, about DES is the fact that we found out about the hazards of DES only because it produces a rare form of cancer at an unusual age. If DES produced breast cancer or lung cancer—something more common—or affected only older women, we might not know about it yet—or ever. DES might still be used in pregnant women. Still it's not enough to ask professional bodies to establish registries: I don't think we can trust them. We need to make provision also for women to receive some sort of card identifying the sonogram she had for future reference.

Mary Jane Gray: I think that's a much more viable option, because until we get to the point where we are comfortable with the notion of having our medical records in a data bank that any professional in any part of the country can tap into for followup, we're not going to be able, on a practical level, to have what I agree it would be splendid to have.

I think it's perfectly possible to have concerned women following their history and knowing what's been done to them and what drugs they've been given.

Elizabeth Kutter: I think to ask any individual physician *never* to use a technique like ultrasound or amniocentesis just because there's not a registry may be a mistake. There are clearly some instances where it may be life-saving or make a very big difference in the outcome. Should we totally eliminate that option?

Robert Murray: I think that one of the problems here is that we haven't presented the literature on the studies of ultrasound. I know that ultrasound has been studied for its effects on chromosomes. To a geneticist, this is one primary concern. We know that, under the dosage levels that we normally use during gestation, there is no *detectable* chromosome damage. That doesn't mean that there might not be some. But then, we're always at risk of chromosome damage from a variety of sources in our environment. So to date we don't have any evidence from tissue culture studies, studies on mice or other mammals, that ultrasound at the level we use it now causes genetic damage. Ultrasound was used for years in attempting to identify liver tumors, brain tumors, and other abnormal growths. The liver is metabolically a very active organ. Its cells are rapidly dividing, and rapidly dividing cells are most susceptible to injury, but there's no evidence that there has been damage in the liver based on very long experience. So we do have some evidence that ultrasound, at the levels used today, is not likely to be damaging.

Then, there *is* the risk–benefit ratio that is subconsciously calculated any time we take a medical action—whether it's taking an aspirin or taking a chest X-ray for a nagging cough. I think that the ethical issue that we're dealing with here is whether a physician—or anybody for that matter—can justify recommending a particular procedure in a pregnant female.

Byllye Avery: We can't look at just the studies, themselves. The people who sell the machines, the people who conduct the studies, are the ones policing themselves. As a health-care consumer, I don't know if I trust the studies any more. You said that 5% of the women who have amniocentesis turn out to have some problem. Do you have a screening process that you could use, so that maybe the women who have no problems would not have to have that test?

Mary Ampola: That's an excellent question, but unfortunately there are *no* known factors other than age that help delineate a "high-risk" group. In fact, all one can do is look at the curve representing Down's syndrome incidence vs age. The risk increases gradually in the early childbearing years, then after age 35, it rises sharply. There's no way we can, or should, test all pregnancies. So one tries to come to some—admittedly very arbitrary—maternal age cutoff. Currently that age is 35. Amniocentesis is an *option* for women. We explain to them, as best we know, what the risk is, and what information we can gain from the test. There is nothing coercive about this.

Byllye Avery: I guess I look at it as, "healthy until proven diseased," and I feel that the medical vision is, "diseased until proven healthy."

Fredric Abramson: We are trying to develop a better definition of "high risk," and then to test only those women.

Jill Wolhandler: It's all very well to say that amniocentesis is simply presented as an option if there's a higher risk. But who is it that presents this option to pregnant women? Bring it down to women's realities, now. It's people such as obstetricians who have great belief in technology. There's a coercive factor in the relationship between doctor and patient. It is not an equal relationship. A woman comes into that relationship in a position of very little power most of the time. And there are many obstetricians who abuse that power. I spoke to a woman last week who is thirty-five and wants to have a baby. Her obstetrician told her not only that she should not have a child because it was "so dangerous" to her, but that if she *did* do it, she *had* to have amniocentesis. I know you're saying that his opinion isn't correct, and I understand that, but this is the way this kind of technology translates into the realities of our current health-care system. We cannot forget that when we talk about it.

Norma Swenson: I support what Jill just said. Some women are routinely scheduled for ultrasound every single month of their pregnancy, through private physicians' offices that are not connected in any way with genetic counseling. It's information the physician wants. Amniocenteses require two ultrasound pictures to be done accurately. It's not necessarily a once-in-a-lifetime event. Most women are not being given informed consent. In a recent Boston television show on the wonders of prenatal diagnosis, a woman was invited to come up from the audience and have this ultrasound beamed on her, and there was the picture of the baby, and it went on and on and on. The FDA is proposing to study and regulate ultrasound use. No one here has talked about the ultrasound issue in terms of amniocentesis. The FDA wants to regulate ultrasound precisely for this reason: that we *don't* know what the long-term effects are. The fact that we don't have any immediate results from those low-level bombardments in adults does not guarantee that the fetus inside the uterus, at adulthood or sooner, will not show some effects. The scale of assessment on these two situations is very different. Animal studies already show changes in cell structures as a result of ultrasound exposure. Women are not being given this information. I don't think we can wait for registries or any other kind of revolution. The first thing we have to press for at the federal level is that there is—in the same way that we're trying to have informed consent procedures built into patient package inserts—an informed consent procedure that precedes any of those tests, and that it is in writing, and it is signed, and women and physicians take responsibility for that. And it should say that the long-term effects are unknown.

Mary Ampola: Until just recently, women 35 years and over have not come for amniocentesis at their obstetrician's insistence. They came referred by the *Ladies' Home Journal* or other women—i.e., some nonmedical source. Obstetricians were generally *not* telling them about (1) their increased risk, or (2) the possibility of amniocentesis. Just recently, a suit was decided against an obstetrician for not telling a woman about the possibility of amniocentesis. All of a sudden, things have shifted. Now I am seeing many women referred by obstetricians. I see amniocentesis as an opportunity for women to further empower their lives and work. Have you ever lived with a Down's syndrome child? I've taken care of these children for 12 years. Have you ever tried to care for one with a profound heart defect, or seen the impact on the other children, or seen the enormous divorce rate? Some families *can* make Down's syndrome a positive experience, but they are a very small minority. If a woman is 35 or older, amniocentesis allows her to say "Down's syndrome is something I *can* prevent, and which I will not risk because I have certain values and certain goals in life. I want that option."

Relative to amniocentesis, coercion is a concept that should be absolutely foreign. Women are helped by obtaining formal genetic counseling before the test. The kind of counseling they get from a genetic counselor who is trying to be sensitive to what the woman wants to do with her life—not to what the doctor or anyone else wants—should be very informative and supportive to her. I think you're right, there is danger of the pendulum swinging toward coercion because the obstetrician's going to say, "What if she has a Down's syndrome child? She'll say I didn't tell her." Because of the fear of law suits, some doctors have already begun having a nurse present as witness, or having women sign forms that state they've been told the risk. But that's all beside the central point, which is that amniocentesis is an opportunity for a woman to add some further control to her life.

Joan Holtzman: I wanted to support something that Mary said, perhaps in a slightly different way. The tenor of the conversation seems to be that only technology has risks. Nature has risks, as well. That is, naturally occurring processes produce error, through no fault of human intervention. Things simply go wrong. What makes this a dilemma, what makes this difficult and not a clear-cut issue, is the balancing not only of risks and benefits, but of risks against risks: the risks of not doing anything against the risks of doing something that may also be harmful. So sitting in the longhouse, we might also want to consider how many generations of people could be affected by a genetically carried disorder that went untreated. To say, "Let's close the book on technology, or wait until all the answers are in," is a very conservative position and it would have very conservative results. I don't mean to put away anything you said about caution and information banks and doing all we can to contain the abuses of technology. We need to do all those things. But we need also to be sensitive to the fact that risks are everywhere, and they're not only caused by technology.

Maureen Flannery: Two comments. First—I would agree with Mary that most genetic counselors give women very clear explanations and choices. I'm concerned that women who get their genetic counseling from doctors *or* from *Ladies' Home Journal* are not being adequately informed of two things. In terms of age-related risk of having a baby with a chromosomal abnormality, there's a big difference between being 35 and being 40. A very careful study has been done in New York State showing exactly how the risk increases after the age of thirty-five. Women who delay childbearing need that information. Recent studies also show that the age of the *father* is also important in a number of abnormalities.

My other concern is that enough information is not given women about the limits of technology and amniocentesis. The facts are that amniocentesis can tell you with pretty good accuracy whether you're going to have a baby with Down's syndrome, but it *cannot* tell you whether your baby's going to be all right. Many women, I think, take it to mean that.

Mary Ampola: That's one point we make very carefully in genetic counseling. A normal amniocentesis does not mean a normal baby. It means normalcy only with respect to what we are able to study.

Maureen Flannery: Genetic counselors give that explanation. But more and more physicians are doing amniocenteses in their own offices, without giving women that information.

Rebecca Logan: Can we have the technology for the three percent who need it, without abuses? These technologies are developed by corporations to make a profit. They can't make a profit without large markets so they spend incredible amounts of money advertising the technology. Thus, in the context of our present society, we cannot have these technologies for the three percent without the abuses for the other ninety-seven percent.

Regina Kenen: I think that's a point of view and a valid one, and one that has to be debated. I'm concerned that if we take your position we'd have to get rid of our whole system. It's no longer just reproduction: it becomes a whole different issue. I teach "deviance," and it's very interesting to note that when someone claims there is a biological cause of deviance, everyone rushes to accept that explanation because they can blame it on certain individuals. But when someone says poverty is the cause of deviance nobody wants to face that kind of issue, because it means a restructuring of society. So I don't think the point you are making can be narrowed to just prenatal diagnosis. It's our whole society and what you're going to do about it and its priorities.

Susan Ekstrom: If we uncritically accept the medical model of birth, we're going to continue to get the kind of pathologically oriented pregnancy and maternal care that we currently do get. I agree with Susan Peterson that this talk of demedicalization really has a lot to do with demasculinization. One of the things that disturbed me earlier in this discussion was the assumption that women should go only to "professional" counselors for counseling. That assumption really continues to discount women's networks. Women are discounted, while also being told, "don't listen to other women, to old wives' tales." We are constantly exposed to the ideology that the physician is the unique, crucial authority capable of making health care decisions. I think one of the ways of altering this view is by strengthening women's networks. And women's networks, unlike some other systems, will reach out to *all* women. For example, there is a study that shows that 25% of the poor women in this country get absolutely no medical supervision whatsoever during their pregnancies. The first time they see medical personnel is when they go to the hospital for labor and birth. Although all women, obviously, should have good medical care, not all pregnancies and births should be highly medicalized. And while working to ensure that all women get good, basic medical care, we also need to utilize women's networks, to get away from this concentration on looking to the "masculine" professional for all of our information. There are a lot of wise women whom we can turn to.

Fredric Abramson: I think there's no question that the support systems for women and for men can come from a community base, from other people. And there is a tendency to discount information that lies in the community. Yet I also think that in regard to pregnancy, for example, prior to the advent of the technology that is being challenged, if women had the answers to the tough questions, "Tell me that I'm going to have a good pregnancy; tell me that I'll have a healthy, normal child," then I maintain that it would have been impossible for that position to be usurped. In any system in which there is a vacuum of information, someone can move in. I would expect to see women gravitating away from sources of less trustworthy information, by whatever values they have, to more trustworthy information, by their standard. One of the things that has helped many women feel more comfortable with their pregnancy has come from a technology base. In a sense you're also asserting the denial of choice because you're asserting that only women can provide information to women.

Susan Ekstrom: I think a lot of the assumptions you're making about community are based on a very masculine view. What I'm saying is that currently women's choices are restricted insofar as women are led to believe that the *only* "trustworthy" information regarding pregnancy and birth must come through "professional" sources based on the medical model of birth. I'm also saying that women, and laypeople in general, have considerably greater competence than is currently recognized under the medicalized model of health care. Certainly women and laypeople should make use of information available from medical professionals. But just as certainly, the information available from these professionals should be critically evaluated. And women's networks can help us to do just that. All you have to do is to look at *Our Bodies, Ourselves.*

Diana Axelsen: With respect to who should do the counseling, my viewpoint is that of someone who is 38, intended to have a child at 30, and since then has been continually making the decision not to have a child. My values shift, and I'm not sure what I will do at 40. In making any decision, however, I'd want the help of counselors whom I considered qualified.

Also, although as an individual I would like to have the option of amniocentesis, I'm not sure that this freedom of choice is justified when we consider the social implications. We should look at arguments for and against amniocentesis, realizing that sometimes society should do things that seem to abridge individual freedom. For example, I'm opposed to using prisoners as experimental subjects. Some prisoners feel that this refusal is a denial of their rights. But I'm not sure we should give prisoners this "freedom" to choose to be subjects. At least, first, we need to change prison conditions so that being a subject isn't an appealing option because of economic deprivation, lack of rehabilitation programs, or other abuses. In general, we need to look at a variety of perspectives before determining what decisions individuals are entitled to make, and what sacrifices individuals must make for the sake of the community.

Margaret Kohn: I wanted to address my remark to the link between legal rights and professional responsibility in regard to prenatal diagnosis. This comment is related as well to all of the other topics that we talked about. Unfortunately in our country there is no right to health care—it is premised on whether you can pay for it. We have failed in this whole discussion to consider sufficiently the behavior of physicians who participate in perpetuating the problem of financial access. For example, ob/gyns have almost the highest average income of all physicians in the country. That is part and parcel of the problem. When we talk about prenatal diagnosis, access to midwives, access to ob/gyn services, we have the problem of physician attitudes and behavior, both on monetary issues, and within their own group, of ways in which they prevent people from getting services by harassing their own, by not policing their own, by developing systems of delivery that perpetuate, exaggerate, and exacerbate income barriers. To bring it back to the prenatal diagnosis question, who's going to get these services? Amniocentesis costs five hundred dollars in a lot of places in this country. If you're on Medicaid maybe you'll get it. If you're of a higher socioeconomic level you may be able to pay for that. Many insurance policies will not pay for that. And we talk about this option as a realistic option. It's not a realistic option for many, many people. If we're going to have services available to people, they should be available to people, to everybody and not to just a few.

Susan Peterson: That was my criticism of the liberal feminist perspective, which says that all we have to do is maximize our choices. The limitation on that is that there are people who are economically disadvantaged, who will not be able to take advantage of these "choices."

Judy Norsigian: I think we should proceed with caution when it comes to advancing new technologies. We've got to expect that widespread abuse will occur with the development of new technologies. This must be considered in all these discussions.

We are bombarded with so many complex issues, with so much information, and yet we can absorb only so much before we become dangerously desensitized. One result is that we find ourselves living in a culture where there's nuclear madness. It concerns me that an inevitable consequence of so many new proliferating technologies is our collective desensitization to some of the most important issues. Maybe we've lost some of the sensibility that Katsi Cook describes, not because we're evil or irresponsible or have something wrong with us, but simply because its just humanly impossible to cope with the present "bombardment." It's a fallacy to talk about this or that "wonderful opportunity," if we're not able or in a position to make an informed decision about whether to take advantage of the opportunity.

Ruth Hubbard: It seems to me that there's a hidden ideology and agenda behind the entire subject of prenatal diagnosis that hasn't come up yet. And that's "eugenics." You can't talk about amniocentesis and similar techniques without putting it in the context of the search for "bad genes." The old eugenics died because it was ineffective. There are now more effective ways of looking for "bad genes." And we must be aware that that is one of the aspects of what we're talking about.

The Neonate

Organized by
Caroline Whitbeck

Introductory Remarks

Caroline Whitbeck

The neonate chapter has three specific goals. The first of these is to share information about neonates, or newborns, and the kinds of impairments they may face, the kinds of medical technology—both high level and low level—that may be used with them, the decisions about the use of this technology, and the influence of social and technological factors on those decisions. Second, we want to stimulate a rethinking of the moral issues involved, as they relate to the individual, the family, and the community. Third, we wish to broaden the awareness of what women do in nurturing and caring for the newborn, impaired or not.

The title originally planned for this section was "The Defective Neonate." Previous literature in medical ethics has focused on the question of what to do about the newborn who is so severely impaired that the question arises whether to attempt any intervention. That is only one of the issues about newborns that we ultimately felt obliged to examine. Birth defects are common, even though the severe impairments that have been the focus of attention are not. About one in twenty children is born with some form of handicap or impairment that he or she will carry through life. We examine the supports and technologies available for coping with the task of rearing a baby who has significant handicaps, whether or not those handicaps are so severe that anyone would consider foregoing all treatment for that newborn.

It is worth bringing to the reader's attention that Helga Bendix, one of the contributors, perceived some time ago at a Hasting's Center workshop, the insufficient attention to the perspective of women, and specifically to the perspective of mothers of impaired children. Her dissatisfaction and that of other women were what originally spurred Becky Holmes to organize this workshop and these books.

We wish to examine the whole issue of newborns, who they are, and what we do with respect to them. We must understand the *difference* between a newborn and a child if we hope to achieve any clarity about what it is for a newborn to *become* a child, about what it is we do in calling forth a newborn into human relationship. It is we women, whether the "natural" mothers or not, who most often do this.

It is an extraordinary task, one of those everyday miracles that women perform. To start with a being that is not a relational being, and to call her or him forth into human relationship has no parallel. There are other activities that may mimic this one, projects in which we call forth others in a way that gives them new capabilities, but bringing a newborn into the world of human relationships is the paradigm of this kind of action.

This calling forth receives no significant representation within our culture. We barely have words for it. The lack of naming is an essential part of the mystification of all work that is women's work. We cannot reflect on our project very easily if we cannot represent it to ourselves. The prevailing fantasy within masculinist culture is that we do not *do* anything. It just *happens,* the way *apples* fall from trees. It does not take a great deal of skill to make cooing noises to a three-month-old, we are told. If we consider individual acts in isolation, it is easy to say "Well, those *little* things don't require any skill," but the point is that we do these things in such a way as to engage the infant, something that takes an exquisite sensitivity. We enter into a very complex dialog that makes the other capable of dialog.

Psychologists tell us that, after all, it is important to have "good mothering." But all that language tells us is that those expected to accomplish this incredible task are the female parents. It gives us no insight into how to do it, and how to describe it and reflect on it. Just as cosmology may tell us about the formation of the universe without telling us *how* to form a universe, developmental psychology views our project from the outside, and describes it in terms of "contact" or "attachment." I do not think that that vocabulary is very helpful. It sounds as though the newborn and the nurturer were billiard balls, equipped with glue or hooks or electrical charge. It does not give us an insight into what the project is or how we carry it out. Developmental psychology does turn up some interesting facts, but it does not give us any insight into our own activity.

By my comments on the vocabulary used in psychological studies, I don't want to create a situation in which we will boo and hiss when someone says "contact" or "attachment." That would be a situation in which *we* do not call *one another* forth, but just shut each other up. It would be a shame if we just set up a new elite which decides on a mandatory vocabulary. We are *all* inarticulate. That is part of our condition as women. We are all struggling to be able to say what it is we are doing, to articulate our values and promote them.

There is even a problem about the word "nurturant." It gives you the idea that perhaps what one is doing is maintaining someone, and particularly maintaining by feeding. Now, I would not want to ignore the issue of maintaining/feeding. I think world hunger is a central problem in terms of women's values. But women do much more than maintaining others. That is why I use the expression "calling forth."

This project of calling others forth is what ought to be, in a moral sense, the central project in human life. When we women do this with respect to each other it's called "sisterhood" and accounts for some of the new ways of being and relating that are among the miracles of the Women's Movement. I take this to be something that we do, not in pairs, but as part of a community—which makes new possibilities available to us all.

This calling forth may be not only a process for effecting change, but, indeed, the end for which we are working. As we become clearer about the project of calling others into being, and the personal, social, and economic requirements of that project, perhaps we can be clearer about which applications of technology further this end—and which, by that criterion at least, are moral. In this way we strengthen one another so that each of us will be better able to resist coercion to support projects of domination.

Neonatology

Directions and Goals

Maureen Edwards

INTRODUCTION

The term "neonatology" was not coined until 1960 when Alexander Schaeffer, in one of the first American texts on the subject, used it to denote that part of pediatrics with special concern for the "art and science of the diagnosis and treatment of disorders of the newborn infant."[1] Neonatal intensive care and neonatology are closely related although not completely synonymous areas of expertise. The subspeciality of Neonatal–Perinatal Medicine was formally recognized as a sub-board of the American Board of Pediatrics with its first examination and diplomates only five years ago in 1975.[2] Last fall was the third year this examination was given.

This slow start may relate to the large health problem for practitioners of pediatrics in the first half of this century of infectious disease associated with high childhood mortality. Although the chance of death has always been greatest for an individual in the first hours and days after birth, the relative impact of neonatal mortality has increased as postneonatal mortality has declined. On the other hand, control of infectious disease has allowed time and effort to focus on another major pediatric risk—neonatal mortality and morbidity. In addition, the overall advancement in modern technology has provided professionals with special concerns for sick newborns with the tools necessary to diagnose and treat them.

WHAT IS NEONATOLOGY?

Neonatology is distinguished from other medical subspecialties by:

1. Its focus, of course, on the problems of newborn infants, particularly prematures and infants with lung disease.

From the medical point of view, about 1% of the newborn infants will require neonatal intensive care: I am talking about the really sick, critically ill baby. Another 10 to 20% of the hospital-born babies may require some special observation in the neonatal period.

2. Its intensive care nature. It requires a 24-hour team of highly and specially trained physicians, nurses, respiratory therapists, laboratory and X-ray personnel, in addition to team members to provide specific family supports. It is reasonably practiced only in larger medical centers, where it requires a broad spectrum of advanced technology adapted to the size and needs of neonates. A typical critically ill infant necessitates an incubator for temperature maintenance; a monitor of heart rate and respirations; a blood pressure device; at least one intravenous pump that can deliver small but exact volumes of fluids; equipment for respiratory support, often a neonatal ventilator with attachments for humidification and warming oxygen, and an oxygen analyzer for exact measurements of inspired gases; an available means of rapidly determining oxygen, carbon dioxide, and pH in the blood, plus a bevy of smaller devices. This plethora of technical "assistants" has burgeoned over the last 10–15 years and is progressing at a rate that imposes perplexing problems for the practitioner. The selection of a truly useful and important, documentedly safe, and cost-effective technology is a daily concern.
3. Its predominantly "academic" setting. Most of its practitioners are medical school faculty members; many practice in university settings. Most combine clinical care with contributions to the scientific basis for that care.

WHAT ARE THE GOALS OF NEONATOLOGY?

The goals of neonatology, as I see it, are:

1. To provide each infant and his/her family with the "optimal" chance for a "happy," "healthy," life together.
2. In doing this, to decrease "avoidable" neonatal mortality and morbidity.
3. To lessen the "negative impact" of neonatal "tragedies" on all involved.
4. To continue to add to the body of knowledge that allows this.
5. And finally, "primum non nocere."

The goals might be articulated in a variety of different ways; they are certainly interpreted and pursued diversely. The subjectivity and spectrum of meanings of words such as "optimal," "healthy," "happy," "tragedy," and so on allow for apparently divergent approaches to these goals. The most easily achieved goal of decreasing mortality may be in opposition to the goal of "lessening tragedy" or of a "happy, healthy life." The conflict between "doing no harm" and advancing knowledge is regularly raised at Human Research Committees. Clarifying the goals is not as easy as citing them; picking a goal in an individual clinical situation is equally difficult. Sometimes we focus on individual successes.

IS NEONATOLOGY ACHIEVING ITS GOALS?

A general trend toward decreasing neonatal and infant mortality and morbidity has occurred in all developing countries. The specific impact of neonatology must be seen against this background. The prejudice of neonatology is, of course, that it is moving in a measurable way toward the goals outlined above. The evidence most available and most often cited looks at mortality rates and quantifiable morbidity before and after the advent of neonatal intensive care in general or with specific modalities. Many centers have reported declining mortalities and, more recently, enhanced outcomes with advent of more sophisticated and specialized neonatal care. These reports include those from the Women's College Hospital in Toronto,[3] the University of California Medical Center,[4] the Vanderbilt University Hospital,[5] the University of Southern California,[6] and the Toronto Hospital for Sick Children,[7] to name a few. Surely, children do survive with handicaps who would have died without neonatal intensive care. But our prejudice and, I believe, the facts substantiate that as more children are surviving, most children are healthy, many of whom would have been handicapped without neonatal intensive care.

But there are many congenital abnormalities that we cannot abate—certain kinds of congenital cardiac disease and central nervous system disorders. There are also some diseases and infections that we cannot treat, e.g., viral infections *in utero.* And there is some lower limit of maturity at which we no longer really have a good chance to save a child. This varies quite a bit from center to center. Most centers are able to give an excellent survival chance to children in the three and four pound range. In the two pound range, survival chances are now often very good, and even for babies weighing less than that there is a measurable survival range and good outcome.

WHAT ARE THE ETHICAL ISSUES FACING NEONATOLOGY?

The commonest "ethical" question facing all those concerned with sick neonates is, "When is aggressive intervention not in the child's best interest?" Specific issues concern whether to resuscitate; whether to stop the respirator and, if so, when; when to withhold surgery—in the brain-damaged baby, the baby with multiple anomalies, or the baby with single organ system failure, such as short gut syndrome or chronic lung disease.

The second and underlying question is, "How are we sure?" The medical *facts* rarely give us an absolute certainty.

The third question is, "How do we decide?" Who has significant input? Who has the ultimate decision?

A fourth question is, "How do we manage a child when withholding life support measures?"

And a final question, "What do we do with limited resources—family, medical, financial, social?"

Neonatology cannot guarantee intact survival, for a variety of reasons. There are great variations in, and a changing definition of, what intact means. Intact does not mean the condition of the baby when it leaves the nursery, but rather what the child's condition may be in school or in later life. Intact may mean quite a different thing to the health professional from what the individual parent takes it to mean, although not necessarily so.

There is a high cost to high technology. The cost is partly in dollars. The equipment at any of these babies' bedsides costs in excess of $20,000. The cost per day of the highest form of intensive care, employing the most expensive equipment, probably exceeds $1000 a day. But there are many more costs than that. There are physical costs. There are psychological costs, which we don't understand completely, and which also weigh heavily.

WHAT OTHER DISCIPLINARY PROBLEMS OF NEONATOLOGY AFFECT ETHICAL CONSIDERATIONS?

The major problem is lack of true understanding of one another's discipline. Unfortunately, the medical realities on which decisions are based are rarely totally clear to the neonatologist because of the tremendous individuality of clinical situations. Her or his conveying of this information to others, parents as well as professionals, is influenced by her or his own bias. A wide latitude of individual, personal interpretation of medical and ethical issues exists among neonatologists and this, I believe, is a great problem for others. The neonatologist's position, as the child's doctor and, perhaps, self-appointed child advocate, may put her or him at odds with more parent-oriented professionals. And, lastly, the doctor as "captain of the ship," the "final authority and decision-maker" may pose problems in individual clinical settings as well as in interdisciplinary discussions.

We do not have available to us the predictors that those who deal with patients later in life have. In only about one-sixth of the neonates can we predict the long term outcome. There are some obvious physical conditions where we can say, for instance, "The kidneys don't work." In healthy newborns the long term intellectual and neurological achievement is unsure, and sick newborns cannot be expected to do better than that. We are left with very few predictors of positive outcome, and those we do have are statistics. That may be fine in making policies, perhaps, and generalized decisions, but it may or may not be very useful to individuals involved with sick babies.

CONCLUSION

Neonatology is not *the* answer to high neonatal and infant mortality in the United States. The difference in infant mortality between Sweden and the US does not have to do with the availability of high technology, but with preventing prematurity. That is the answer, I believe, to lowering newborn mortality, not taking better care of them with high technology. However, the premies who are already here ought to be well taken care of.

I would just like to pose a couple of policy problems in closing. How can high technology, if valuable, be distributed to consumers who both want and need it? That is one of the problems of the regionalization of neonatal intensive care. The other problem a neonatologist faces is, "What do we do with the health dollars?" In Washington, DC, for instance, we have lots of neonatal intensive care, yet half of our preschoolers are not immunized against serious childhood diseases.

I went to the Emily Dickinson House during the Workshop and bought a book of her poems. When I opened the book, Emily said to me:

> Faith is a fine invention
> When gentlemen can see
> But microscopes are prudent
> In an emergency.

I'd like to have a microscope available for your sick baby if she or he needs it.

Perfectability and the Neonate

The Burden of Expectations on Mothers and Their Health Providers

Wendy Carlton

It has been a long time since I was a three pound, seven month "premie" and spent the first month of my life, so my mother tells me, in what would today be called an intensive care unit. The summer before I went to college I had a routine eye examination, and the next thing I knew I was told I was going to have surgery forty-eight hours later because my retinas were detaching. Because of that routine examination, which was a low technology occurrence, and because of the availability of high technology, I can see you. And for that, I am grateful.

The definition of what is normal is socially shaped. That means that your notion of what's normal—such as the assumption that you have two eyes and two arms and two legs, and that you have a certain kind of fundamental intelligence, and that you can understand 20% of what you hear—is a normative definition.

Historically, the definition of who is a person has changed radically. One day slaves were not people, and the next day they were. What happened? A biological revolution? When agricultural territories sought to qualify for statehood, women became enfranchised because the men needed their numbers to gain the vote. On the east coast with an ample supply of males, women lagged behind in becoming enfranchised and, in a sense, in becoming civil persons, to use technical language.

Although I could elaborate on the so-called relativity of these definitions, I just want to point out to you that trying to define criteria of personhood that will allow for a line of demarcation between the "nonperson," who is still an organism and a member of the human species, and the human species member who is a person, is a distracting device. It allows us to avoid asking questions such as "How do we, as a society, create a definition of a person based on the notion that if you look different from me, there's something wrong with you." If the difference is a physical handicap, we know from many academic studies that any such difference is much harder for the person to overcome; for such individuals it is much more difficult to become integrated into a social group because other "normal" people feel much more discomfort. In this circumstance, it often becomes better to have some horrible problem with your kidneys, so that you are not constantly flashing your difference, forcing people to confront it, and thereby being labeled as a deviant.

We have to be aware of that tendency, and avoid wasting time deciding whether we should hand over to the physicians a list of criteria that says, "In *this* situation, this entity is a person and you should commit resources, and in *this* situation you should not."

As a medical sociologist, I spent nine long months following medical students around, day and night, weekends, weekdays, trying to find out how they dealt with ethical issues in the clinical setting. For the sake of brevity, I will simply say that it became a systematic study of avoidance behavior. I could elaborate somewhat as to how they decide to avoid, obfuscate, deny, reconvert, translate, and avert their eyes from ethical issues—including issues found in the neonatal nursery. I spent a month there. It was probably the most enjoyable month I spent. I know that sounds strange, but it was a great team of people. I learned a lot, and in their own way they realized that I learned a lot, because as I was leaving the service, they congratulated me on all the medicine I had learned. And it so happens that, indirectly, I learned a lot about how they thought as physicians, how they act as physicians, how they dealt with parents, what they *said* they did, and how they actually acted. Each month a medical student informant would say, "You wait and see. We'll be ethical." And I'm still waiting. Forever.

You'll notice that originally the panel was supposed to be about "defective neonates," and the title was struck from the program because the term sounds so horrible and objectifying. That is why physicians often use that language—because it helps control some of the stress of the situation. You can see a lot of things and feel a lot of things, but you need some handles on your own anxiety—and let me tell you: medical students, in particular, are very anxious people. Without realizing it, they use objectifying language and turn people into things. They are really saying in a fairly subtle way that they suspect that people who do not have the potentiality, as *they* see it, to grow up and become medical students, are somehow inferior people. If your whole self-identity as a physician is tied up in your quickness, your ability to solve difficult problems, your capacity to abstract, then you begin to think that anyone who does not have an IQ of 160 is really missing out on something.

Now, I think we should be sensitive to why this behavior occurs, as distasteful as it may be, because they, too, are victims of the system. We could easily fall into the trap of blaming the victim and, as women, we all know what it is to be blamed as victims.

Having run around after physicians—they told me that I was pretty good running down the stairs, but I wasn't so fast running up the stairs—I learned that you need the constitution of a workhorse to be able to serve on a clinical service day in and day out and not keel over. I once did an informal study in which I asked physicians what things would be worse than death, and they said things like, "being paraplegic," or having visual or hearing impairments, or not having both your arms. These findings are appalling, and I believe they suggest that the problem of defining normality is greater than the misuse of technology. Once the technology is out there, people feel a compulsion to use it. So I think that medical students and physicians, and many of us who do have reasonably high IQs and do have all our bodily parts, tend to be overly invested in our identities, because that is how we see ourselves. And some of us who have been a little bit more limited in our social experiences sometimes think that that is all we are. We spend a long, painful, adolescence trying to reattach, or reassociate, these bodies and these minds. Physicians and medical students lead very warped lives, and it comes out in terms of their policy considerations regarding defective neonates.

I teach these people, and their lives are so narrow; and they will continue to be narrow. By the time they get to the end of their residencies they become bitter; they say, "I've been short-changed. I've spent all my life at this." It all goes back to when they were trying to get that "A" in high school so they could be admitted to the right curriculum package. Basically, they are faced with two dilemmas: they can go into specialized medicine, because they have been told, "Good physicians use their smarts to work on physical problems that those dumb-dumb local physicians can't handle," and that any attempt to look at more general problems is a waste of their education and time. Or they can take on those general—so-called primary care—problems and worry that they are going to be bored because they were not trained all this time to look at runny noses and migraine headaches, and to listen to middle-aged black ladies saying that they are tired and weary. Professional dissatisfaction leads to impatient physicians who are quick to show irritation with your "insignificant" medical problems. I do not expect you to get out your handkerchiefs for them, but they *are* in these binds.

We should take note that there has been no mention of the increasing difficulty that poor women have in getting into medical school, because they lack both the financial and the emotional support to take on that horrible situation. Minority enrollments in medical school are falling—I should say plummeting—even though the enrollments of women seem to be holding their own, or are in many places still growing.

We, as women, have to ask how women can get on the boards of admission that make the decision that the only person who can be a good physican is someone with a 4.0 average in biomedical sciences.

Until women can get tenure in medical schools and universities in general we will still have an educational process that is dominated by men who foster the sexism and racism we constantly fight. As far as I am concerned—if I am ousted from that system I can not say anything to my pre-med students with their incomes of $30,000 who have never had a woman faculty member teach them anything they feel is valuable, and who do not understand why I bring my baby into class, and how I combine a career and motherhood.

Women are continually placed in no-win situations. That is, if you like, they're damned if they do, and they're damned if they don't. Psychologists call this a double-bind. Let me give you a couple of examples, because in medical services, women continually confront double binds.

If a woman does not accept that fact that her newborn infant is severely handicapped, because she says she cannot cope with the lifelong burden of caring for that child, she feels that she is a "bad woman"—i.e., a bad mother—and there is something terribly wrong with her. And she takes that to heart, you can be sure. If she does take this child and tries to raise it as best she can, and in the course of doing so she wants services, she wants assistance, she wants friendship, she wants comfort, she wants support, she is labeled neurotic and bothersome to health professionals. Women always have this problem. They are then told that they are overly invested in this child, that they are neurotic, that they can not get their own act together.

This is all the more ironic because we, as women, have continually been blamed for failing to execute our responsibility, and I think we will see this more and more in regard to antenatal testing. At some point there is a limit to how much you solve on an individual self-responsibility basis. We can see this also in contraception, and in terms of prenatal care. We have to be aware of the fact that individual responsibility can be very burdensome. Women can now fail at giving birth because they did not successfully use Lamaze; they did not breathe the right way; they asked for an anesthetic; they screamed in pain; they did not have an immediate loving attachment to this tiny thing that has torn them up inside and out. I do not mean that in any kind of cynical way. I think it is unfortunate that we should put women under this pressure to be perfect.

The other double bind I want to point out is one we can all too easily fall into from our positions of relative well-being. It also has to do with self-responsibility. We continually hear that we should take responsibility for our health. And, to an extent, I really agree with that. However, if we who can opt out of this conventional medical system put all our energy strictly in the alternative service, then we allow physicians to continue to serve the *status quo,* and we let our less able sisters—and brothers, for that matter—suffer the consequences of poor medical practice. I think it is unfair to place another burden on people who are already disabled for reasons of finances, geographic location, whatever: for them to feel guilty that they cannot successfully manage, co-opt, or in some way manipulate the system to serve their self-interests is intrinsically unfair and unrealistic.

Decisions About Handicapped Newborns

Values and Procedures

Diana E. Axelsen

Margaret Mead, in her autobiographical *Blackberry Winter,* commented, "There is hope, I believe, in seeing the human adventure as a whole and in the shared trust that knowledge about mankind, sought in reverence for life, can bring life." The scientific investigation of human reproduction has raised serious questions about whether our advancing knowledge is in fact encouraging reverence for life. New technology in the areas of prenatal screeening and abortion has led to questions concerning the morality of ending the lives of the unborn when handicaps are detected. The availability of more life-preserving technology has led to the question of whether its use for handicapped infants is always morally appropriate. In focusing on decision-making concerning handicapped newborns, I would like to use as a background Margaret Mead's suggestion that we view the human adventure as a whole. Thus, we shall raise specific issues within the context of general ethical analysis of scientific knowledge and its applications.

Decisions that we shall consider include whether to use medical means to try to remedy handicaps with which an infant is born; whether simply to maintain life by providing minimal care; and whether to hasten death with the intent of alleviating suffering. We shall first consider who should have the responsibility for making these decisions; I shall suggest possible modifications in the decision-making process, as part of a concept of interdisciplinary approaches to ethical issues in medicine. I shall also discuss the "right to life" as it relates to decisions concerning handicapped newborns.

RESPONSIBILITY IN DECISION-MAKING—TOWARD THE INTERDISCIPLINARY TEAM APPROACH

My fundamental position is that maternal and parental autonomy should be the foundation of responsible decision-making concerning newborns. There are important roles for physicians willing to help without insisting on control, for structured support teams, and for informal interaction with families and individuals who have faced similar dilemmas. I will discuss some of the considerations behind this perspective, and will suggest that medical criteria alone are inadequate as a basis for decisions about neonatal care.

Some distressing reports of the results of emphasis on medical criteria appear in Rosalyn B. Darling's study, "Parents, Physicians, and Spina Bifida."[1] Physicians who attempt to base the decision whether to treat a newborn with spina bifida on strict medical criteria, often define a life as "intolerable," and influence parents to accept their judgments as physicians. Even physicians whose criteria for treatment are much more liberal find themselves, in those cases in which treatment seems inadvisable, choosing between active euthanasia, which is illegal, and vigorous treatment deemed medically inappropriate. Although such physicians "believe strongly in personally discussing the prognosis in great depth with the new parents and allowing them to make the final decision," some also recognize that parents are strongly influenced by the way in which the physician presents the medical background. This is evidenced by the widely varying proportions of newborns treated by different physicians. For example, one doctor reports that he treats 90% of the newborns with spina bifida whom he sees, compared with 25% for a physician whose treatment philosophy differs.[2] Yet both physicians have carefully analyzed the values they regard as relevant to the decision whether to treat. The kinds of cases do not differ enough medically to account for this variation; rather, the physicians' views on the appropriateness of vigorous treatment differ. These views seem to influence parents strongly; the data support Darling's conclusion that "parents are generally unaware of the bias behind the physician's recommendations."[3] They are thus in no position to make an independent judgment.

Sometimes the influence of medical values on parental decisions is less subtle. Jane J. Stein[4] describes a case in which a couple first consented to corrective surgery for their son, Jason, who was born with Down's syndrome, but later changed their minds after receiving further negative information concerning his prognosis. The day after reaching this decision, made after consultation with a member of the clergy, the parents visited Jason in the nursery. The mother commented, "The nurses stared at us with resentment and anger. They were trained to save lives, and they couldn't do anything for Jason because of our decision." The case eventually went to the Georgetown University Hospital ethics committee, which upheld the parents' decision, though some dissenters wanted to charge the parents with child abuse. The parents and many others involved felt that their decision was a responsible one, based on love for the infant and concern about his possible future happiness. Yet in addition to the stresses of decision-making in a painful situation, the parents had to confront the conflicting values of both medical and nonmedical personnel, and even a possible court case. At the same time, it is important not to ignore the dilemmas faced by individual medical personnel, who seek to act on their own moral values and who have a basic commitment to the patient. The solution, it seems to me, is not the indictment of individual physicians and nurses, or of individual parents, as inadequate decision-makers. Nor is the solution to be found in any generally applicable guidelines for specific situations. Rather, it is the entire process of decision-making, and the associated power structures, that must be examined and modified.

A central problem, then, is to determine what persons are entitled to be involved in the decision-making. In thinking about this question, we might want to distinguish among three sorts of situations: (a) cases in which death is almost certain, and there seems to be no possibility of temporary or permanent improvement; (b) cases in which the short-term and long-term effects of the handicap are uncertain (e.g., Down's syndrome); and (c) cases in which treatment can eliminate or minimize the handicap (e.g., phenylketonuria, PKU). In the third situation, the primary concern seems to be to make screening and treatment readily available. Such cases seldom raise dilemmas peculiar to neonatology, though they pose problems when parents oppose all medical intervention on religious grounds. The agonizing decisions that we are currently confronting involve primarily the first two sorts of cases, and it is these with which we shall be concerned.

Who might be included in decision-making concerning the handicapped newborn? The obvious candidates are the parents, the primary-care physician, and medical specialists. Others are nurses who have cared for the newborn, a nurse-midwife, if one assisted with prenatal training and/or the birth, a representative of the hospital administration, a patient advocate who might be viewed as a representative of the newborn, a psychological counselor, a social worker, and a member of the clergy, preferably one trained in medical chaplaincy. In view of the many parents whose religious faith will be an important factor in their decision, I would stress the hospital's responsibility for taking the initiative in seeing that the parents have the opportunity to discuss the decision with a member of the clergy, if they desire. Although I personally do not believe that any body of religious teachings, in itself, contains answers to all the questions raised by modern medical technology, I do believe that involvement of the clergy may sometimes be crucial if the parents are to reach a decision with which they can be at peace. I am reminded of the lines in Psalm 139, "O Lord, . . . thou didst form my inward parts, thou didst knit me together in my mother's womb." Jane Stein illustrates the relevance of religious beliefs, in mentioning a sign, "Please be patient—God hasn't finished me yet," placed by the mother of a premature infant on one baby's Isolette in a neonatal intensive care unit.[5]

Two other possible members of the decision-making team might be, first, a bioethics adviser, and, second, a representative of the state. A bioethics adviser could help to organize the issues for the family in a nonthreatening and supportive way. Such a person could play a potentially very central role in the decision-making process, especially if his or her role is defined as one of clarification and support, not as one of advocacy. Finally, one might consider the possibility of including a representative of the state. For me, the undesirability of this step makes it imperative to attempt to reach a consensus, and to support parental decisions even when they conflict with the values of some of the other individuals involved in the decision-making process.

MATERNAL AND PARENTAL AUTONOMY

Given the possibility of an interdisciplinary team approach to decision-making, are there arguments to support the claim that normally the ultimate choice should be made solely by the parents? We shall leave aside such problematic cases as ones in which grandparents will assume major responsibility for the child, or in which the father will leave primary responsibility to the mother. We shall look at the role of parents in the simplest case: one in which both partners in a marriage have planned a pregnancy, have chosen birth rather than abortion, and have agreed on the decision they would make about their handicapped newborn. (For some couples, abortion may have been rejected after explicit consideration, perhaps following amniocentesis; other parents may simply have given no thought to the possibility of having a handicapped child.) I shall argue that the importance of maternal attitudes in determining the future of the fetus, together with the psychological link between the mother's feelings about the fetus and about the newborn, provides a reason for claiming that the decision of the mother (and hence, in this case, of the parents) should be the final basis for determining what treatment the newborn should receive.

A central element in my argument for ultimate maternal authority is the claim that every pregnancy is a unique psychological state, in ways that are profoundly relevant to moral evaluation. I have never been able to dismiss as morally irrelevant the difference between one woman's perception of her pregnancy as a disturbing state that she must confront, and another woman's perception of herself, sometimes from the presumed moment of conception, as existing in a unique relationship with another living being. This personal variation seems to lead to differing attitudes toward the newborn. What is morally relevant in the case we are considering is the unique bond that I presume to exist between the mother and the newborn whose birth was chosen. (This is not to say that the bond may not exist in other situations as well; but the clearest case for maternal authority seems to be inherent in a situation in which pregnancy and birth were chosen and there is no conflict between the parents.) Stress resulting simply from the event of unexpectedly having a handicapped child does not count as an "automatic disqualifier" with respect to decision-making; the woman who is truly incapable of responsible consideration of alternatives would be the exception in the sort of case we are discussing.

The physical state of pregnancy need not be present for a woman to feel herself in relationship to another being. Just as the pregnant woman seeking an abortion may *not* feel that she "contains" another entity, so the woman who uses birth control may feel herself related to a baby whom she chooses not to have. Anne Kent Rush comments on this phenomenon in *Getting Clear: Body Work for Women.* In the chapter "Childbirth, Children, . . . and You," she discusses abortion and the Gestalt technique called "goodbye," in which the woman is encouraged to talk to the unborn child. Rush suggests that:

> . . . one way to explore your feelings about your unborn child and your unexperienced motherhood is through a Gestalt technique of talking to the child as though it were there . . . I do a variation of this Goodbye exercise because even though I have never been pregnant, I am aware that I am continually choosing not to have children now. I feel mixed about that. When I acknowledge my sadness I am brought more fully into the present.[6]

Parents, too, may grieve for "a child who was never born." The crucial point here, from the moral standpoint, is that the variation in psychological states calls for an acceptance of different moral decisions concerning the same kind of biological events.[7]

If we look at linguistic usage, we find confusion over whether the fetus—and sometimes even the neonate—should be called "he" or "she," on the one hand, or "it," on the other. Also different cultures accord different ontological and ethical status to both the fetus and the neonate, as do different members of the western culture. Again, this seems to support the claim that there is a place for ethical relativity of a limited sort.

Possibilities such as artificial insemination or the implanting of a fertilized egg in another woman's body reveal to us how different our concepts of biological and psychological parenthood are. An especially troubling example involves a case in which one woman agrees to bear a child "for" a woman who is unable to conceive, with the first woman being impregnated by the second woman's husband. Biological facts do not seem to settle the question of who is the "real" mother, at least in cultures where this is not a common practice. In commenting on "surrogate motherhood," David Zimmerman quotes a psychologist as saying, "The biological mother is apt to feel a sense of loss, and the emotions of the adoptive couple can range from affection and gratitude to anger and resentment."[8] This is further evidence that the psychological dynamics related to reproduction make it important to respect individual feelings when moral decisions are made.

At this juncture, the importance of using the team approach to decision-making becomes even more apparent. There may be great variations in the kinds and degrees of support that family and friends can offer. Persons other than the physician are often in a better position to aid in assessing the overall impact on the individuals, the marriage, and the family as a whole. The opportunity to talk with parents of children with similar handicaps can also be extremely helpful to parents attempting to make a decision; yet too often in the modern hospital, peer counseling remains a neglected resource.

THE PRINCIPLES OF "RIGHT TO LIFE" AND "RESPECT FOR LIFE" AS A CONTEXT FOR DECISION

I turn now to the question of what ethical principles are relevant to the actual decisions. Much of the discussion of such decisions has centered on the "right to life" of the newborn. However, this focus on rights is misleading, because it suggests that if something or someone does not have a right in a certain situation, then no one else has any moral responsibilities with respect to that person or thing. There seems to be an unarticulated fear that to deny rights to such entities as fetuses and newborns is to give everyone else license to behave on the basis of individual preference. This fear lies, I believe, in an inappropriate extension of the contractual model of correlative rights and obligations to our thinking about our moral responsibilities related to life and death. It is important to recognize a principle slightly different from the one embodied in the notion of a right to life. I shall call the related ethical responsibility "the duty to respect life." As I interpret it, the principle of respect for life can express itself, for different persons, in such varied ways as a rejection of abortion; in the refusal to condone euthanasia for handicapped newborns; in concern for the survival of animals and plants; in opposition to environmental pollution and nuclear power; in a moral commitment to vegetarianism; in an absolute or relative commitment to pacifism; in a rejection of capital punishment; and by the condemnation of all forms of genocide, including such practices as encouraging the purchase of food products that are life-threatening in some cultural environments (e.g., powdered milk formula for infants in developing countries). It is by seeking how all these issues are interrelated that we can best see the moral issues raised by the handicapped newborn in proper perspective. We sometimes lose sight of the holistic nature of all questions involving life and death; but by acknowledging the principle of respect for life, and by recognizing that it may be expressed in a variety of ways, we can approach the moral dilemmas raised by decisions related to human reproduction in a more responsible fashion.

This sort of perspective seems essential to me because I have found that there is no generally satisfactory way to make morally relevant distinctions among such entities as the zygote, the fetus, and the newborn. Let me use several examples in the area of reproduction that illustrate the sources of my perplexity.

In an article on abortion, Judith Jarvis Thomson refers to the sense of indecency we would all presumably feel toward a woman who had an abortion in her seventh month to avoid postponing a trip abroad.[9] There is something wrong with the woman's decision; but I do not think that an explanation is provided by a principle such as "Only reasons that society at large considers nontrivial can justify late-term abortions." Two other hypotheses come to mind. First, the woman may simply be generally irresponsible in her decision-making. Second, she may have a respect for life, and be able to make responsible decisions, yet she may not feel that respect for life rules out *her* abortion at *this* time. She may be having severe psychological problems, and have come to see her trip as a way out of an otherwise impossible situation. (It is hard to imagine why someone not under stress would postpone the decision for so long.) Similarly, I am not prepared to say that a parent who chooses not to have surgery on a handicapped newborn, but who is a consistent pacifist, is more or less moral than the person who regards some wars as justified, but who would never sanction anything other than vigorous treatment for her newborn. If we lose sight of the broader context within which we raise these individual questions, we may forget that a crucial issue is always the *intention* of the decision-maker. Certainly we should express respect for life, and strive for consistency in application of the principle to our actions; but I do not think that we can go much further in specifying a behavior for every situation that is the only appropriate method for expressing that respect. Another contrast that supports this view is that of the committed vegetarian, on the one hand, and that of the person who kills animals for material and ceremonial needs, but who also expresses a respect for the wholeness of nature through specific religious practices.[10]

With these thoughts about respect for life in mind, let us consider how one physician sees the differences between his views and actions and those of another physician:

> . . . with equal conscience and good will Dr. L . . . and I treat widely different numbers of patients. I fail to believe that either of us is unethical. And yet, we both can't be right—or can we?[11]

If what matters is that each doctor take decision-making seriously, that he or she exhibit respect for parental autonomy, that each be aware of the need to utilize varied resources to assist the parents in reaching a decision, and that each act on the principle of respect for life as he or she interprets it, then two doctors whose practices differ radically may indeed both be right ethically. In our evaluations, we should consider the process by which the decision is reached, the respect for life evidenced by all those involved in the process, and the support provided for parents who reach their decision responsibly.

SOCIAL RESPONSIBILITIES

What, now, of society's responsibilities? One under-utilized option is to match parents who decide that they do not wish to assume responsibility for care of a handicapped newborn, with individuals or couples willing to adopt the newborn and assume primary responsibility for his or her care. The presence of an opportunity for immediate adoption would spare parents the agonizing choice between institutionalization or death for a child for whom they feel they cannot care; it would eliminate possible periods of maternal deprivation; it could alleviate some of the problems inherent in the foster care program as it now operates; and it would be a social demonstration of concern for life. Moreover, it could help to reduce the number of "unadoptable" children, since prospective adoptive parents might well be more willing to assume responsibility for a handicapped child when they can work with him or her from birth and be sure the maximal support is provided from birth onward.

Finally, in order that we move away from the view of the birth of a handicapped newborn as an unusual and tragic crisis for which few parents are prepared, I urge that sex education and prenatal care include counseling concerning the possibility that a child may be born with a wide variety of physical or mental differences. A trained counselor should make prospective parents aware of the possibilities, without exaggerating the problems or the risks, and without attempting to push the parents toward any particular attitude toward various contingencies. Such assistance not only should be an adjunct to genetic screening and counseling, but also should be available as a routine part of prenatal care. However, great caution should be exercised to prevent prospective parents from feeling that they have an obligation to undergo prenatal testing. The aim of this general information, like the aim of providing data on genetic screening, should be to make parents aware of choices and to help them prepare themselves and their families for possible challenges, not to exert any pressure of the sort we associate with eugenics movements.

In this connection, the representation of women and ethnic minorities on policymaking boards is of special importance. Statistics by race and sex of the composition for 1978 of the 166 public advisory groups serving the National Institute of Health indicate serious problems in this area. Out of a total membership of 2218, in 1978, 0.2% of the members were Native Americans or Alaskan Americans; 2.6% were Asian Americans; 3.5% were Blacks, and 1.3% were Hispanics; 17.1% of the members were female. These advisory groups are responsible for recommendations on key legislation concerning screening, counseling, and treatment of genetic diseases, such as Senate Bill 2598, an amendment to Title XI of the Public Health Service Act, or the "Genetic Disease Amendments of 1978."[12]

It seems especially important both for minorities and for women generally to be sensitive both to the source and nature of legislation and to its implementation in this area. Monitoring is needed to see that services are equitably and responsibly provided; it is also needed to ensure that support is given to those parents who choose to risk the birth of a handicapped child, or who opt for aggressive treatment in the case of such a birth.

A utilitarian position that emphasizes the cost to society of providing for handicapped children is beginning to pervade the legislation in this area. Without minimizing such concerns, I strongly question whether this should be a dominant social priority; especially I am concerned that freedom of parental reproductive choice may be compromised by the allocation of funds for health care. The principle of respect for life requires vigilance, too, in cases where newborns are kept alive only for experimental purposes, but the issues involved there are beyond the scope of this paper.

Only when our entire concept of human life is altered, so that we cease to look upon the birth of a handicapped newborn as a catastrophe, will parents be able to make decisions that are truly free. As a society, we must abandon the attitude that the birth of a "less than perfect" child is an event for which we cannot prepare and which we therefore contemplate with fear. By eliminating such attitudes, we can create a social environment that will foster humane decisions about the treatment of handicapped newborns. Such a social environment can be expressive of genuine respect for life as well as of respect for individual differences. We need not and should not allow medical and economic criteria to settle issues concerning the treatment of newborns—issues that are of fundamental importance to us as mothers, parents, citizens, and as the ancestors of future generations.

Response

Caroline Whitbeck

When we consider decisions about the care of severely impaired newborns we are dealing with a situation that requires more than getting *informed consent.* In *my* view, what is required are skills in fostering people's development, "calling forth," as I termed it earlier. Informed consent may be sufficient in other situations.

When Helen Barnes was talking about informed choice concerning contraception, that seemed appropriate because the people making the choice are not under unusual pressure; they experience only the stress that usually attends a visit to the physician. It is not the kind of catastrophic situation that is faced by the parents of a severely deformed newborn.

Calling forth pcoplc in catastrophic situations requires a good deal more than just providing information. It is not enough for people to have all the facts. People must have special support to reach a considered decision under these tragic circumstances.

I think it is interesting that one of the people who opened up the subject of making decisions about severely impaired newborns— Raymond Duff, a pediatrician at Yale-New Haven Hospital and co-author of *Sickness and Society*— is a person who is extraordinarily skilled at enabling *other people* to come up with decisions that they can live with. When a man has those skills, the sort of skills expected to be natural in women, either of two things happens. If he is seen as having high status, he is described as "a saint" or "enlightened." If the man is of lower status, then he is regarded as "a fool." And, indeed, I have heard both sorts of terms applied to Duff, depending on the relative status of the speaker. In both cases what they say serves to excuse or justify others for not behaving similarly. The behavior is viewed either as beyond the capabilities of ordinary men or as stupid and irrelevant to a physician's real task.

There is a final problem that bears mentioning: that is, medical interventions with newborns whom no one expects to live very long, but who are kept alive just to be studied. You can see from my previous remarks that I am very much against viewing physicians as mad scientists. The problem of interventions that serve only medical curiosity is a real one. One case was that of a newborn without kidneys who was kept alive for two weeks in intensive care because people wanted to see what would happen to her. Her flesh became necrotic—that is to say, she rotted before she died. There was no hope for her, and it would have been kind and merciful to have let her die quickly and painlessly. I think that the people who have vigorously advocated the sanctity of life have ignored this kind of case, where the motives for keeping someone alive may be just curiosity of the most inhumane sort.

Rights of a Handicapped Neonate

What Every Parent and Professional Should Know

Helga M. Bendix

INTRODUCTION

The birth of a child identified as having a life-long handicap presents problems of varying degrees and kind. The immediate reactions of professionals and parents go a long way towards the acceptance or non-acceptance of the newborn and his or her handicap. Usually the parents have had little or no experience with handicaps and realize that the handicapped infant is not what had been hoped for or dreamed about for nine months. Therefore the hospital professionals set the tone for the handling of the crisis. Because the hospital professionals have a crucial role to play, it is incumbent upon them to be most informed about a variety of matters. For this, an interdisciplinary team should be immediately available to analyze jointly with the parents all the aspects that such a birth brings to bear.

One perspective that must be shared and be part of the professionals' information bank is the tremendous change in the perception of the place of the handicapped in our society today. The thrust today is to mainstream the handicapped wherever and whenever possible. There has been a great emphasis on the human and civil rights of the handicapped. Major laws have been passed to effect what good intentions never did. A handicapped neonate is to be seen as a person with special needs whose needs are to be fulfilled. Once born, such an infant has a "right to life" and it is necessary for society to enable the individual to lead the best life possible. Because the adults involved are of a different generation and were probably raised with a different outlook, there may exist a gap between the adults' viewpoints and the intent of recent legislation. It is my purpose to share some of the legal developments of the past decade and to encourage their use to achieve the good life for those not made so perfect.

In recent years, the handicapped have visibly, and sometimes militantly, emerged from the closet. The civil rights movements to attain equality for blacks and women began with public consciousness-raising and were later punctuated with supporting judicial decisions and legislative responses. Almost the reverse process occurred with the handicapped: disabled individuals and parents of handicapped children learned from the successful strategies of the blacks and women and joined forces at the beginning of the decade to push for successful litigation and favorable legislation. Thereby the public education aspect was left undone, to be done now as we all proceed to implement favorable judicial decisions, statutes and accompanying regulations and guidelines. The legal entitlements and rights to services have been more or less spelled out, to the consternation of some, especially the personally unaffected public.

For those who wonder about the relevancy of laws to a discussion of ethical issues, let me explain my perspective. Laws are perhaps the culmination of innumerable discussions of many aspects including relevant moral and ethical issues. Sometimes a moral principle has to be formalized in a written document, as is the case in all civil rights legislation. For some people, the passage of a law is the end of an endeavor, but for others it is only the beginning. Implementing a law is not easy and the law is occasionally subject to amendments and interpretations because the legislators were unclear or had not foreseen all possible circumstances. Nowadays it is important to know relevant legislation because legal tactics are being used to achieve accountability and equal opportunities that should have been part of moral behavior all along.

LEGISLATION AFFECTING NEONATES

Because decisions of varying magnitude need to be made from birth on, it is important to remember constantly the affected individual and to accord him or her all of his or her entitlements. The handicapped neonate is a person with special needs for whom the opportunity to equal access must begin in the crib.

> The denial of services in life-saving situations occurs when the disabled person is an infant or is unable to consent for himself. The parents or the professional involved often feel they have the right to make such a decision on behalf of the individual. The courts have said that this is illegal; that the individual has a right to be represented when a life-saving decision is to be made.[1]

The following basic legal principles come into play in medical decision-making[2]:

1. Parents have no legal right to make decisions which are harmful to their child.
2. Courts will intervene to protect the children who have been denied medical services.
3. In an emergency, medical services may be provided to a child without parental consent.
4. The willful taking of a child's life is an unlawful homicide.
5. Court orders may be obtained to prevent denials of medical services to handicapped individuals.
6. The prospective "quality of life" of a handicapped person is not a legally relevant factor to be considered in determining access to medical services.
7. Denial of medical services to handicapped persons may result in criminal and/or civil penalties.

Whatever other patients' rights that exist for the hospitalized would have to be extended to the handicapped as well.

The President's Committee on Mental Retardation's *Century of Decision* Report, 1976, enunciates some principles in this area:

— The right to be free from the arbitrary denial of lifesaving medical services.
— The right to medical and medically related services on an equal basis with other citizens.
— The right to be protected from unnecessary and experimental research procedures.
— The right to health services necessary to prevent or control mental retardation.
— The right to have access to all available social services which facilitate the retarded person's adjustment to society or which facilitate his development.

Although the above is written with respect to the particular handicap of mental retardation, its thrust is applicable to all the handicapped.

Once medical details have been dealt with, other questions demand answers. The nature of the handicap requires explanation. The future must be predicted with a degree of uncertainty given the educational opportunities delineated below. There should be no reservations about where may be the best place of residence for the child. The child is to be in the "least restrictive environment," and that would have to be defined in the first instance as the natural family. The love and care that parents can learn to give their less-than-perfect child outweigh all else.

Current emphasis on the development of community services argues in favor of family support services and against the foster care system or putting the handicapped child up for adoption. Furthermore the foster care system itself needs improvement, as indicated by reforms proposed at the national level and for my state (New York). It may even be illegal to recommend institutionalization so early in an individual's life, if ever. Court decisions, such as the Willowbrook Consent Decree in New York State and the Pennhurst decision in Pennsylvania, practically preclude the option of institutional placement. With the emphasis on preschool and school age services to the age of 21 and with the primary responsibility with the Local Education Agency, it is unnecessary to make lifetime decisions or predictions for adulthood while still rocking the cradle.

LEGISLATION AFFECTING CHILDREN

Until this decade most legislative items affecting the handicapped usually addressed the provision of services in piecemeal fashion. In the 70s the thrust has broadened to human and civil rights and an attack on discrimination, with emphasis on the individual. The most all-encompassing statement is Section 504 of the *Rehabilitation Act of 1973* (P.L. 93-112):

> No otherwise qualified handicapped individual in the United States, as defined in section 7(6), shall, solely by reason of his handicap, be excluded from the participation in, be denied the benefits of, or be subjected to discrimination under any program or activity receiving Federal financial assistance.

The above is the civil rights focus of the activists of the handicapped movement and was the backdrop for the angry and determined demonstrations in HEW offices in the major cities in spring 1977 when Secretary Joseph Califano of HEW appeared to delay signing the implementing Federal Regulations.

> The language of section 504 is almost identical to the comparable nondiscrimination provisions of title VI of the Civil Rights Act of 1964 and title IX of the Education Amendments of 1972 (applying to racial discrimination and to discrimination in education on the basis of sex). It establishes a mandate to end discrimination and to bring handicapped persons into the mainstream of American life.[3]

"Accessibility" and "reasonable accommodation" have become key implementing words. The concept of physical accessibility was previously embodied in the *Architectural Barriers Act of 1968* (P.L. 90-480) whose thrust was "to insure that certain buildings financed with Federal funds are so designed and constructed as to be accessible to the physically handicapped." Section 504 regulations give guidelines for "program accessibility" and "reasonable accommodation" to better help the integration of the handicapped into the mainstream of life.

Accessibility of education for all was achieved through the *Education for All Handicapped Children Act of 1975* (P.L. 94–142).

> It is the purpose of this Act to assure that all handicapped children have available to them, within the time periods specified in section 612 (2) (B), a free appropriate public education which emphasizes special education and related services designed to meet their unique needs, to assure that the rights of handicapped children and their parents or guardians are protected, to assist States and localities to provide for the education of all handicapped children, and to assess and assure the effectiveness of efforts to educate handicapped children.

This right to education was achieved by arguing from the XIV Amendment to the Constitution of the United States which entitles citizens to "due process of law" and "equal protection of the law." A specific law was necessary because our history has many examples of exclusion from schooling based on handicap. Of further interest are two definitions from P.L. 94-142:

> The term "special education" means specially designed instruction, at no cost to parents or guardians, to meet the unique needs of a handicapped child, including classroom instruction, instruction in physical education, home instruction, and instruction in hospitals and institutions.

> The term "related services" means transportation, and such developmental, corrective, and other supportive services (including speech pathology and audiology, psychological services, physical and occupational therapy, recreation, and medical and counseling services, except that such medical services shall be for diagnostic and evaluation purposes only) as may be required to assist a handicapped child to benefit from special education, and includes the early identification and assessment of handicapping conditions in children.

Another change is a redefinition of education with implications primarily for the severely handicapped who traditionally were closeted or warehoused.

> Not all children can be educated as we usually think of the term "education,"—grade school, junior high school, et cetera. The diagnosis of Tracy Ann's condition is "psychomotor, growth and developmental retardation with seizure disorder." Such a child requires another kind of "education,"—how to hold a spoon, feed herself, dress herself, toilet training, et cetera, in addition to speech

therapy, psychiatric and psychological treatment, et cetera—all these and more add up to the education of this and other mentally retarded children, and they are entitled to be so educated.

(In the Matter of Tracy Ann Cox, No. H-4721-75, N.Y., Fam. Ct. Queens County, April 8, 1976)[4]

Educating all handicapped children will hopefully become a reality in these United States in the near future. Emphasis has been on finding handicapped children, serving first the unserved and then the underserved. There have been great fiscal laments regarding the implementation of this law and Section 504 which are intertwined in regulations. The Federal Government acknowledges in the Federal Regulations for Section 504:

> ...the fact that ending discriminatory practices and providing equal access to programs may involve major burdens on some recipients. Those burdens and costs, to be sure, provide no basis for exemption from section 504 or this regulation: Congress' mandate to end discrimination is clear.

These requirements to educate all handicapped children must become broad knowledge. In particular it should be known to hospital personnel when counseling the parents of a handicapped newborn. In some instances the child may be immediately eligible for some educational services. The Federal law begins at age three unless state law mandates otherwise. In New York State some deaf and blind infants are eligible under a special law and other handicapped children may receive funding for preschool education if their parents petition Family Court.

Another gradual change is the rise in expectations and real abilities of handicapped children as they are given the opportunity to learn and grow up in a stimulating environment. Not long ago Down's Syndrome children were expected to function no higher than the "trainable mentally retarded" level; today, with better education, this once-standard "plateau" has been pushed upward to at least "educable mentally retarded." The deinstitutionalization process is showing us that individuals who had been given up as lost causes learn and develop self-help skills in their new homes, the community residences.

The young handicapped child has a much better future ahead than existed for the child of yesteryear. This optimism, this change, these rights must be conveyed as part of the prognosis given to parents. Hospital staff should take affirmative action and be instrumental in linking up the child and the parents to agencies and parent groups outside of the hospital setting so that no time is lost in obtaining services and so that parents can communicate with someone who is familiar with their problem and needs. If the hospital staff does not know where to turn, one suggestion is to go to the home school district because all school districts must have some handicapped children for whom they are responsible. The staff could accompany the parents initially to help advocate for appropriate services. These comments apply even when the child is profoundly multiply handicapped. The "least restrictive environment" is now considered to be the desirable setting with the emphasis being on participation in "regular educational programs" when considered appropriate. Only time will tell how different the next generation of handicapped adults will be, but this emphasis on education and mainstreaming should help both the handicapped and the nonhandicapped.

Another legislative landmark is the *Developmentally Disabled Assistance and Bill of Rights Act of 1975* (P.L. 94–103). It proclaims that:

> Persons with developmental disabilities have a right to appropriate treatment, services,and habilitation for such disabilities.
>
> The treatment, services,and habilitation for a person with developmental disabilities should be designed to maximize the developmental potential of the person and should be provided in the setting that is least restrictive of the person's personal liberty.

Some of the requirements for a state under this legislation are:

1. To establish a Protection and Advocacy system "to protect and advocate the rights of persons with developmental disabilities."
2. To have a state plan designed "to eliminate inappropriate placement in institutions of persons with developmental disabilities."
3. To "provide for the early screening, diagnosis, and evaluation (including maternal care, developmental screening, home care, infant and preschool stimulation programs, and parent counseling and training) of developmentally disabled infants and preschool children, particularly those with multiple handicaps."
4. To "support the establishment of community programs as alternatives to institutionalization and support such programs which are designed to provide services for the care and habilitation of persons with developmental disabilities, and which utilize to the maximum extent feasible, the resources and personnel in related community

programs and to assure the provision of appropriate supplemental health, education, or social services for persons with developmental disabilities."

5. To require the drafting of individual habilitation plans for a person with developmental disabilities.

The above described major pieces of legislation apply to all 50 states. There is much more at the Federal level, including amendments to the above, but the other items are often for a particular handicap or for a particular situation. The above is a mere overview intended to convey the intent of enacted legislation about which all people involved with and working on behalf of handicapped individuals must be knowledgeable. Familiarity with state laws is also helpful.

CONCLUSION

Living with an impaired child is not a bed of roses, nor is it necessarily so when all children are "normal." Life brings both good and bad, but we usually try to look for the silver lining. Life should not be painted all black when a "disaster" has occurred. In fact, such a "tragedy" can bring unique rewards. Today's world, armed with the clout of laws, can bring about changes to benefit all people. What is needed is an army of advocates marching on discrimination. The ethical issue is not whether to end discrimination, but rather to ask why we ever had it and why it is so hard to eradicate. Even our traditional moral leaders, the religious institutions, have been remiss vis-à-vis the handicapped and their families, and are under pressure to make their buildings and their programs accessible to the disabled and to close the gap between their teachings and actions. It is therefore our collective responsibility to see to it that the human and civil rights of our handicapped neonates are protected and that they are given the opportunity to pursue life, liberty and happiness.

Living With An Impaired Neonate And Child

A Feminist Issue

E. Virginia Sheppard Lapham

The issues raised by feminists during the last two decades have risen from a belief in the value of women as "people in our own right."[1] Betty Freidan wrote eloquently of the feminine mystique that defined woman "solely in terms of her three-dimensional sexual relationship to man: wife, mother, homemaker—passively dependent, her own role restricted to timeless, changeless love and service of husband and children."[2]

Nowhere is this three-dimensional sexual relationship more obvious and more exploited than with women who bear a baby with birth defects or have a child who develops a handicapping condition.

Prior to the feminist movement there was enormous reluctance in our society "to bring into public view anything that had to do with the private lives of women."[3] Such topics as contraception, rape, abortion, amniocentesis, incest, and spouse and child abuse were taboo. Childbirth was shrouded with both mystery and anesthesia, and motherhood was elevated to sainthood. The woman whose child was "different" was considered most saintly (and pitied) of all as she either followed the professional advice to "put her child away for the sake of the other family members," or made extraordinary efforts to be teacher, therapist, recreation director, and so on, as well as parent. Often she was also isolated and provided with little support or time off from child care. In spite of this many women have found the strength and resources to rear children with handicaps and find satisfying life styles.

Some of the systems affecting women who live with a handicapped child are the major socializing forces affecting all women with children, namely the family, the educational systems, and religious institutions. Additionally, the woman with a handicapped child is impacted in special ways by the medical/rehabilitation system, the mental health system, the community, and the political/economic system.

It is my intent to examine the roles of women with handicapped children within each of these systems in terms of feminist issues such as: use of language, information provided, who does the decision-making, whether or not a support system exists, attitudes toward women and their children, possible alternatives, and values of persons involved. I argue and demonstrate that these women are oppressed by our society, and that they have internalized societal attitudes of being of little worth by virtue of having a child of "little worth." Nor have they been helped by the feminist movement. Furthermore, professionals in many of these systems continue to oppress even as we attempt to help these women. Professional women and men with a feminist "ethos" will sometimes find it conflicts with our professional "ethos." There are also times when the rights of women who have a child with a handicapping condition conflict with the rights of the child.

Readers may be wondering by this time why the word "mother" has not been used. Along with Angela Barron McBride, I believe "mother" to be an emotionally loaded word in our society, which precludes us from objectively examining the many roles of a woman who happens to include parenting among them. In speaking of the motherhood mystique Ms. McBride says:

> I have already suggested that a world beyond the motherhood mystique might conceivably not include any mothers. It would be peopled instead by female parents and male parents . . . I have already spelled out many of the reasons why one should do away with the word "mother." The word no longer refers to a woman, but describes some imaginary element of nature in female form, who unconditionally affirms the child's life and needs. Mom is expected to be everything her children and her child-rearing "experts" want her to be. She has come to mean a person "destined" to live vicariously; her only hope for "fulfillment" is in finding a penis substitute, a baby. Mother in our society has also become so equated with failure that it is questionable whether any self-respecting person would want to assume an identity riddled by so much guilt or responsibility. It is no wonder that Shulamith Firestone (author of *The Dialectic of Sex,* New York, Bantam Books, 1970), "looks forward to childbearing being taken over by technology."[4]

Technology is already able to intervene in the processes of child bearing from conception and gestation through birth and lactation, to the benefit of the child, the parents, and society, or to the detriment of one or all. In the end, however, it is the woman bearing the child who is expected to bear the consequences of the technological intervention, second only to the child; and I would argue that sometimes the woman is most affected.

Let me make it clear at this point that I do not see all women who have a handicapped child as being equally affected by the various systems. Each woman brings to every child-bearing and child-rearing experience her own personality and previous life experiences and present environment. Some of these variables include self-esteem, education, health, ethnic background, socioeconomic status, composition of present family including other children, marital and significant other relationships, and expectations about the unborn child. Another very important variable becomes the nature and degree of the child's impairment, or birth defect, or handicapping condition.[5]

Since the medical system is generally the one in which a child is initially identified as having a handicapping condition, we will begin there.

MEDICAL SYSTEM

An estimated 250,000 babies are born each year in the United States with congenital birth defects.[6] It is unlikely that many women would deliberately bear a handicapped child if they had a chance not to do so.[7] Following genetic counseling or amniocentesis, some women do choose to bear a child knowing there is an increased risk of the child's having a birth defect. It is highly probable that even these women hope to "beat the risk" and have a nonhandicapped child.

Researchers have found that, whoever they are, women who have a child with birth defects want to be told about it as soon as possible, with sensitivity, and in language they understand. They want the child's father to be present when they receive the news; they want information about what the impairment means, what the alternatives are for treatment, and what to expect in the future. They want to be involved in decisions made about their child; they want to know where to find community resources, what are the costs of medical rehabilitation care, and what kind of financial help is available.[8]

Women with handicapped newborns reported that at the time of their child's birth physicians used technical language that they did not understand. Their child was referred to as a neonate, a fetus, or an "it," all object language that possibly helped the professional remain objective, but dehumanized the child and conveyed that to the parent. Women have commented that condescending attitudes are also expressed toward women in hospital settings.

> In the hospital we are depersonalized . . . We lose our identity. We are expected to be passive and acquiescent and to make no trouble. We are expected to depend not on ourselves, but on doctors . . .[9]

Feminist women feel that their value systems are different from those of obstetricians. "We emphasize teaching ourselves to participate wisely and strongly in our childbirth experience. They emphasize 'what might go wrong' and make us totally dependent upon them."[10]

When something does go wrong and a baby is born with birth defects, situations become confusing. The doctors and other hospital personnel are ready to provide treatment to the child using very sophisticated technical equipment and expertise.[11] The woman who has never thought beyond "what might go wrong" may now be asked to make life and death and disability decisions when her physical and emotional energy is at its lowest. She may not have sufficient background to make fast decisions even when information is provided. She also may not be provided with much information.[12] She may also not be consulted at all, in an effort by professionals and/or family members to protect her. It is as well a most difficult time for physicians who are faced with taking action or inaction on the basis of incomplete or inadequate diagnosis, especially when there are multiple defects.

In this crisis period parents and professionals must deal with the question: in what form is life worth living? It is no problem if all agree that life in any form is worthwhile including lifelong dependence on technical support systems. The only question then becomes the cost and availability of equipment. Anything short of that requires decisions that women who have never thought through what to do "if anything happens" are ill-prepared to make. Sometimes the technology further impairs the child even as it saves his or her life. An example of this is the use of fresh oxygen to save the life of a premature infant, which then causes blindness.[13]

This period is very important for women who live with a handicapped child. It is often remembered later with laments that begin, "If only I had known," or "If only I had been told," or, "If only I had been asked." This period has enormous psychological impact upon the woman and is remembered as the beginning point in living with the child. It is recognized that the right to medical treatment of the infant and the rights of women may conflict at this point.

One child-rearing system that was available until the last few years was institutions for severely handicapped children. Recently, recognition of the rights of mentally retarded children and adults to the least restrictive environment has resulted in a trend toward deinstitutionalization that has made this option unpopular and almost non-existent. It has served to correct the routine manner in which some professionals recommended and some parents sought institutional care for children thought to be mentally retarded. In so protecting the rights of children, the alternatives instead of the parents rearing a severely handicapped child have become practically nil. Foster care and adoption are available in some situations,[14] though generally not sanctioned by society. In extreme cases, babies are abandoned while in hospitals or child care agencies at a cost in 1977 of $73,000 per child per year.[15] There are now few alternatives but for the mother to take on the major responsibility of rearing and socializing the child. This is not to imply that most women would choose otherwise, but that choice is seldom a factor; the difference becomes doing what one must, rather than what one chooses, even though the outcome would be the same most of the time.

THE FAMILY SYSTEM

The isolated nuclear family is not an adequate social unit for human satisfaction or child rearing even if its maintenance tasks can be carried out.[16]

If the nuclear family that has emerged from our industrial society is inadequate for child-rearing in general, the additional demands placed upon it by the birth of a child with handicaps can be staggering. And the person upon whom the major responsibility falls is generally the female parent.

When a father is part of the family, the extra costs of medical/rehabilitative treatment may necessitate his working longer hours or more than one job, thus further isolating the woman from adult company. If this is a first child and the woman has worked outside the home she may experience an abrupt social discontinuity. There may be little continuous support if the extended family lives at a distance. Even child care may be a problem. The *New York Times* quotes one father of a severely brain-injured child as saying, "Try to get a baby sitter for a few hours. Even family members don't want to baby sit. They admire the job you do, but don't get them involved."[17]

Some women have been able to build a network of unrelated persons to provide a kind of extended family. Or, the presence of older children may be helpful to the woman in caring for the handicapped child. A woman whose sixth child was handicapped found her life style, child rearing, and community volunteering changed very little as the older children assumed some of the child care responsibilities.[18]

The presence of other young children may necessitate a juggling act if the handicapped child requires extensive care at home and if multiple visits to medical rehabilitation and social agencies are required. If these activities deprive the other children of whatever level of care the woman deems adequate she may then feel mutually exclusive demands placed upon her time and energy.

Most women cope with the multiple demands of child rearing in a nuclear family, and the presence of a handicapped child changes their concepts and habits very little.[19] By the same token, a woman who mistreats and abuses any child in the privacy of her home for whatever reasons of having been abused, of being overwhelmed with problems, may abuse her handicapped child as well.[20]

EDUCATIONAL SYSTEM

Going to school is the first major step away from home on the road to independence for children in America. It is thus both symbolic and realistic for women with handicapped children to ask even in the first few months, "Will my child be able to go to school?" Until the Congress passed legislation mandating the states to provide education and related services to all handicapped children, the answer was "no." Prior to this, Congress found in 1975 that half of the nation's eight million handicapped children lacked appropriate education for equal opportunity.[21] The state and the local school systems not only denied education for any number of programmatic and prejudicial reasons, but many of the women accepted the denial without protest, having internalized the societal view that their child was not worth the expenditure of educational resources. This situation changed only a few years ago when women's consciousnesses were raised by the black civil rights movement of the 1960s and the women's movement that followed.

Women who know about the rights of their children to be able to attend school may feel some reassurance about their continuing there. In the past private and public schools who accepted handicapped children often had expectations about what parents should do to effect educational carry-over. The educators may or may not have considered what else was going on in the family and how the parents might be able to incorporate their suggestions, but they expected parents to follow their advice. The parents tried, because to do otherwise might have resulted in their child's termination from the program. This control that schools once had over the lives of the parents is also addressed in current legislation. Children may no longer be terminated from an educational program without parental consent or a due process hearing.

The tension between parents and teachers of handicapped children may also be a women's issue. Teachers (mostly women) choose to teach handicapped children after several years of preparation. Parents (mostly women who have the most involvement with the schools) did not choose to parent a handicapped child and had little or no preparation.

The daily responsibilities of the teacher are for a six or seven hour period with mandated relief periods; the remainder of the child's day is the responsibility of the parents. The teacher may also choose to teach other children or no children, while the parents' responsibility to the child is lifelong.

The blurring of roles, in which teachers fill a nourishing, parenting role, while parents are expected to teach their handicapped children, has often resulted in a competitive relationship between parent and teacher, each blaming the other when progress is slow. Sometimes it is the parents who encourage the school to take on a parenting role. On the other hand the schools may ask for followup work at home, potentially "an intrusion into family living."[22] At the same time professional educators may also hold "the impression that parents of handicapped children are guilt-ridden, anxiety-laden, rejecting beings who are inclined to be troublesome to professionals in clinics and schools."[23] This impression may be responsible for some of the tensions between parents and teachers. In any case, the right of the child to attend school is also helpful to the women who parent them in providing time and space for those women to pursue their own interests.

THE MENTAL HEALTH SYSTEM

The unfortunate labeling of women who have a handicapped child came out of research that was undoubtedly intended to assist in the process of understanding the problems women experienced and how the professionals could be helpful. The results, however, have been to create a set of labels that assume that the problems are internal, the fault of the woman. A woman is said to reject or overprotect her handicapped child; to deny the child's condition or to have unrealistic expectations; to be unconcerned or overinvolved[24]; to create a "cycle of infantalization."[25] There is no middle way, no "normal" way for a woman to respond to a handicapped child. A review of professional literature in the mental health field included such comments as: "Guilt, overprotection and resentment seemed to feed upon each other in a never-ending cycle."[26] Sometimes the labels are extended to other family members: "a family in which there is a handicapped child becomes a handicapped family." The high divorce rate among parents of cerebral palsied children "illustrates the devastating effect of the cerebral palsy child on many families."[27]

Believing that women responded in one or another of the categories of pathologies described, I reviewed the literature several years ago to find the best methods of intervention to help these women deal with their internal problems. I found that, in spite of the labeling, in spite of the lack of support and resources and services, most women were managing quite well in rearing their handicapped child in ways similar to the way they raised their "nonhandicapped" children. They were not guilt-ridden, anxiety-laden, over-protective, rejecting parents, and their life styles were varied.[28] I also found that until the 1960s social workers, and probably other mental health professionals, provided limited services to retarded persons and their families. "Since social agencies and social workers were convinced that retarded individuals had little chance of improvement, mental retardation became synonymous with hopelessness."[29] Is it any wonder then that researchers found that parents of handicapped children availed themselves of therapy less frequently then the general population?[30]

RELIGIOUS INSTITUTIONS

Catholic, Protestant, and Jewish congregations have begun to open their doors to handicapped persons.[31] These recent changes reflect "a passage from charity, condescension and custodialism . . . the conventional wisdom of an earlier era . . . to one of partnership with disabled persons in a common quest for independence and self-realization."[32] Religious institutions are also supporting community change for and acceptance of handicapped persons, and some are sponsoring group residences for handicapped persons, providing parent advocacy groups, adapting buildings and programs to the needs of handicapped persons, and providing counseling and outreach to parents.

An effect of this new openness upon women with a handicapped child is that acceptance of the child in the programs and activities of the religious institutions also allows her to participate in adult activities of her choice instead of baby sitting during this time. Another effect upon women is that theologians are taking a new look at the many Biblical references to handicapped persons out of which came the views that handicapping conditions or blemishes were a punishment for sin or wrongdoing, or a sign of being possessed by evil spirits. The doctrine of predestination and fatalism resulted in many women considering a handicapped child her "cross to bear" or her "punishment from God for some real or imagined deed of omission or commission."

Theological changes away from this position may not be welcomed by some women who have placed the responsibility for a child's handicap on a divine being.

THE POLITICAL/ECONOMIC SYSTEM

The costs of diagnosing, treating, rehabilitating, caring for, and educating a handicapped child are so high that even middle-class families with jobs and insurance may be financially devastated by the hundreds of thousands of dollars required for adequate services for their child. It has been estimated that a nonhandicapped baby costs society 10 years of nonparticipation by its mother in the labor force; a second child costs three years and a third child costs two years.[33] The woman with a handicapped child may be out of the labor force 30–50 years or until she dies. One writer has concluded "we generally offer helping services not because an individual needs them, but because it is part of a business transaction. Health restoration and care are profitable to doctors, health insurance groups, hospitals, nursing homes, limb-makers and hearing aid dealers."[34] Because of our racism, "poor and non-white women have greater difficulty in getting accurate information and adequate health care, and have most often been mistreated."[35]

A final part of the political/economic system at which we will take a brief look is the emphasis on the mother as a cause of birth defects, which is only now starting to change. The major focus in the last two decades has been on the ways in which the diet and lifestyle of a woman in the childbearing years affect her offspring. The disabling effects on the fetus of maternal rubella, smoking, alcohol consumption, and drugs have all been fairly well documented. Women were the only ones studied, so it was a matter of finding out how she was responsible for having children with birth defects. Researchers are now reporting a new area of inquiry, the effects of male lifestyles on their offspring. One example is the study being made of children with birth defects born to men exposed to a defoliant "Agent Orange" while stationed in Vietnam. Another example is found in that male rats given heroin, caffeine, morphine, lead, and thalidomide for several days prior to mating had progeny with decreased birth weight, litter size, survival and learning ability, and altered behavior.[36] The research shows that we not only need to seek true answers to old questions, we must also learn to ask the right questions of both women and men.

CONCLUSION

Each year 250,000 women hear the news that their newborn child has birth defects. When a child is born with a birth defect, the values of the professionals may be imposed upon the woman by not using life-sustaining measures to "allow" the child to die or by using artificial life supports without consulting the woman, or by withholding information needed to make a conscientious decision. A conflict of values may also occur between the child's right to medical treatment and the woman's right to live a life free of continuous and lifelong care of another human being.

The irony of the feminists' concerns about childbearing and child-rearing responsibilities is that the concerns are epitomized in women whose children are severely handicapped, yet this subject is seldom mentioned in feminist literature. This may reflect the concern that having a handicapped child is more to be feared and avoided than death and dying.

A brief look at several of the systems that impact upon women who live with a handicapped child showed a consistent pattern of enormous responsibilities being relegated to women who bear children with birth defects; ambivalent if not negative attitudes displayed toward them for having the "different" child; assistance provided to women and handicapped children at financial, emotional, and time-consuming costs to the women; and a low value placed upon the work she does. She is additionally labeled as pathological. Society loses creative talent and energy when the major responsibilities of rearing a handicapped child are enforced by the lack of alternatives rather than assumed willingly by the woman.

The task we have, as women concerned about women who have handicapped children, is to begin a strategy for a process that would:

1. Deal with society's negative attitudes toward women whose children are born with or acquire handicaps.
2. Bring into public view the private lives of women who are rearing handicapped children—not all roses, but satisfying in some ways when responsibilities are shared.
3. Develop a support system for women who have a child with handicaps.
4. Get beyond the "if something goes wrong, but don't mention what" mentality and help women of childbearing age prepare in advance for decisions that might have to be made if a child is born with birth defects.
5. Accept persons with handicaps in our society in a mutual exchange, because accepting differences in others helps us to accept our own differentness.

Neonate Discussion

Moderated by
Catherine A. Musemeche

Hilary Salk: There are two levels of decision-making concerning handicapped newborns. One is on the individual level and may require making a decision whether a particular infant's life should be continued through the use of the complicated technology we have heard discussed today. At this level, I feel that the decision should be in the hands of the parents of this baby since they will ultimately have most of the responsibility and emotional connection to the child. On a policymaking level, I would agree that we probably have enough financial resources to support this technology if we diverted some of these resources from military spending. However, if it presently means that the creation of such elaborate machinery requires diverting resources from nutrition, childbirth preparation, and other forms of preventive care, I opt against the decision to allocate resources for such elaborate technology. Right now I am depressed by the sight of all the machinery when I know that many pregnant women and newborns are not able to obtain adequate nutrition.

Presently it seems that on the individual level parents do not control decisions about their children. In Massachusetts, the state has seen fit to grant the decision of the medical expert greater weight than that of the parents. In the case of Chad Green, the state took custody of the child when his parents decided against the medically advised treatment for his leukemia.

Beth Shearer: They did not say they would not have the chemotherapy. They said they wanted to have laetrile and megavitamin therapy along with it, and Massachusetts General Hospital could not deal with that.

Mary Ampola: A point of information: the parents were refusing chemotherapy. In fact, Chad Green's particular form of leukemia now has a 25% survival rate. It was *not* a hopeless case. I think one could argue strongly that the parents were not meeting their parental responsibilities and that the state had an obligation to the defenseless child to give him a chance to live. That was the grounds on which the state won the case.

Kristin Luker: I have a colleague at the University of California, San Diego, who's studying deinstitutionalization, Andrew Scull. One of the points he makes is that in a capitalist society it's too expensive to keep people in institutions. So we are finding that institutions are closing, and they're moving their patients to minimal profit-making enterprises, usually run by poor people, such as the board-and-care homes for mentally ill people. And one of the things I'm told from research on neonatal intensive care units is that parents have *only* the option of taking their children home. It's not really an option to leave the child in a hospital or in an institution.

I have another colleague, Diane Beeson, who's studying amniocentesis; she finds that the more traditional the division of labor between husband and wife, the less likely the husband is to permit a selective abortion. My colleague suggests that since he doesn't have to take care of it, he can afford to be "moral." But when husbands and wives share childcare, the cost of keeping a damaged or handicapped child at home is assessed differently. One of the things that we haven't really talked about is who takes care of these newborns when they go home.

Barbara Andolsen: The medical facilities with which I am familiar are tertiary care centers. When a severely ill child is born anywhere in the region, the baby is transported by specialized ambulance to the receiving hospital. In some cases, such as spina bifida, decisions to treat or not to treat must be made within a short time. However, the mother, still recovering from a difficult birth, may remain in a local hospital many miles away. The father has to make those decisions himself, alone, and he is not the person who is going to bear the major strain of caring for this child. Maureen, is that a problem in your hospital, and have you found any effective ways of involving mothers whose children are brought in from a distance?

Maureen Edwards: In my hospital, babies are inborn, but I have worked in hospitals with that problem and it's difficult, for a couple of reasons. One is that the mothers who have sick babies are often sick themselves. So even with optimal interrelationships, her ability to involve herself in the decision-making process, physically and emotionally, may be difficult. Some decisions cannot be postponed. The things that can be done are: familiarize the mother as much as possible with the baby, prior to transport; it is particularly important that she see the baby, that she understands as best she can, in her own way, what the baby's conditions are. Most transport teams spend time with mother. Fathers usually come along with the baby to the referral center where more information is given. We encourage him to go back and as best he can, in his perhaps biased way, to relate to mother and to have mother's input. We hope to have a decision that families are making together. And I don't think in the long run it will go well if parents are forced into a stance where one or the other gives in.

Helga Bendix: Has transporting the mother along with the child ever been considered, in the same or in a second ambulance?

Norma Swenson: A lot of us have fought for that very hard, without very much success, both at the level of the national health planning guidelines for neonatal care and also at the local planning level. So far there are no requirements that mother and baby be transferred together.

Helen Swallow: University of Connecticut, Farmington, replaced their single van, that was only able to take one baby at a time, with two vans they call the "White Whales." And they transport, ideally, mothers with risk babies still inside. If not possible they delay the transfer until the mother can come. They recognize the problem; it doesn't always work, but it's possible.

Maureen Edwards: In many geographical locations the children's hospitals do not have the facilities for mothers' care. If we were planning regional neonatal care starting from scratch, we wouldn't be in this situation.

Margaret Steinfels: Maureen Edwards points to an issue that has wide ramifications for childbirth in general. That is the national plan to regionalize newborn care in order to maintain scarce resources in central locations. This will have an important effect on prenatal care, labor, and delivery. Given the lowered birth rate, local hospitals are not delivering the number of babies they once did. As a consequence, many community hospitals are closing their maternity wards and pushing people on to central and more technological settings. We can see the way in which a variety of circumstances are drawing people into more technological settings—many of them inappropriately. I am impressed with what Maureen had to say about that technology saving lives and preserving health, but we need to understand that this technology and this regionalization are also affecting the care of normal healthy mothers and infants.

Norma Swenson: People interested in the regionalization issue can read the last appendix of the current edition of *Our Bodies, Ourselves.* In it I summarize a kind of political analysis of regionalization, partly in terms of the emphasis on prevention and partly in terms of the motivation of planners. In addtion to that, the National Women's Health Network and our collective and about eight other national groups got together and put out a national mailing to all of the health planning agencies in the country, trying to give them our feminist/consumer analysis of regionalization as a perspective on the report, *Toward Improving the Outcome of Pregnancy* [National Foundation/March of Dimes]. The establishment itself has not criticized the concept of regionalization much until recently. Fortunately, the medical establishment has now produced some literature that does contradict the claims for cost and outcome that were made on behalf of regionalization. If any of you are interested in that, you can write to us and we can arrange to get that packet of materials to you for a nominal sum. One of the major points we raised is that not only is more prevention possible but much psychological damage can be prevented if mothers and babies are transferred together.

Diana, in light of the incident that you reported where there was the threat of child abuse, in light of the Chad Green case that Hilary brought up, and in light of the fact that we have documentation now that at least three women have been forcibly removed from their homes during labor and taken by police into the hospital to give birth, what do you mean that a representative of the state be a member of one of these decision-making committees? I liked your list until you got to the state.

Diana Axelsen: I meant *possible* members. The hypothetical decision-making team could include a representative of the state, but I am firmly opposed to that. My position is that we should get rid of the medical hierarchy in which the physician has so much influence in decision-making involving issues of human values. Instead, we need a decision-making situation in which an interdisciplinary team assists the parents in reaching a decision, and supports them even when consensus is not reached. The first priority to me is involving the parents in a basic way; but I also am concerned with the interaction of the parents with medical personnel, nurses and midwives, religious advisors, and psychological counselors. Such support would help move us away from the kinds of state intervention I oppose.

As I see it, there are two possible interpretations of the Chad Green case. One is to say that the parents were denying their child medical treatment. The other is to say that they were asserting their right to choose the kind of treatment their child would receive. Part of their reasoning, as I understood it, also had to do with their son's reactions to chemotherapy; they were arguing for the importance of quality of life. They also wanted to rely on more "natural" forms of treatment, which is not the same as doing nothing at all. I realize that parents abuse children, but that's different from allowing parents to choose unorthodox treatments that they regard as in their child's best interests. I find the Green case a frightening example of the power that both physicians and the state are ready to exert over even well-intentioned parents.

I think that it's really important to bear in mind that at this point there is an alliance, a *de facto* alliance, between the state and the monopoly that is allopathic medicine in this country. And if we don't bear that in mind then we have really misunderstood, quite fundamentally, how inappropriate it is for a hospital to be the custodian of a child.

Dorothy Wertz: I think that one of the basic issues that this conference is going to have to face is at what point does the mother have the final responsibility to make decisions, not only for herself—I think that she should always have responsibility for herself—but for the potential child or the actual child, and at what point does the state have the responsibility to step in to protect a child or potential child. This is a very difficult issue. Suppose that a woman who is having one of the few percentiles of high risk births, risks a ruptured uterus that would kill her, but also would usually kill the child, then insists upon having a home delivery. Should she have to right to do so? Now I would say, very reluctantly, and I have problems with this, that if the child is not yet born, she should have the right to make that decision.

Suppose a woman who is having an Rh baby does not want an *in-utero* transfusion that would save the baby: should she be able to say, "No, I have my own beliefs about health, and I will not have this transfusion?" I think she should have the right to make the final decision, but that we also have a moral obligation to present her with information on the risks and benefits of various alternatives. As long as the child is not yet born, though, the decision must be hers. After the child is born she is in practice allowed to make a life or death decision only in cases where there is severe genetic defect or damage that medicine cannot change. She is not really given the decision if there is simply a low birth weight baby that may or may not have brain damage. You just heard Maureen say, "If it looks as if it might be healthy, we go ahead and resuscitate." Suppose the mother says, "No, I don't want a brain-damaged child, I don't want to take *any* chance." Now at this point does the state have the responsibility to intervene? This is a difficult question.

What about a child like Chad Green? (I think this case is very relevant.) His parents insist upon the right to free choice in health care and really have very good intentions. Do they have the right to make the final decision or does the state have the right to step in, in the interest of protecting the child? I would, with some qualms, say that at this point the Commonwealth of Massachusetts had the right to step in and insist that the boy be given chemotherapy. There are problems with this because I think that the treatment that's given against the family's will is less effective than it would otherwise have been. But I think the time comes when you have to say that at this point the mother or the family can no longer be given the final responsibility. These are tough questions, and I think we are really going to have to deal with these issues.

Janet Farrell Smith: I hope also that this conference can come out with some kind of resolution on decision-making processes with newborns and with genetic counseling. Some people have spoken of our conference here as professionally or academically weighted. It is less so than the conference I attended in May 1979 in Boston on "Genetics and the Law," sponsored by the American Society for Law and Medicine. Most of the speakers were MDs or JDs. However, there was in that conference a general tone of criticism about moving medical decisions into the court system. MDs are very concerned about this trend. Furthermore, at that same conference, Joseph Fletcher, a leading theologian and professor of Christian ethics respected by many, came out strongly with the position that people who have genetic defects should not be allowed to reproduce. He took this position openly to a somewhat receptive audience. At least there was not a general outcry against him. His remarks were the only ones reported in the *Boston Globe.* It is important that we here know what others are saying about the same issues we are scrutinizing.

Susan Bell: I've been struck over the last couple of days and again today about two issues. One is the narrow focus on physicians as providers of care. Particularly in high technology medicine, there is a retinue of people who provide care. The issue that Wendy brought up needs to be extended to all the other providers. The other issue is eugenics. Once again the notion of perfection has been raised: how to produce "perfect" babies through neonatal care, or how to prevent "imperfect" babies through sterilization. I would like to see this issue addressed critically.

Caroline Whitbeck: We *haven't* talked about the rest of the health care workers. We should realize that most health care is given by women, women who are in low status positions, such as nurses and nurses' aides. If we want to bring about any major changes in health care, we've got to be working with and supporting those women. One of the issues that has divided us is "professionalism." Nurses very often speak about being professionals and being recognized as professionals, meaning to draw attention to the importance of their work and the importance of their skills. There is a faction of critics who, when they hear the word "professional," say, "Oh, well, that means nurses want to be a part of the establishment, want to buy into this, want to sell out to that, and just want to be mini-doctors." That's *not* what the nurses are saying. Also, unfortunately, division between professional and so-called "nonprofessional" nurses is often fostered by this talk of professionalism. The people who are LPNs or LVNs are afraid that they're being told that their work is unimportant. LVNs and LPNs know all sorts of very important things, but they don't get them from their training programs. They brought them with them from women's culture. What I learned about breastfeeding I learned from an LVN; what she transmitted to me was a part of women's culture.

Susan Ekstrom: It's difficult to refocus people's attention from the physician as the primary caretaker to all of the women "under" him. One of the things that is particularly clear to the women going into hospitals for the birth experience is that decision-making power lies with the physician. If you can't negotiate birthing practices and procedures with "him," no matter how caring and nurturing the nurses are, they have no power to change the doctor's "standing orders." People get co-opted by this; the nurses fall into this co-optation. They have a conflict: their caring is for the patient, and yet they are responsible to the physician.

Caroline Whitbeck: I'm talking about supporting the nurses in their attempts to change medical care from *their* perspective. I think that actually it's the nurses who run a hospital: if the doctors didn't make rounds one morning people would notice, but nothing would happen. If the nurses didn't show up, the hospital would cease to be a hospital. What I'm suggesting is: there is tremendous skill and power there, and helping the nurses to organize themselves is an important thing to do. We can't just focus on the physician. It's nice when you have a physician like Duff who knows that he needs to listen to everybody—the housekeepers, the dietitian, everybody—because he knows that they are the only people who can really hear what some of the patients are saying. Well, that's lovely, but it doesn't happen often enough. We're not going to change physicians overnight. We also need to work to strengthen the hand of the nurses.

Susan Ekstrom: Well, I think that might happen if we work, for example, to support nurse-midwives with childbirth education groups. But simply giving emotional support women-to-women is not enough, although necessary since the nurses do get poor treatment.

Regina Kenen: I visited a tertiary care neonatal unit. It was so incredibly good that I wondered if this was typical of these centers or whether we were shown a "Potemkin Village." I expected to see upsetting technology; what I did not expect to see were mobiles, decals, and shades with little pictures of things and children in bright colors. One baby in an incubator had a quilt made by her mother. I saw the same incredible love and care shown by the staff, the nurses and the residents, equivalent to what the nurse-midwives have described here. This was a referral center and nobody was denied access for lack of money. In fact, a great percentage of cases came from low income families because of poor nutrition and prenatal care.

The nurses within the team were given a large role in the decision-making, because it was the nurses who watched the baby minute by minute for the entire day. Their evidence was highly valued, and they were very concerned about the future of these babies: what kind of home would they be going to, what kind of care would they be getting, would they be abused? The team discussed the cases with a social worker. The facility seemed too good to be true, and that's the question I throw out: Is this a typical center?

Gerene Major: I worked for a year and three months in an environment such as Reggie just described, and I think there are problems under that facade. Some of the nurses—particularly young ones who have never been married and who want to be married and to have children—have theories about mother-infant bonding. Some identify with mothers, and if a mother does not bond the way the nurses think she's supposed to, they convey quite damaging nonverbal messages.

Maureen Edwards: In intensive care nurseries, the most important professional player is the nurse who is a nurturing person. And I agree that raises a lot of difficult problems: who is the nurturer of this child? The aim is to create a nurturing environment for the child. It sometimes may be misguided. There is a very heavy emphasis on nurturing activity for a variety of strictly medical as well as psychosocial reasons.

Wendy Carlton: The nurses get a little jealous that the mothers want to come in and claim the babies, because after all, they've been there much more than the mothers themselves. The other thing I can't restrain myself from commenting on is the bonding literature. Despite our great criticism of Freud for giving us only six years to screw up our children's lives, the bonding people seem to give us anywhere between the first five minutes to the first three hours of life. And I think that should be taken with a note of caution.

Caroline Whitbeck: Having worked with a neonatal group in Texas, I agree that there is a problem about the attachment of the nurses and physicians to the infants. The nurses and physicians do raise concerns about the kind of home life that the infants will have. I think that's okay. It would be much worse if people didn't care about the babies. (It would be a serious problem if the nurses and physicians were suing for custody of the children; that isn't happening.) The staff has to be attached to the infants whom they are calling forth as people. If that means that there is going to be some problem with grief and concern when the baby leaves the hospital, then we should just see to it that the staff has an opportunity to work through those feelings.

Catherine Musemeche: Before further discussion I want to say a few words from the medical student's point of view, specifically from a woman medical student's point of view. Also, just because I'm a woman, I don't pretend to know what every woman feels. And I don't think I can assume that, when I get my MD, I'm going to be able to relate to all women. The women in the health collectives know women and it's my obligation to learn from them; why should I expect them to "educate me to take their money?" I just want you to know that I've heard the critique of the profession. I have really heard it. And it's hit me hard and people have told me not to take it personally. Well, I'm sorry, I do, and I'm glad that I do because I don't want to be like those people who don't hear you and don't respond to you. So I just want to thank you for being open and honest with that criticism because I've learned a hell of a lot and I look for more.

Renée Jenkins: I can appreciate your comment, but I also have a response, as a female physician. During this conference I've tried to be open. And I really learned other perspectives on things that I take for granted or that I do for which I have not, in an ethical sense, considered the long term effects. And I appreciate that. But I also have been a little bit embittered by comments from people who say they represent what a woman's response is, and who have lumped together physicians in such a fashion that they come out from identical templates—"This is a physician; a physician behaves this way." Just as different people who are feminists have different roles, there are also different physicians who practice medicine in different ways. Essentially to decide and to state that all physicians behave alike, I think, is really demeaning. It's making a judgment that you don't want anyone to make about you. The physicians who are here obviously don't have the same views that you are attributing to all physicians. And I would like you to open your minds and give your time to speak to us so that you can get some different perspectives on how physicians behave.

Susan Bell: One of the issues that's been brought up is the relationship between the institutions, institutional roles, and the people who fill those roles. To what extent do people carry out the goals of an institution and to what extent do they make individual decisions? For instance, some medical students struggle against the institution and institutional roles. Some give in to institutional roles and/or don't think about the medical system they're becoming part of. I like to confront medical students in a responsible way to stimulate them to think about why they're learning what they're learning.

Joyce Berkman: Helga, as I've listened to your litany of laws I've grown increasingly depressed because I know that few of those laws are being enforced. Chapter 766 of the Massachusetts State law that regulates special education is defied flagrantly with no punishment whatsoever. The profound taxpayers' revolt in this country makes me pessimistic that any of these laws having to do with special education and rehabilitation can be implemented. In Amherst, people in revolt against 766 are insisting that every parent who has a child who's handicapped should meet at least 50% of the costs. They say it's an unfair burden to place on the community to have to pay for those kinds of needs, especially since the classroom teacher is overwhelmed by special needs students and can't attend to the "normal" youngsters. There is very little sense of the reciprocity that has to go on in a community between different kinds of people and little appreciation for what youngsters can learn from interacting with special needs children—that's education too. I want to caution against any complacency because I think, in fact, that we are moving backwards rather than forwards.

Helga Bendix: I couldn't agree more with you, but if I gave up and was too pessimistic I'd stay home instead of trying to have the ideals implemented.

Sex Preselection

Organized by

Janice G. Raymond

Introduction

Janice G. Raymond

Sex preselection and the technology that is now being developed to implement it demand a profound and searching woman-centered analysis. Cultures and individuals have always preferred male children, but the technological means of assuring this preference have only recently been contrived.

Papers, responses, and discussion at the sex preselection session made clear that many of the conference participants were affected by this presentation in a way that was distinct from their responses to other sessions. Women had listened to several days of how we have been victimized by a whole spectrum of reproductive technologies, from contraceptives to sterilization abuse. Yet the impinging reality of sex preselection moved our discussion of manipulative medical technologies into the realm of *previctimization,* i.e., the spectre of women being destroyed and sacrificed before even being born. Previctimization is analogous to Mary Daly's notion of the *prepossession* of women. "This is possession before a woman's original movement in be-ing can break through to consciousness. It involves depths of destruction that the term *possession* cannot adequately name. For someone to be possessed, she must first *be.*"[1]

The topic of our panel cannot be separated from a larger sex selection system that is operative in all facets of a patriarchal world, and that promotes "different nurturance of children and different roles offered to children." Adequately confronting the technology of sex preselection means centering on an "ecology of femaleness" that examines the total patterns that exist between women and a man-made environment.

Ruth Nentwig presents an eminently clear account of the technical aspects of sex preselection. The earliest researchers in this area focused on procedures that would separate X- and Y-bearing sperm before conception. Electrophoresis, the acid-alkali process, centrifugation, and antigen–antibody reactions are the main procedures that have been studied. After conception, amniocentesis has been the main procedure used in detecting fetal sex. Used initially to determine genetic defects, amniocentesis came to be employed by many physicians solely for the detection of sex. Couples may then choose to abort if the revealed sex of the fetus is not the preferred sex. Since amniocentesis cannot be performed until the second trimester of pregnancy, the risks of an abortion at this point are greater. Therefore the Anshan aspiration method was developed in China to be used during the first trimester of pregnancy. This procedure involves insertion of a suction tube into the cervix and aspiration of fetal cells sloughed off into the cervical canal. In the Chinese study of this method, 100 sex predictions resulted in 30 abortions, and of these 30, 29 aborted fetuses were female.

Roberta Steinbacher presents the futuristic implications of sex preselection, implications that, one might say, are not all that futuristic. She takes exception to those researchers who conclude that, given its development, sex preselection technology would be infrequently used and its effects mitigated by the incidence of unplanned births. She reviews much of the literature dealing with parental preference in sex control and finds that son-preference clearly outweighs daughter-preference for both women and men. Steinbacher concisely outlines the psychological costs to a woman that accompany sex preselection, the fact that the physiological risks are almost entirely borne by the woman, and the ultimate political effects of such procedures, which will literally be beyond female control. Calling for women to no longer cooperate in our own oppression, Steinbacher concludes that all women must insure the strong survival of women and, ultimately, "test whether sisterhood is powerful or just a good idea." In the final analysis, she maintains that only women who truly esteem themselves will want to reproduce themselves.

From the outset of her presentation, Tabitha Powledge makes clear her opposition to "picking the sexes of children no matter what the means." Her concern is whether one can or should translate this opposition into public policy. She begins by making one policy recommendation of spending no more money on any further preference studies since, among other things, they tell us what we already know. Furthermore, they cannot answer whether or how much the sex ratio will change and do not help people assess the likely consequences of sex choices. In her opinion, "speculations can be either apocalyptic or playful, but they are still just speculations." Unfortunately, as Powledge argues, "the implication of my conclusion is that we will have to develop the technology, turn it loose, and see what people actually do with it . . ." Moreover, to legally prohibit the choice of sex through technological means is to chip away at women's hard-won gains of reproductive control. Although Powledge believes that technologies for sex preselection should not be financed, developed, or used, the outcome of preventing their use through legal regulation opens the door to legally restricting reproduction in general. Powledge's conclusion is that we should not underestimate the value and power of moral education and exhortation.

The concluding responses to these papers make a still wider range of points. Is this a relevant issue for women of all races and classes? Why is it that although women have had little to do with the development of these technologies, women are encouraged to deliberate and share the burden of deciding what to do with them, once they have been developed? And, finally, how are the findings that even women would choose sons related to the reasons why women learn to prefer men in many other contexts, even though their primary and life-giving relationships may be with women?

Technical Aspects of Sex Preselection

M. Ruth Nentwig

Historically, parents have preferred male children in order to continue a family line, manage property, work in the fields, and fulfill the father's image of potency and manhood. Accordingly, very early men of science were interested in the area of sex selection and prediction. A Chinese manuscript 4400 years old deals with the subject at length. An ancient Egyptian document states that if the face of a pregnant woman has a greenish cast, she is certain to bear a son. Hippocrates believed that females developed in the left uterine horn and males in the right. Therefore, Aristotle advised women to "think male" and lie on their right sides after intercourse to increase the amount of "generative heat" that he thought was the chief cause of male children.[1] The list of myths and advice to women is endless and spans all of history owing to the great economic and social value placed on having male heirs. Within these primitive cultures, the burden of producing sons lay solely with the wife; if she gave birth only to daughters, her husband had the right to divorce her and marry another woman.

It was discovered much later that sex determination resided with the male rather than with the female. Cells in the human contain 46 chromosomes, two of which are sex chromosomes. Males possess an X and a Y chromosome, while females have two X chromosomes. During the development of sperm and ova, the germ cells undergo a reduction division resulting in a halving of chromosome number. A mature ovum therefore has 23 chromosomes, one of which is an X. Mature sperm also have 23 chromosomes, but the sex chromosome in a given sperm can be either X or Y. When the ovum and sperm unite, the resulting zygote will be female if fertilized by a sperm containing an X chromosome (called gynogenic sperm) or a male if the sperm has a Y chromosome (called androgenic sperm).

Armed with the knowledge of chromosomal differences between sperm, early researchers in the twentieth century turned their attention to developing separation techniques to segregate androgenic and gynogenic sperm. One of the earliest processes involved the use of electrophoresis, that is, separation of materials based on differences in electrical charges. The pioneer work in this field was done in 1932, by a Soviet biochemist, V. N. Schröder,[2] who discovered that rabbit spermatozoa placed in a vessel with a positive electrode at one end and a negative electrode at the other migrated in each direction or stayed in the middle. (Normally in electrophoresis, materials move to either one electrode or the other.) When sperm collected next to the positive electrode were placed in the reproductive tract of a female rabbit, all the resulting offspring were female. Sperm obtained at the negative electrode produced mostly male offspring, and those remaining in the middle yielded equal numbers of males and females. Dr. Schröder and her colleagues continued these tests with rabbits for the next ten years and were reportedly successful in controlling sex of the offspring 80% of the time. Duplication of these studies by American researchers met predictions less accurately and the method was abandoned.

The next technique to appear in the 1930s was the acid-alkali process developed by Ünterberger in Germany.[3] He observed a high correlation between alkaline vaginal secretions and the production of male offspring. Women previously shown to be sterile because of highly acidic vaginal secretions were treated with alkaline douches and subsequently gave birth only to males. Ünterberger reported that 53 out of 54 females treated over a ten-year period had babies, all of which were male. The one exception reportedly did not follow her doctor's prescription. Once again, interest in this as a technique for sex preselection faded because repeated tests and experiments by other researchers failed to substantiate earlier results.

Differential centrifugation arrived on the scene in the 1950s. Since the X and Y chromosomes differ in size, with the Y chromosome being smaller, it was believed that the sperm bearing the two types would be of two different weights and could therefore be separated physically according to density. A centrifuge is routinely employed in the laboratory to separate materials from a mixture by spinning a solution at high speeds to produce a faster settling out or precipitation of heavier materials from lighter ones. Differential centrifugation is a more sophisticated form of this process that allows separation of several materials at once into a number of layers. In theory, the gynogenic sperm should precipitate out as the heavier layer, but in practice it was found that female-determining sperm were more sensitive than the male ones and were damaged in the centrifuging process. A number of animal breeders with high hopes of obtaining the sex of their choice by using the separated spermatozoa for artificial insemination were terribly disappointed when the results showed an overall decrease in fertility. Studies with bull spermatozoa showed the number of male offspring was higher than normal, but the mechanical damage of centrifugation interfered so greatly with fertility that this method was also abandoned.

However, a modification of this process is now being used in fertility clinics in San Francisco and Chicago. After centrifugation and the accompanying destruction of most of the gynogenic sperm, the resulting solution is placed in a test tube containing human serum albumin, which is difficult for sperm to swim in. The lighter androgenic sperm happen to be the best "swimmers" and make their way to the bottom of the tube. These sperm are then introduced by artificial insemination and guarantee male children 65–90% of the time. The technique was developed and patented by Dr. Ronald J. Ericsson[4] of Gametrics Limited of Sausalito, California. Only couples desiring male children will be served by these fertility clinics.

The major sex preselection technique of the seventies involves antigen–antibody reactions between sperm and egg. Since sperm are foreign bodies introduced into the female reproductive system, a slight immune reaction occurs when the ovum is exposed to cells unlike its own. Gustaaf van den Bovenkamp of San Francisco developed a technique to isolate the separate antibodies produced by the ovum to both gynogenic and androgenic sperm. These antibodies can be injected into the female to produce either a male or a female child. For example, if antibodies produced against androgenic sperm are injected, only the gynogenic sperm will be capable of fertilizing the ovum and producing a female. Bovenkamp patented his technique, so that further details of this method are not available.[5]

A positive and simple approach has been reported that utilizes a more natural system, one that can be controlled for the most part by a woman and eliminates the need for artificial insemination. Dr. Sophia Kleegman[6] of New York University found conception of females about 80% of the time when intercourse had occurred 36–48 hours prior to ovulation. This method involves very careful charting of the menstrual cycles for several months and daily temperature monitoring. A woman's body temperature generally rises one degree on the day of ovulation. According to Kleegman, if copulation occurs at this time chances are four to one in favor of conceiving a male. Thus the method involves defining the time of ovulation very precisely and working forward or backward from that in attempting to select for the sex of the child.

Another technique that is said to yield 80–90% selection for female babies was developed by Landrum Shettles[7] now at Gifford Memorial Hospital in Randolph, Vermont. This simple procedure makes use of the functional differences in androgenic and gynogenic sperm. It is known that gynogenic sperm are slower swimmers and live two to three times longer than the faster swimming androgenic sperm. In addition, the gynogenic sperm are less inhibited by the acidic environment of the vagina, but are negatively affected by the alkaline environment of the cervix, uterus, and fallopian tubes. To select for a female child, Shettles recommends an acidic vinegar douche preceding coitus, shallow penetration of the penis to ensure delivery of the sperm only in the vagina where acidity levels are high, use of the face-to-face missionary position of intercourse, and avoidance of orgasm, since this increases the alkalinity of the uterus. By reversing these conditions, a male child can be conceived.

Thus, it is clear that technology has progressed to the point where researchers are getting patents on their methods and using them in fertility clinics to allow couples to select the sex of their child. Because these preconception techniques are new and not yet foolproof, methods of determining the sex of a young fetus have been developed as a by-product of other basic research.

One of the earliest techniques developed for detecting fetal sex was amniocentesis, a procedure whereby a long hollow needle is inserted through the abdominal wall of the mother into the amniotic cavity surrounding the fetus. By aspirating a small amount of amniotic fluid, a number of fetal cells can be obtained for biochemical and microscopic analysis. The technique was originally developed as a diagnostic tool about ten years ago to screen for possible genetic defects. Since the procedure could be done during the 16–20th weeks of pregnancy, the couple could choose to abort in the event of serious defects. A number of genetic disorders are sex-linked, resulting from a gene on an X chromosome. Generally they are more common in males in whom a recessive gene on the single X chromosome will be expressed. As a result, detection of fetal sex was a by-product of amniocentesis.

As this procedure was perfected, its cost decreased and usage increased. Many physicians used it solely for detection of fetal sex in cases where no genetic or physical abnormalities were suspected. A great moral and ethical controversy arose within the medical community regarding this possible misuse of technology and is still raging. However, of greater concern is the fact that amniocentesis cannot be done until 16–20 weeks of gestation. The additional 3–4 weeks required for biochemical and chromosomal analysis make abortion, if selected, a risky procedure, since this is now a second trimester abortion, which yields statistically 18.6 maternal deaths per 100,000.

A possible solution to the difficulties presented by amniocentesis may lie in non-invasive sampling of chorionic villi (fetal cells) sloughed into the cervical canal during the first trimester of pregnancy. According to an article in the Chinese Medical Journal,[8] physicians at the Hospital of the Anshan Iron and Steel Company were able to detect the sex of an embryo as early as 47 days after conception. The procedure involves insertion of a suction tube into the cervix and aspiration of sloughed-off fetal cells. Fetal sex can then be determined by chromosome analysis. The Chinese predictions of sex proved to be 93% accurate when compared with actual figures at birth or after abortion. The chilling fact of this "Anshan aspiration" technique is not its accuracy in prediction, but its possibility for control owing to its low risk and simplicity. Of 100 experimental sex predictions in the China study, 30 resulted in planned abortions. Of those 30 aborted fetuses, 29 were girls! According to a report in Medical World News[9] US researchers have begun to utilize and extend this technique. At Indiana University, a study performed as a diagnostic aid to prevent risks from sex-linked disorders such as hemophilia and muscular dystrophy yielded very high levels of accuracy with a modification of the Anshan aspiration technique. Women who participated in this project were not informed of the results until after the 20th week of pregnancy to prevent any possible abortions based on sex preferences.

The latest procedure for sex determination involves finding fetal cells in maternal peripheral blood.[10] Swiss scientists reported 86% accuracy rates for their technique, which involved culturing fetal blood cells and staining with quinacrine, then looking for the fluorescent Y chromosome. However, this method cannot be used until 14–18 weeks of gestation when fetal blood cells have begun to differentiate and some have crossed the placental barriers into the mother's circulatory system.

In summary, we possess a variety of emerging techniques for sex preselection before conception either through artificial separation of androgenic and gynogenic sperm and subsequent fertilization by artificial insemination, or by timing the occurrence of intercourse and making use of functional differences between the two types of sperm. We also have at our disposal techniques allowing determination of fetal sex as early as 47 days after conception, allowing the possibility of abortion in the event the fetus is not of the gender of the parents' choice.

The implications of our scientific advances are frightening and must be dealt with. As a result of changes in our culture that produce a more liberal attitude toward abortion while at the same time clinging to the belief that having sons yields the greatest fulfillment for both mothers and fathers, physicians and researchers are presented with great moral and ethical dilemmas. Some individuals have capitalized on male preference by seeking patents on their techniques that ensure male children to couples at fertility clinics. Other researchers are torn between their pursuit of a natural scientific interest and the implications of that work for society as a whole. On the international level, the medical community has taken a stand. A world conference held in Stockholm, Sweden, on Prenatal Diagnosis of Genetic Disorders of the Fetus reported a general lack of support of prenatal sex determination with the objective of aborting the fetus if it is not of the desired sex. These procedures were not deemed justified merely to satisfy parental curiosity. These professional affirmations do not resolve all the dilemmas confronting a physician around this issue. For example, a pediatrician at a large medical center saw a pregnant woman and her husband who came with a family history of hemophilia. After amniocentesis, the pediatrician informed the couple that, since the fetus was a girl, they had no worries about a sex-linked disorder. At that point the parents-to-be replied that they were off to get an abortion because they really wanted a boy and made up the hemophilia story in order to have the amniocentesis done.[9]

Perhaps the issue to be concerned with is that people can feel so strongly about the gender of their unborn child as to abort the unwanted sex. With all our available technology and scientific advances, we would be wise to consider the process of conception, birth, and child rearing for what it is: a natural, normal biological occurrence.

We cannot ignore the preference for males that was so prevalent in the past and still exists today, but we can give our daughters and the other females in our lives support and encouragement in finding their own sense of self-worth to the extent that they would want to reproduce their own sex and possibly even convince the fathers of their children that gender in and of itself is not the major issue in life.

Futuristic Implications of Sex Preselection

Roberta Steinbacher

A review of the current and proposed methods of sex preselection provides ample evidence that technology has far outdistanced conceptual and applied work on the human and ethical effects of this technology. It is only a matter of time before the most effective of these methods will be available for widespread use, perhaps as easily acquired as a bottle of aspirin. Given the status of women in this nation and in most countries throughout the world, unless we make our voices heard now we will be faced with a range of outcomes that could make the label "second class citizen" a given reality. What are the implications of being second born, and knowing at some early age that you were planned-to-be second? How many female fetuses are now being aborted so that couples might have a firstborn male? What happens in an already male-biased world when the sex ratio at birth increases? Will the cost of achieving population stabilization be the elimination of a disproportionate number of future females? These and other questions surrounding the issue of sex preselection must be addressed if we as women are to have any control over this life and death matter.

Here, I will attempt to analyze the future implications of sex preselection in light of present sociopsychological and demographic findings. It should be noted at the outset that I take exception to the conclusion of those researchers[1] who believe that sex preselection techniques would be infrequently used, and that given the "considerable incidence of unplanned births in the United States... the effects of sex preselection would be further diluted." Rather, I believe, the patriarchal values in this society will continue to dictate that: if it's inventable, invent it; if it makes money, market it; and if women get hurt in the process, systemic male bonding will save one from prosecution.

Also preceding any analysis of the implications of sex preselection, the historical reality of son preference throughout the world must be recognized. Nancy Williamson[2] in her insightful review of parent preference in sex control admits that there is *no* evidence that son preference is declining, either in the United States or in developing countries. Although Williamson summarizes her review of the sociopsychological and economic background facts by stating that men "tend to prefer boys more than girls," Lolagene Coombs, citing data from the National Survey of Family Growth, gives us more discouraging information[3]: "one-half of married women have an underlying preference for sons, one-third prefer daughters and only one-fifth have a clear preference for balance."

When we add to the literature on son preference the findings on firstborns and firstborn male preference, the information is devastating to women. That there is a strong preference for firstborn males on the part of both parents has been abundantly documented.[4–8] The reported percentages range as high as 79% of the women tested preferring a boy to 12% a girl, and 80% of the men preferring a boy to 4% a girl.[7]

That firstborns have distinct advantages over later borns has been well-documented for years. In general, research strongly supports the fact that the firstborn is more intelligent, more achievement oriented, more successful, and more affiliative compared to later borns. Specific research on second-born women indicates that a woman from a two-child family tends to disparage herself more if she has an older brother than if she has an older sister, i.e., she has lower self-esteem.[9]

The serious implications for women in relation to these findings *combined* with the availability of sex preselection methods are unmistakable. The *de facto* second class status of women in the world would be confirmed *in fact, by choice.* In addition, male egos (already inclined to be relatively inflated because of "superior" status) would clearly receive an even more powerful message.

This message is translated into reality when selective abortion is utilized as the method of preselection: the availability of abortion for poor women in this country is already severely restricted; the number of firstborn males will rise among the *privileged* and remain unchanged among the lower socioeconomic classes, thereby insuring that increasing numbers of women in the future are locked into poverty while men continue to grow in numbers in positions of control and influence. Whatever selection method is utilized, the end result will carry with it the lasting opportunity for institutionalizing sexism in birth order. And Margaret Mead's statement that any females who are born will at last be wanted is small consolation when being wanted secondarily is the actuality.

It is alleged that one societal consequence of widespread use of sex preselection techniques is that higher sex ratios would occur at birth.

Various authors have predicted both the occurrence of a higher sex ratio and possible consequences of this alteration [1, 5, 6, 10–15]: surplus of males, increased crime, wars, polyandry, women as a rare commodity, and so on. More optimistic predictions would concentrate on population limitations, i.e., if parents could choose the sex of their children they would complete their families with the second or third child. Coombs, in analyzing the 1965 National Fertility Study, concluded that second parity couples with children of only one sex are more likely to say they want an additional child than those with a child of each sex.[16]. At second, third, and fourth parity, mothers with children of the same sex are more likely to expect additional children than mothers with both sexed offspring.[17] The research in this area of the interaction between sex preselection and population limitation is limited at best. At worst, predictions tend toward Postgate's scheme to save the planet by eliminating most of the women in third-world countries,[15] and May and Heer's solution to the population problem[18] in India as the "reduction of family size required to assure son-survivorship."

Fewer firstborn females, a higher sex ratio at birth, more poor women in developed countries, and elimination of women in the third world are indeed devastating outcomes of sex preselection for women.

After intensive research into the area of sex preselection and its effect on women, Williamson has concluded that there are some positive, but minimal, outcomes[19]: individual women would have more choice and less uncertainty; there would be fewer children of the "wrong" sex; sex-linked disease for some women would no longer be worrisome; and single women who prefer a female child would feel freer to become pregnant. In summary, women would theoretically have more control over their bodies and their lives. Williamson adds, however, that the costs far outweigh the benefits of this control.

There are many *psychological* costs accompanying sex preselection: mutual decisions and potential conflict with a husband over the "right" sex and birth order; the possibility of a mistake in selective abortion; the need to protect a husband's ego around artificial insemination, etc. In addition, *physiological* risks are disproportionately, or in most cases entirely, borne by women: amniocentesis with abortion in the second trimester (six times as life threatening as first trimester), temperature watching, timing of intercourse, and so on. If, in fact, a pill becomes the most marketable method of choosing the sex of offspring, it could be predicted that it will be made *by* men *for* women, not for men, as is the present case with "The Pill." And did we learn from the pill? Who invented it, who manufactured it, who licensed it, who dispenses it? But who dies from it?

Politically, women are at a decided disadvantage in sex preselection technology as in most other cases. We have little control as a statistical majority; as a minority the picture will become even more grim. Unlike cloning, where, in a Lysistratan sense it could be possible for women to control their own ova, or in parthenogenesis where we have no need for men, there is no specific possibility of control by women in the area of preselection in sexual reproduction. We are grossly underrepresented in the biological and health sciences—we are grossly underrepresented in policymaking positions, and as a group we have been grossly unaware of the potential results of this technology.

In addition, we have not learned how to build a constituency so that our needs will be met—we often do not know who the enemy is *or* who our friends are—the rage that we feel about our oppression is all too often turned inward to each other. We must refuse to cooperate any longer in our own oppression—instead we must learn that we have to engage all women in a serious political and ideological struggle that will ensure the strong survival of our half of the human race.

In effect, we must test whether sisterhood is powerful or just a good idea.

There are steps that can be taken to prevent our lives from being controlled by technologies that will not be stopped or reversed, or by male physicians unaware or uncareful of the effect of these technologies on women, or by husbands demanding firstborn male heirs, or by drug companies capitalizing on the market, or, in the long run, by the Federal government itself. These steps and others for which we have yet to develop strategies are critical not only to the survival of women but also to the survival of the species.

First, we must make sure, by whatever means necessary, that women are an integral part and have voice and vote when policies are made concerning all aspects of sex preselection research. Second, we must take a hard look at educational policies and demand that universities (especially our own state universities supported by our tax dollars) actively recruit women and give scholarships to poor women in the biological and health sciences. We must also scrutinize our elementary and secondary school policies regarding counseling of our daughters and the kinds of career choices laid out to them. Why is it, according to one study,[20] that among elementary school pupils little boys prefer boys and little girls prefer girls as their offspring when they grow up, but by junior high teen-age future mothers have a strong preference for boys?

Third, we must educate (in the best sense of the word) ourselves and our sisters in the wholeness and the politics of self-esteem. According to the data cited earlier in this paper, an alarming number of women prefer male children. Why *don't* all women want to reproduce themselves? Perhaps we should ask ourselves this question in our attitudinal research rather than those questions that solicit ideal size, composition of the family, and firstborn preference. Asking women "Do you hope that your first child is a boy or a girl?" is quite different from "Do you want to reproduce yourself?" At least by asking ourselves why we *would* or *would not* want to reproduce ourselves we might gain additional insights into our self-perception as women. Every new insight can in some way contribute to greater self esteem, and every woman who truly esteems herself will want to reproduce herself—eventually first among her children.

Unnatural Selection

On Choosing Children's Sex

Tabitha M. Powledge

It is important for most discussion purposes to underscore the distinction between techniques of sex choice that involve the abortion of a fetus already conceived, and preconception techniques such as the sperm separation and artificial insemination methods being done in Chicago now.[1] There is, obviously, an important moral difference between attempting to conceive a child of a particular sex and aborting such a child. There are also other differences, such as the increased risk to the mother in an abortion.

But although I believe that distinction is important for some purposes, it is irrelevant for the ultimate argument I wish to build around the general question of whether people should choose the sexes of their children. I will say at the outset that I oppose picking the sexes of children no matter what the means. I will also say that I am, and have been for the several years that I have been thinking about this problem, quite uncertain about how—or even whether—my opposition should be translated into public policy. I base my argument against the use of these techniques partly on the likely consequences, to many of which Dr. Steinbacher alluded, but I want to make an ultimate argument from principle that, for me, overrides any argument about consequences. I think it is possible there would be some "good" consequences of sex choice, but my argument from principle is intended to take precedence even over those.

The chief argument about consequences has always been the question of whether or not techniques of sex choice would alter the present sex ratio. (The sex ratio is the ratio of males to females, with the numbers of males always being stated first.) Before I discuss that ratio I would like to discuss the implications—or, actually, what I believe to be the *lack* of implications—of the sex preference studies that undergird all the arguments about whether or not there will be alteration of the sex ratio.

To my mind, these sex preference studies—which have been going on since the 1930s—are an excellent example of extensive social science research that gives us a thundering confirmation of something we all know anyway. No reader should be surprised by the news that people (even female people) prefer males to females.

Furthermore, these studies present many methodological problems. There is no time here to explore them in detail; let me briefly mention two. One is that even those studies that have been done on married women have almost never also surveyed their spouses. It will be a very rare woman who will take a decision like that upon her own shoulders; she is, at a minimum, likely to consult with the prospective father of the child, and in many cases his preference will be exceedingly important to her. For a lot of women it may even be decisive. The fact that this is really a joint decision has been ignored in most preference studies, and it is a major failing of them.

The second one has been pointed out by the economist Thomas Schelling:

> The sex of children is a question about which most people are unprepared, especially people who have not yet had their first child. Nobody would dream of making a decision within the short time the interviewer will wait for an answer; and no couple is going to attempt to reconcile any differences they have, or even delicately explore each other's preferences, for the sake of providing a hypothetical statistic in a survey.[2]

This leads me to one policy recommendation I can make wholeheartedly. I see no point in spending one single dime on any further preference studies. I think they are worthless. They are worthless because (a) they tell us that people prefer boys, which we already knew; (b) they cannot answer the question of whether the sex ratio will change, or how much; and (c) partly because of (b), they cannot help us assess the likely consequences of sex choice. Unfortunately, the implication of my conclusion is that we will have to develop the technology, turn it loose, and see what people actually do with it before we have any reasonable sense of what the outcomes might be.

Most things that have been written about sex choice assert that the sex ratio is roughly equal, but in fact that is not the case. Many more males than females are conceived; the latest conservative estimate is 120 : 100.[3] But an appreciable portion of those fail to make the nine-month journey to the delivery room. At birth in the US right now, we get between 107 and 104 males to every 100 females.[4] More boys than girls die in infancy and childhood from both disease and accidents, so by reproductive age the ratio is about equal. But males continue to die more frequently than females, and that trend accelerates throughout the remainder of life; there were only 72 men for every 100 women over 65 in 1970.[5] The greater survival of women is, by the way, a recent trend, essentially confined to the developed nations. I do not suppose we have any way of knowing what sequence is indeed the "natural" sex ratio. Certainly the extreme disparity in the ratio over 65 is not "natural," because what is "natural" is for us all to be dead long before that. One of the unpleasant consequences of improved sanitation, better nutrition, and the conquest of infectious disease (which have made such major contributions toward the lengthening of life) is to condemn many heterosexual older women to lonely lives. A remedy for that situation is one of the few "good" consequences that I have been able to adduce might result from a dramatic alteration in the at-birth sex ratio in favor of males. They would, of course, still die at a greater rate than females, but because there would be many more of them, more would survive to older ages.

Many things can and have altered the sex ratio at various ages in times past and will do so again. There are ethnic differences: blacks have a lower ratio at birth and lower overall population ratio than whites.[6] Cultural practices can, of course, work dramatic alterations, both against males (in the case of war) and against females (in the case of infanticide). Because it fluctuates so much, it is not clear to me that the sex ratio is sacrosanct. On the other hand, as long as we are ignorant about what the natural ratio is, and even more important, about what its function is (something, I might point out, that nobody really knows), I should think we would want to be very cautious about deliberately altering it. Until we know what it is for, we probably ought to leave it alone.

There has been much speculation about what might be the consequences of a massive alteration in the sex ratio in favor of males. Many of you may be familiar with Etzioni's well-known article of ten years ago speculating that such a move would result in the demise of both organized religion and the Republican party (women being the bedrock of both), an increase in crime, and a kind of pervasive, strident locker room atmosphere.[7] Postgate has speculated that women, being scarce, would be hidden away, consigned to a form of purdah.[8] I suppose it is wise always to take the pessimistic view for strategic reasons, but it is conceivable that it could also have the opposite effect, at least in some countries. It might be that if women were in short supply they would also be in great demand; they might be more courted, more coddled, more nicely treated, each of which has some pleasant aspects—although doubtless it would not be good for our characters. My point is that the speculations can be either apocalyptic or playful, but they are still just speculations.

The mention of Postgate brings me to my other "good" reason for proceeding with sex choice, or at least proceeding with development of what he calls The Manchild Pill, a cheap, simple, easy, pre-conception way of assuring that it will be a Y-bearing rather than an X-bearing sperm that fertilizes the egg. He thinks this would be a good idea because it would enormously increase the effectiveness of population limitation programs around the world. The argument goes this way: The Third World is in a terrible population bind partly because in poor countries, people have to rely on their children for support as they get older. They therefore seek to have enough sons to assure their futures; in those countries you cannot count on your live-born children reaching adulthood, so you have to over-produce to be on the safe side. People therefore go on having children until they get the number of sons they want. If that number could be assured at the outset, Postgate argues, final family size would be reduced. And since the number of females in the next generation would also be dramatically reduced, population would plummet further in a secondary effect, because the limiting factor on population growth is the number of available uteruses. Nobody knows, of course, whether or not that would be the result, but the argument is exceedingly plausible—and distressing for that reason.

With the exception of the population reduction argument, I think it is fair to say that virtually all the social consequences we have imagined might follow a major alteration in the sex ratio sound either unpleasant or uncertain. They seem not worth risking, particularly since (again with the exception of the population argument) virtually the only benefits from this technology will be the satisfaction of individual desires. (I am excluding here the use of occasional prenatal diagnosis for sex followed by abortion in the case of sex-linked disease, which I find marginally acceptable.) Although such satisfaction is an important value, it is not an absolute one. It must on occasion give way before other more urgent, more profound social needs. The possible social dislocations are serious enough that private desires here are simply not worth the risk.

On these consequentialist grounds alone, it is possible to build a strong, tight case against sex choice. But as I have already said, I do not want to rest my argument there. I want to argue that we should not choose the sexes of our children because to do so is one of the most stupendously sexist acts in which it is possible to engage. It is the original sexist sin. This argument applies to both pre- and post-conception technologies. To destroy an extant fetus for this reason is more morally opprobrious than techniques aimed at conceiving a child of a particular sex, but they are both deeply wrong. They are wrong because they make the most basic judgment about the worth of a human being rest first and foremost on its sex. I think prenatal assessment techniques—early or late—should not be used in this fashion. Furthermore, I think we should not put public money into the development of pre-conception sex choice technology, even a Manchild Pill, and I believe that such technology, if it does become available, should not be used.

I arrived at this position some years ago, and then I found myself—to mix an androgynous metaphor—on the horns of a feminist dilemma. I wish to share that dilemma with you, and indeed ask your help with it. Although I believe these technologies should not be available (or, if available, should not be used), my dilemma is that the price of preventing them from being available and being used is higher than I want to pay. Let us ignore for a moment the question about whether or not regulation of these technologies is a practical possibility. That does not mean I do not think it is a serious question. But even assuming we could find a way around the practical difficulties, it seems to me there are very great dangers in doing so. To forbid women to use prenatal diagnostic techniques as a way of picking the sexes of their babies is to begin to delineate acceptable and unacceptable reasons to have an abortion. Though I think there are good reasons and bad reasons to have abortions, I do not think I, or the State, ought to be in the business of deciding for other people what they are. To make it illegal to use prenatal diagnostic techniques for sex choice is to nibble away at our hard-won reproductive control, control that I think most of us believe is the absolute rock-bottom minimum goal we have got to keep achieved before we can achieve anything else. I do not think I need to belabor that point for this audience, though I am often amazed at how many people—including some women—do not quite understand how fundamental that issue is. This reproductive freedom I am talking about, of course, extends beyond abortion. I do not mean only that women must have the right to choose when and if to abort. They must also have the right to choose when and whether to become pregnant in the first place, and that is why my argument against legal restriction of these technologies applies as much to pre-conception as it does to post-conception ones. I hate these technologies, but I do not want to see them legally regulated because, quite simply, I do not want to provide an opening wedge for legal regulation of reproduction in general. There is a certain amount of irony—not to say annoyance and frustration—in the fact that I have arrived at these mutually exclusive positions through a commitment to feminist goals, but there it is.

It is important to point out that this technology is already being regulated, though not by law. It is being informally regulated by the medical profession. Prenatal diagnostic techniques are today being performed largely in major medical centers. Many physicians and other medical people involved in this technology will not use it for sex choice, although others have begun to do so, particularly if the woman presents with a reason that they find particularly compelling. One hears anecdotes, for instance, of pregnant women who come to the prenatal diagnostician saying they already have three daughters and they are going to abort unless the doctor can tell them it is a boy this time. In this case the doctor feels he may be saving a life if he performs the prenatal diagnosis, and some have succumbed to that argument.

But this technology is beginning to move out of the major medical center and into the private obstetrician's office. More and more doctors in private practice are learning how to do amniocentesis and then send the fluid out to commercial laboratories for culturing. Even though women may occasionally find doctors refusing to perform these tests for sex alone, today a determined woman will not have too much trouble eventually locating someone who can help her. And tomorrow it will be easy. Furthermore, if we develop diagnostic techniques that are adequate in the first trimester,[9] or that, like fetal cell sorting,[10] do not directly invade the uterus, we may see a quantum leap in the uses of these techniques for sex choice. This lends a certain urgency to this discussion. And even though at the moment we do not have any good pre-conception techniques, when and if they arrive... well, quite frankly, I think the floodgates will be open.

So here we are, with a perniciously sexist technology the regulation of which appears to me to also be perniciously sexist. What, then, should we do? We may want to turn to such time-honored measures as boycotts, and putting pressure on funders not to underwrite such research. We may also want to give some attention to a mechanism that appears weak, but may be undervalued: moral exhortation. We must say over and over again to friends and neighbors, in the pages of magazines and newspapers, on television and radio, that this technology, even if available, should simply not be used. We sometimes underestimate the power of such exhortations to influence behavior, particularly in a matter like reproductive behavior. I strongly suspect that most people have just simply never given serious thought to the implications of choosing the sexes of their children. I believe (or perhaps it is just that I hope) that there are many couples who, once they understood what was really at stake here, would simply decide against the use of this technology. I do not think, of course, that it would work on everybody, but perhaps it would at least improve the situation.

On other occasions where I have made my arguments against sex choice technologies, people have asked whether I would make the same argument if the technologies were likely to be used more against males than against females. In reply, I point out that my argument rests quite explicitly on the assumption that men and women should not be differentially regarded on the basis of their gender, and therefore, I would *of course* object to the use of this technology selectively against males. Women have (regrettably, in my view) tended to build arguments against this technique on the knowledge that it will be used mostly against *us.* But it is just as wrong and just as immoral to abort a fetus because it is male as to abort one because it is female. I have heard women who call themselves feminists say they would welcome this technology because it would give them a chance to bear only daughters and to raise them "right." A woman who believes that is, in my view, incapable of raising a child "right," if by "right" she means anti-men. That is why I am dismayed by the talk here about "reproducing ourselves." The work of the past ten years, and the work of our grandmothers and great-grandmothers, will have gone for nothing if all we want to do is take revenge and reverse the oppression. Foolish and unfashionable as it may seem, I am working for a nonsexist world. I have no interest in doing battle with the bad guys if the victory means that I will simply reverse the process, adopt their discriminatory values, and in so doing become a bad guy myself.

Response

Martha Mathis

Fewer first-born females, higher sex ratios at birth, more poor women in developed countries, and elimination of women in the Third World are, indeed, devastating outcomes for women. If you are feminist women of the majority, the concerns about sex preselection must be frightening—and frankly, politically, your loud voices are being heard in whispers.

For those of us of the minority, I question whether the idea of sex preselection is relevant at all—*now*. Not that the issue is not relevant in terms of all women becoming concerned and educated about the future of this topic, and other health topics, but is it relevant, and realistic for minority, Third World, and all women of color? Is this an issue for poor welfare recipients? Is this an issue for lower-middle-class blue collar workers, who have survival issues to deal with daily—whether they have male children first or female children first?

As a minority educator and community-oriented professional, I am very concerned that there are two distinct groups who are involved with this issue. The first group—the socioeconomic group that I am assuming will be seeking facilities that will encourage preselection—are clearly women of groups that have political, religious, and economic reasons for their choice. The second group—the socioeconomic group of women that I am assuming will *not* be concerned with this as a *top* priority—are those women that see no economic, political, or religious gains from having either sex.

Should we not be examining our motives for having children in the first place, and not necessarily what gender we will be having? As a minority woman, I am more concerned that thinking about the issues of contraception information and options, birth process, and childbirth be encouraged. The issue, as I see it, is how many children to have, when and how to have these children, how to provide care for the numbers of children that one already has, what and where are the health-care facilities—not which gender will I keep, or which gender will I abort.

The issues facing women of color are broader and need more attention, such as: How do I stop having children?

Another broad issue is: What are my health-care responsibilities? We here know the questions to ask our physicians. We know when to tell them that we want this particular medicine, or we do not. Please keep in mind that there are still many women, many, many women in different socioeconomic groups that are still looking at physicians as god-like and as total healers. I think that crosses status and race borders.

A third question is: How can I become involved in some of the grass-roots concerns of women and their health care responsibilities? I think we really need to start considering what we can offer people in the community, to help them take charge of their own health care. I urge those of us do who have more good and valid choices to become more concerned about those women who are being abused, owing to poor or nonvalid choices in health care, *and* sex preselection, if you will.

A fourth question is: Can I enjoy, and be encouraged to select no children? In a society that is still motherhood-oriented? There is a high expectation for the women of many socioeconomic groups and of many cultures to continue to reproduce. Question number four is something that we should keep in mind while we are wondering about sex preselection. There are some of us who have opted to have no children in a culture that makes such a lifestyle quite difficult.

I also have to include, in question four: Is this an issue for women of all races and status who cannot or should not have children at all? Can those of us who have fertility problems, for example, really understand the needs of sex preselection research and study and funding?

Although I find the topic of sex preselection a valid radical feminist concern (and I like to think that I am one), I am also concerned about another list of questions that we need to ask ourselves because we are feminists, and because we are truly concerned about different levels of health care.

For example, who are the women using the least effective birth-control, if any? Another question to ask yourself: Who are the women being abused by Depo-Provera and sterilization? Who are the women who mastered midwifery hundreds of years ago, and then not until the 1960s or so were allowed to have their children, by choice, in a hospital, unless it was a segregated type of situation? Who are the nonwhite or the "unknown" women in the studies and the research that we heard about DES? Who are the women who benefit from conferences, from conferences of this type, first? Who are the women who assume political power, over other women? I think so many times we lose sight, when we gather like this as women, and think that it is only men who control the political and the financial power: Where I'm from, that's not necessarily always so.

Who are the women who despair over money, proper medical referrals, proper physicians, care, etc.—when confronted with prenatal and neonatal problems? What group of women would you identify with that?

And, lastly, to tie this into the subject matter: Who are the women for whom the question of sex preselection is being researched, funded, and realistically answered?

Response

Denise Connors

I think we have realized how important it is to see all of the issues that we have been discussing in context. And when we look at the issue of sex preselection, we certainly cannot avoid this contextual approach. Historically, it has been demonstrated that, when the so-called "first wave of feminism" crested in this country, the profession of gynecology simultaneously was receiving recognition. The "second wave of feminism" has also been met with an escalation of gynecological intervention, such as unnecessary surgery, DES, and Depo-Provera, to list only a few examples that have been addressed here. From this perspective, it makes sense that sex preselection be the next approach in the effort to be counterrevolutionary to women's interests. Perhaps making women a scarce commodity will be a more efficacious way to maintain and/or purify patriarchy.

As men begin to recognize that women are waking up and becoming aware of our own power—in terms of the birthing process and in terms of our Selves—they are seeking to increase the technological control of who will, in fact, exist.

Susan Cavin, a lesbian feminist sociologist from Rutgers, has studied sex ratio distribution. From her extensive research, she found that when there are near-equal and high male sex ratios (which are results of patriarchal manipulation) these have proven to be the source of a dangerously high rate of rape, child molestation, and violence against women and children.[1] This information lends itself to further speculation about the possibility of maleness as a mutation.

There have been some prophetic statements made about the kind of technology prevailing today, and I'd like to share them with you. In 1899, Sir Theodore Fox stated: "We shall have to learn to refrain from doing things merely because we know how to do them." From Valery: "One can say that all we know—that is, all we have the power to do—has finally turned against what we are." From Mary Daly: "When technical knowledge is separated from ontological reason, the science which it dominates becomes dogmatic, manipulative and destructive."[2]

We have seen that many of the technologies discussed here have to do with a philosophy or rationale that what we *can* do implies what we *ought* to do. This way of thinking cancels out the possibility of women's autonomous choice. Choice is intrinsically connected with the *power* to choose, and this power is systematically undermined by patriarchal values. The fact that women "choose" male children in a culture where women are programmed not to value themselves can hardly be termed choice.

Misleading scientific and professional legitimations have made it possible to "answer" questions about the potentially destructive effects of medical and technological intervention by saying, "There is *probably* not much danger, and we *hope* that there really isn't anything to worry about." This "scientific" mentality is based on an endless chain of inconclusive studies that serve to validate the continual ruthless experimentation on women and animals. This system assures itself that all the information will never be in, and, therefore, nothing will be proved to those who do not want to know.

This lack of definitive information also enables men to erase their responsibility. It is interesting that although women rarely have anything to do with the invention of these technologies, we are encouraged to deliberate and share the burden of figuring out what to do about them once they have been initiated.

Women must be made aware of the trap of reinforcing the phenomenon of expectancy verification that was mentioned earlier here. Teach us to think of ourselves as "high risk," and we function to make that a reality. Teach us to fear that our bodies are potentially lethal, and that fear, alone, will function as an AMA-approved justification for mastectomy and hysterectomy.

The language of medical technology deserves a much more extensive analysis. I think all of us have realized the limitations of language as we have listened to one another share common concerns. Gena Corea noted the war terminology that is used in much professional jargon, for example, "target population." Another example frequently observed on medical charts is the habit of referring to operations as "surgical attacks." "Invasive" procedures are distinguished from "non-invasive" procedures, when in reality the distinction is between visible and invisible invasion.

Susan Peterson spoke of the tone, the body language, and the emphasis on disease that prevails in the medical profession. Selective perception results in blaming women for everything. A classic example is the notion that when a woman is over 34 years old, her offspring will have a higher incidence of congenital defects. What is erased from this is the fact that women often marry men who are older than they are.

What about the older men's sperm having something to do with the congenital defects?

Julia Stanley, a feminist linguist, has described one malfunction of language that she calls "agent deletion."[3] All of us can think of examples of this in the other papers in this book. We hear about things being "acceptable," but we don't hear *acceptable to whom.* We hear about technology, but the underlying question of *whose* technology is not answered. It has been "proven." It is "known." Then there is the familiar phase "cost-benefit analysis." Deleted from this phrase are the questions: Whose cost? Whose benefit? Whose analysis?

In the course of this conference we have begun to trace the threads of connectedness among the atrocities committed against us (a process of analysis well developed in Mary Daly's book, *Gyn/Ecology*). As we have discovered these threads, we have experienced the power of what Adrienne Rich has called "thinking through our bodies." This process brings us back to our senses, enabling us to recognize that everything *is* connected to everything else. It is a woman-identified, woman-affirming, biophilic process.

Sex Preselection: A Response

Janice G. Raymond

In responding to the papers, I want both to address the issues raised by the speakers and to push some of their ideas in different directions.

First, what we are witnessing with the advent of sex selection technologies is not an isolated phenomenon. Sex selection takes place everyday in this society without a specific biomedical technology. These procedures merely carry out, on a technological level, what happens on other levels. Preference for males is evident in much more than just the studies that bear out that *even* women would choose male children, given the technology.

This brings me to my second point. Tabitha Powledge and Roberta Steinbacher make clear that it should come as no surprise that the studies reveal that both women and men would select for male children. But the studies do not tell everything. And one thing they do not explain is the social context in which women *learn* to prefer men in lots of different ways, even though many times their primary emotional and life-giving relationships may be with women.

I am going to put forth an assertion here, and it is this: given a different social context in which women were empowered with a sense of strong selfhood and where the primary bonds were with women, most women who wished to have children would prefer daughters. In fact, I think most women already do. But I also think that that preference has been smothered and buried in many ways.

What gives impetus to this assertion about daughter-preference is that in the same way that women have been forced into denying their primary relationships with women as friends, as life-mates and companions, and as lovers—in the same way that these relationships have been castrated, extinguished, silenced, and put out of sight—women have denied their preference for daughters, even going to the extent of *saying,* and perhaps *believing* themselves, that they would prefer a male child. The statement that most women prefer male children has the same obscuring function as the statement that most women are heterosexual—i.e., it functions as inevitable, and it requires no explanation. As Adrienne Rich has written: "To acknowledge that for women heterosexuality may not be a 'preference' at all but something that has had to be imposed, managed, organized, propagandized, and maintained by force, is an immense step to take if you consider yourself freely and 'innately' heterosexual." Yet, as Rich further commented, "refusing to examine heterosexuality as an institution is like refusing to admit that the economic system called capitalism is maintained by a variety of forces, including physical violence and false consciousness."[1]

Powledge concludes that women who want to bear only daughters would simply be turning the tables. There are so many issues to address here. I get frustrated with "reverse discrimination" and "turning the tables" arguments, because they always abstract from a social context of who is really doing what to whom. They are also, in my opinion, utterly ahistorical. It is not women, or a female-dominated system, who have invented sex selection technology, and it is not women/wives who are placing pressure on men/husbands to prefer daughters.

The "turning the tables" argument does two things in this context. It shifts the focus off the fact that anti-feminism and woman-hating is all around us, and that the real threat is male preference for boys. But it also implies that any woman-directed and woman-controlled action, from lesbianism to daughter-preference, has to be labeled as anti-male, rather than as pro-woman. This point needs a more subtle clarification.

Woman-identified women are *anti-male* in a sense that goes far beyond the meaning of that label as it is used by those who attack women who are clearly and outspokenly feminist. We truly abhor what men individually, collectively, and institutionally have done to women. However, this anti-maleness cannot simply be equated to men's anti-femaleness. Men have hated women so as to deprive women of life, health, creativity, and well-being. As Pat Hynes has phrased it, men have hated the very facticity of female existence.[2] The anti-maleness of feminists has not spawned any institutions comparable to footbinding, witchburning, or sadistic gynecology, to name but three atrocities. To attack a woman-centered vision of the world, which would foster the existence of lesbianism and daughter-preference, as "turning the tables" or as "anti-male," is muddle-headed and/or deceptive. As Mary Daly has written: "The courage to be logical—the courage to name—would require that we admit to ourselves that males and males only are the originators, planners, controllers, and legitimators of patriarchy."[3] Therefore, women who affirm that they are anti-male are really affirming that they are not afraid both to see clearly and to name specifically the true agents of an anti-female, gynocidal, and woman-hating society.

My third concern is to expand a bit about the Postgate material, which suggests the use of a man-child pill to solve the world population problem. It is important to understand that Postgate is talking about using this in what he calls "under-developed, unenlightened communities," i.e., among African, Asian, Central and South American peoples where, again in his words, the prejudice to breed male "amounts to an obsession." In brief, Postgate is talking about the obliteration of third world women, for "humane" reasons, of course.

Postgate's article appeared in *The New Scientist* about six years ago. It included suggestions for what would happen to those few women who would be left.

> All sorts of taboos would be expected and it is probable that a form of *purdah* would become necessary. Women's right to work, even to travel alone freely, would probably be forgotten transiently. Polyandry might well become accepted in some societies; some might treat their women as queen ants, others as rewards for the most outstanding (or most determined) males.[4]

Clare Booth Luce has been the most recent popularizer of a man-child pill. In her words "a pill, unguent, or injection which, taken prior to coitus, would assure that the birth of a son would come as *man-ah!* from Heaven." To quote her further: "What theological objections could the Pope himself raise to a birth-control method that simply permitted parents to choose a son in preference to a daughter? After all, God did."[5]

Thus we have futuristic fetishism of the first order, under the guise of concern for the ecology of the planet. The rhetoric of global concern disguises the smallness of the solution. The solution of a man-child pill is so ultimately non-ecological that it is devoid of any personal and social meaning for over half the population of the planet.

It is only within the last century that anti-feminism has taken on a biomedical imperative and has been given a scientific-therapeutic rationale. Women have always been expendable—witness the history of footbinding, clitoridectomy, witchburning, rape, and woman-battering. Yet something quite different happened with the rise of gynecology and obstetrics in the nineteenth century, and, most currently, with the rise of the biomedical sciences for the engineering of human reproduction in this twentieth century. The classic perception of woman as *Matter* becomes even more reified and objectified, because women are now biomedically manipulable. Postgate's solution of a "male-child" pill signals a view of women where we are not only medically manipulable, but where we are *Matter to be totally dispensed with,* devoid of spirit, and totally viewed in the perspective of ability to produce more *Matter.*

Ivan Illich in *Medical Nemesis* has spoken most directly about the *medicalization of life*—the notion that more and more areas of living have been colonized by medical intervention and investigation and staked out as medical territory.[6] As Mary Daly has pointed out in her most recent book on *Gyn/Ecology: The Metaethics of Radical Feminism,* nowhere do we witness this medicalization more than in the establishment of the specialties of gynecology and obstetrics in the nineteenth century. Although certain aspects of men's lives were medicalized with the emergence of modern medicine and its specializations, women's lives were *totally* medicalized. As Barker-Benfield notes, this total medicalization of female existence is attested to by the lack of a corresponding field of medical *andrology* for men.[7] The female body was analyzed, quantified, qualified, and integrated into the sphere of medical practice by reason of a perceived pathology intrinsic to it—i.e., its ability to reproduce.

The engineering of human reproduction made possible by technologies of sex selection, test-tube fertilization, and the like can only add to the persistent medicalization of women's bodies, and thus to the biomedical management of women's lives, even to the point of encouraging women *not* to reproduce themselves.

Whether it be sex selection, test-tube fertilization, or other modes of biomedical engineering, woman is still the experimental object. What is ultimately involved in the engineering of human reproduction, and the sciences and technologies that it develops, is the reproduction or the elimination of women according to biomedical standards.

Sex Preselection

Discussion Moderator's Remarks

Emily Erwin Culpepper

I want to make it clear that I attend this conference as a Lesbian and that I speak from a Radical Feminist perspective. This includes, first of all, the feminist insight that "the personal is political." In bringing up "the personal is political," I want to clarify that this is not simply anecdotal; nor is it about making absolute-truth claims on the basis of our personal history. Rather, it means we recognize and value our experience as *one primary* source of information that we bring to all questions that affect women.

Here, since this is a workshop on sex preselection, I therefore want to offer you some facts of my history and hence a part of the perspective I bring to these issues. I was a planned child and a first-born daughter. As a firstborn daughter I bring a special interest to looking at the literature about sex preferences in this country and in many countries where the norm for families in the minds of many people is a firstborn son. There have been many interesting sociological studies claiming all kinds of things about firstborn daughters; for example, that we are more likely to be prostitutes and strippers! I first ran across this when I entered college and thought, "Well that's not where I think I'm headed."

Another bit of personal history I want to share with you is that before I entered Harvard Divinity School, where I am now a doctoral student, I was a Massachusetts State Adoption Social Worker. I did home studies on people wanting to adopt children. There I ran into very explicit statements of sex preference from people who had the opportunity through adopting to consider whether they wanted to make a sex preference statement or not. I am sure you can imagine a lot of what I ran into. A male first preference was highest for middle class protestants. Also, I did find some revealing exceptions to this—older, catholic [lower case intended] couples, and white people adopting mixed racial children were the main groups with girl preference.

From the traditional point of view, a feminist perspective is really an interdisciplinary or transdisciplinary approach. What this means for me as a feminist is not a fragmented, but a wholistic approach from an acknowledged point of view, seeing threads of connectedness between things that often are regarded separately. Dr. Janice Raymond referred to the phrase "metaethical," meaning that we are not accepting traditional definitions even of what ethics is. To that end, I would like to recommend to you a recent book by Dr. Mary Daly entitled, *Gyn/Ecology*. This is written with a slash: gyn/ecology, because she is not talking about just one discipline, gynecology, but about the ecology of femaleness. The subtitle of that book is "the Metaethics of Radical Feminism," and there is a chapter in it particularly relevant to this conference as it looks at the medical profession.

A final point is that there already has been and *is* a sex selection system operating in many direct and subtle ways—through infanticide, different nurturing of children, different roles offered to children. This already existing system is enforced with rewards and punishments. Here we focus on the attempts to expand and enforce this condition technologically. I also hold up to you an interest in some other kinds of "technology." In particular, Lesbians and other women are interested in the possibilities of parthenogenesis and in the fact that women might be able to affect our fertility and perhaps sex selection psychically or through other internal mechanisms. I definitely do not see this topic as just limited to the technical means now in traditional medicine.

Sex Preselection Discussion

Moderated by Emily Erwin Culpepper

Sandra Serrano Sewell: This whole topic is one that I find very moving. I wanted to say something about Tabitha Powledge's paper. I didn't connect with a lot of what you were saying—probably about 99% of what you were saying. One thing that you said really disturbed me, as a parent. In replying to Roberta Steinbacher's paper, you stated that if one wanted to reproduce one's self, then you're not a fit parent. I feel that's an unfair statement. You don't know any of the folks in this room. You don't know me. I very much wanted a girl child first. But that didn't make my ability to be a parent any more or less fit.

Tabitha Powledge: Would you have used the technology to achieve the girl child first?

Sandra Serrano Sewell: You know, I never even thought about that. I don't know now.

Tabitha Powledge: It may be the phrasing I objected to. Children are individual persons, and I am distressed by the notion of anybody using the phrase, "I want to reproduce myself."

Laura Punnett: But in your objection, you seriously misinterpret Roberta Steinbacher's point. She made a powerful statement about the problem of societies in which women learn not to value other women and therefore don't want to reproduce women. When we look at other women, we also see ourselves reflected in them; if we truly value ourselves, then we will value other women as well. The desire to reproduce ourselves, to give birth to other strong and independent women, is a healthy way of affirming our self-worth as women rather than denying women's worth, as most of us have learned to do.

Tabitha Powledge: But, if we think about reproducing ourselves on the basis of gender, we are morally no better than men who are hipped on the subject of sons. I want more progress than that. I want children to be valued for their individual selves, not as extensions of their parents.

Barbara Andolsen: Tammy, I heard you saying something different when you said "reproduce youself" than I heard the people over here say. I heard them say that women should value women and therefore feel very comfortable about having a daughter.

Tabitha Powledge: I assume everybody realizes that I agree.

Barbara Andolsen: Now—I heard you saying that when parents feel that they can tailor-make a child prenatally to fit some predetermined image—the "acceptable" child—there's a tremendous burden on the child to live up to all these parental expectations. I would like to have a daughter. I know that one reason that I want to do this is because I have a mental image, not just of *a* daughter, but of a precise kind of daughter, and that could be very damaging to the female person born to me. What we have been discussing links up with the problem we talked about yesterday—coping with children born with handicaps. It also connects with contraception. I am concerned that the more we control our reproduction through contraceptive technologies, the higher expectations we will have of our children. If I have only two kids, they've got to be the brightest young feminists that anybody ever had. If one of them has a mental or physical handicap, then perhaps I won't cope as well as my mother, who had ten children (one of whom had a severe handicap). There's no way, when you have ten children, that all of them are going to turn out according to your model. So you've got to learn to accept differences. But if you have one or two kids, you may be determined to turn them into what you want. The issue of shaping our children to meet our desires runs through contraception, through dealing with defects, through sex preselection.

Laura Punnett: I want to clarify the implications of Roberta's statement. The concept of women identifying positively with women as a group, and caring about our collective survival in the present and future, is potentially revolutionary. It is also one of the special contributions of feminists to the discussion of the uses of reproductive technologies.

Barbara Menning: I want to speak to another way children come into our families—and that's by adoption. I have three adopted children, and it might interest people to know that when couples are given a choice of sex, they choose girls over boys, two to one. In fact, it is very hard to place little boys—especially little boys from some cultures—in homes. One argument that's been made about adoption, and I don't think there's been enough research in this area, is that perhaps there's a certain devaluing of the adopted child and, the rules of primogeniture and heredity following in the male line, we prefer to bring female children into our homes. I do not think that explains why we really do, two to one, select little girls over little boys. In my own experience with adoption, I made no sex selection of the first two children because I wanted it to be at random, just as if it were a child born to me. I got two little boys, and on the third time round, I insisted on a little girl.

Emily Culpepper: I did home studies on people who wanted to adopt children, and I feel that those statistics really have to be broken down. I found very great differences in terms of who was comfortable expressing what they really felt to the social worker, for one thing. By class, race, and other factors I also found sex preferences different. It stood out to me greatly that white, upwardly mobile, protestant adopting families did request, first, boys.

Yvonne Brackbill: Emily, are there more girls available for adoption?

Emily Culpepper: Not so much, although the whole adoption picture is changing drastically with the essential non-availability of children of any race under about two-and-a-half, and white children under about six.

Yvonne Brackbill: Saying you can't determine people's sex preferences for children is a good example of why it's always dangerous to say something *can't* be done. As soon as you say it, somebody comes along and finds a way of doing it. It certainly is possible at the present time to find out how many couples in the United States would like to have boys only, or first-born boys, and so on. Polls use very sophisticated research techniques to yield accurate estimates within a fraction of one percentage point of error on either side.

Tabitha Powledge: Irrespective of the methodological questions (and I think there are still arguments to be made about that), it's not clear to me that even if we have a perfect handle on everybody's preferences, that would give us any handle on what the social outcomes or dislocations from those preferences would be. We don't know whether people would in fact act on those preferences.

Norma Swenson: I am aware, now, on a more than intellectual level, of women in other parts of the world. Their status and survival as women is frequently attached to their production of a male child. I think even in our culture women can get more attention, more respect, more money—perhaps—if they produce male children. So even though preference for males may not be conscious, I think there are a lot of practical reasons why—depending on which ethnic group is involved—people exhibit some of those preferences. It makes a very real difference to a woman's life, to the extent that she's dependent on the males around her—her father, her husband, and her son.

There's something else I want to say that goes along with what Barbara Andolsen said. We didn't get a chance to do much analysis on some of the things that are happening in childbirth and obstetrics, but one thing that is really clear about the physicians' dilemma—apart from how they're behaving—is that parents are saying, "I'm only going to have one child. I have to justify being pregnant, and I have to justify having more than one child at all." That's one of the reasons for the scale, intensity, and aggressiveness of the interventions that are going on right now in obstetrics. Not only has that baby got to survive, but that baby has got to be perfect. Sex preselection is part of this same mentality.

Mary Jane Gray: One of the things that I want you to think about is what the effects may be of knowing—from sixteen weeks on—the sex of the child you're carrying and the effects on the role development of that child afterwards. Are we going to reinforce stereotyped roles by having women know the sex of the child they're carrying?

From this, I'd like to get some of the panel's reaction to a dilemma that obstetricians find themselves in right now. When we're doing amniocenteses for genetic reasons, one of the side effects is that the geneticist almost always reports back, along with the other information requested, the sex of the fetus. Should this information be passed on at that time to the woman, and what effect is passing that on going to have?

Tabitha Powledge: One anecdotal example—a thirty-seven-year-old woman learned through amniocentesis that she was pregnant with her fourth daughter. She wept at the news that it was female, but she proceeded with the pregnancy, because it would never have occurred to her to do otherwise. She ended up feeling that knowing the sex had been a very positive experience. Aside from the fact that it solved practical problems, such as picking a name far in advance, it made her feel much closer to that kid. This baby, in contrast to her other three, was a person to her long before birth.

I gather that it's standard practice, when amniocentesis is done, to be asked whether you wish to know the sex of the fetus. It's your choice. I guess I view that as morally appropriate, because I want to push for an acknowledgment that people own their own medical information. I don't want doctors keeping things secret from us. They've done that far too long. I also believe that a doctor's legal obligation is to provide you with that information. They cannot, as I understand it, legally withhold it.

Denise Connors: I think it's interesting that the question is even posed that it's the doctor who would have the information about what the sex of the child is. It assumes that a woman, being in touch with herself, would not know that on her own. Again, the whole idea that medicine is going to reveal these things to us is something else that should be looked into.

Tabitha Powledge: Are you saying that women know what sex fetus they're pregnant with?

Denise Connors: I'm saying that I think that's something that should be considered as a possibility.

Tabitha Powledge: In 50% of the cases, that's probably correct.

Emily Culpepper: I don't think Denise is saying that's necessarily the case right now, but that might be a potential we have within us. I think that's an important open question.

Renée Jenkins: I want to pick up on something Norma said about the studies on sex preference, and what Emily said about some of the factors for adoption. I don't know what your figures bear out, but as a member of black culture, I think that females, for a long time, have been the preferred sex—because of the known risk in producing a male and the adverse kinds of things he would have to face in society. In fact, females much more easily graduated up the scale and had many more educational opportunities. So there appears to be a very strong feeling in the black community that females are a preferred sex. I would like to hear more from people who know more about matriarchal structure, because I'd like to hear what we're expecting that will be so much better from a matriarchal situation. As you know, even in the subset of black culture that's historically matriarchal, there's a high crime level, high violence level, and I think we've got to get more at what the factors are that contribute to these outcomes, that are not sex-related.

Byllye Avery: I want to echo that point, because that was one point I really wanted to bring up. When I was growing up, girls were always the preferred sex, and we felt that we could go out and do whatever. Girls were mobile in black culture because we could get jobs easier than black men, and since women were more responsible for children, emphasis was placed on the education of girls.

I want to focus on something else. There are questions women ask in pregnancy. "What will the sex of my child be?" and "Will my child be all right?" The questions may not arise in that order. I find that among midwives the answers to "What will my child be?" vary from "The heartbeat seems strong, it might be a girl"—on one prenatal visit—to "It sounds like a boy"—on the next prenatal visit—to "It might be either one" on another. The answers to the other question are usually, "Well, everything seems all right. We did the measurements. How are you feeling?"

At Birthplace, we don't tell women they're going to have boys, or they're going to have girls. I mean, every question we ask ourselves as we live in this culture is not something that can be answered, and they're not things that deserve to be answered. Like, people who came to this conference knowing what the answers ought to be. So therefore, when it's not moving in the direction you think it ought to move, you think it ain't goin' right!

Joyce Berkman: I think the term "black matriarchy" is most unfortunate. It was proselytized under the Moynihan report, with damaging results on black families in this country. I urge any of you to accept that description of the black family with great caution.

Also, from my reading of what's been happening in the past several years in the mid-East and near-East, I gather that societies such as Kuwait have a higher percentage of women lawyers, women engineers, and women doctors than the United States. The Third World is highly heterogeneous. Although there are areas that would be very sympathetic to "annihilating" women, there are many areas that prize women far more than we do in our country. I've been very uneasy about references to the Third World or "underdeveloped" world as a sort of passive homogeneous vessel for experimental products.

Betty Hoskins: What would a world and social context with women-generated values be like? I'll start by asking Jan: if somehow we evolved, or leapt to, a social context in which we had pride and self-esteem, in which we had males and females who were androgynous or—much better—gynandrous, or even better, who live with an ethic of integrity, why would we then want to choose one or another sex as better? You said we would then prefer daughters, and I keep visualizing (as I try to grope toward an answer) that one thing we would stop would be that patriarchal, hierarchal "I'm better than, because I'm this kind or that kind." Why would we not simply value whatever people happened?

Janice Raymond: Well, of course, ultimately in a gender-free society that would be the case, Betty. But I'm talking about the blueprint for getting there, before the goals you're projecting are ultimately achievable.

Betty Hoskins: That seems to me to continue to participate in a male model of rank ordering, better-worse dichotomies, which automatically makes judgments and choices.

Janice Raymond: I don't think it's a rank and order model. I think it's a priority model. I think priorities are important, and I think priorities are necessary. We're used to perceiving priorities in terms of a rank and order model, but I don't think we have to see them that way.

Betty Hoskins: I'm saying that in a technologically conditioned society, we often leap to making priorities when we have no need to. We could say both choices (female and male) are important, and we refuse to choose between them. Can we push toward that?

Janice Raymond: I guess I'm not that much of a liberal, Betty.

Diana Axelsen: I'd like to go back to the term "reverse discrimination" used in response to the notion that a lot of men have preferred men children, so why don't we women prefer women? Could you explain what you were attacking when you said you didn't like reverse discrimination?

Janice Raymond: I was trying to point out the insidiousness of the "reverse discrimination" argument. The terminology of "reverse discrimination" once more puts the blame and the burden of oppression back on the oppressed. It distracts and abstracts from the real context of who is doing the "discriminating" and who is being "discriminated" against. A better wording, if we want to play the jargon game, might be to call any meager benefits that do accrue to women (such as two faculty positions out of forty in a department!) "compensatory justice." However, I don't like that term either. But at least it signifies that those gains, few as they may be, are rightly our due. I think much of our reality is determined by the language we use. Those who use the term "reverse discrimination" focus on quite a different thing from those who use the word "justice."

Diane Axelsen: My basic question is whether, given a social context that encourages men and women to prefer male children, what should women's response be? Is the right answer really women wanting daughters, rather than both parents deciding that they will educate their girl and boy children to have a feminist, humane outlook? I have some faith in our ability to counteract sexist influences in raising children of both sexes. Is it clear that persons who prefer daughters will really be better parents? Some people may choose girls in order to raise "little ladies," not feminists!

Janice Raymond: Because of some of your statements and those of others, I want to make it very clear that I am not advocating sex preselection technology to breed females. But if the technology is turned loose, I would turn it loose among women who would opt for daughters—as a pilot program, of course. Otherwise, I would propose taking all of the money that would be spent on sex selection technology and giving it to self-help centers, birthing centers, and alternative forms of healing research.

Judy Norsigian: Unfortunately, it's very clear from this panel that the technology's here and it's being used and abused. I'm surprised to find myself reacting more strongly to this presentation than to any of the others, and feeling threatened in a way that I haven't been by anything else. If we focus public debate on this topic, it might give lots of people ideas about choosing male children over female children, especially at a time when the devaluation of women is already so pervasive. Some issues being raised here—like reverse discrimination and male influence on women's choices—seem to me possibly counterproductive "distractions."

Caroline Whitbeck: I want to respond to what was said on the issue of a women-centered society. I don't think we've really seen women-centered values even where we see women in a strong position in a subculture. If we had a society that placed central value on nurturance, and what I call "calling forth," we wouldn't find violence. We have to recognize that violence as a result of oppression. One thing that I would suggest is that there's a significant violence done to the psyches of male children, in that the project of nurturing and "calling forth" is one that they don't identify with, since they usually receive this care only from women, with whom they are not encouraged to identify. How are we going to bring forth a generation that really cares about nurturance and "calling forth"? I would start by making sure that every infant got a fair amount of that care from someone of the same gender. Why gender? Because in our society at least, infants learn gender so early. The evidence is that a child's gender identity is set by seventeen months. If a child's gender is misidentified at birth, it turns out to be disastrous to reassign the child's gender after seventeen months. Children learn gender—not necessarily genital differences, but gender—very early. I think that if each child is going to learn to identify as a person who nurtures and calls forth others, if each child is going to learn to form relationships of *mutual* caring, rather than learning ways to dominate and control someone who will nurture them, they need to be "called forth" by someone whom they, and the society, perceive as being like themselves in a very fundamental way. The problem is: Where are you going to get many men who can nurture and call forth male infants?

Janice Raymond: The question I have to Caroline's question is: Are women, then, going to be not only mothering children, but mothering men to mother children?

Caroline Whitbeck: No, I am not suggesting that. I am suggesting that as long as the society puts a primary emphasis on competition and domination, we women have to take special steps to see that our nurturing and "calling forth" are not used to serve the interests of domination. We women must think about finding ways to refuse to cooperate with domination just as pacifists see to it that they don't cooperate with the institution of war, and abolitionists refused to cooperate with the institution of slavery.

Maureen Flannery: I'm feeling uneasy about this discussion, and the reason is that I think we're looking at this in a very male way. To me, the basic questions here are the ones that Byllye Avery mentioned that women ask in pregnancy. "What sex is my baby going to be?" and "Is it going to be all right?" Those are the questions that women ask. My feeling is that women have had, in the past, ways to answer those questions. We've lost them, and we're buying into a system where male professionals magically give us answers to questions that we could answer ourselves, as Denise Connors said. Two examples are not as complicated as sex preselection, but illustrate this better. One is early diagnosis of pregnancy. People are working on radioimmunoassays to diagnose pregnancy early—before the first missed menstrual period. That's an irrelevant test. That's something that men developed. Women know when they are pregnant. A woman who's in touch with herself can tell. What we need to do is help the women who don't know—like teenagers—get that kind of self-knowledge.

Much of the technology we are discussing here purports to answer that question: "Is my baby all right?" Women know that, too, and there have been studies demonstrating that a woman's perception of her baby's movement in the latter part of pregnancy is more accurate than fetal monitoring in determining whether that baby is all right. But a woman is invariably discredited when she says to her physician: "My baby isn't moving much." The doctor listens with an instrument and says: "Everything's O.K." He uses technology to reassure her, and she learns to ignore her own intuition. In the same way that women know of pregnancy and their baby's well-being, I think that women have ways of determining the sex of their baby prior to conception, and of knowing what sex baby they are carrying. What we have to get in touch with is the wisdom and power that women used to have, instead of buying into male technology that promises to give us answers.

Sandra Serrano Sewell: I'd like to explore a little bit the issue of who's really using technology. I brought this up with respect to DES the other day, and somebody said that this was one of the times when you were lucky to be a minority, because statistical information regarding minorities and DES could not be found. I thought to myself, "Ha, ha, ha—that's because society could care less if minority women miscarried."

I want to ask, again, "Who's going for these tests [to determine the sex of the fetus]?" I know I'm not going, and I know my friends aren't going, and I know the women in my community aren't going.

Tabitha Powledge: I'll tell you who's going. Doctors' wives are going. They know the ropes, and they know what to say to get the tests.

Janice Raymond: I don't know who's seeking it, Sandy, but I know who has expressed considerable research interest in the topic. For the most part, it's some population groups.

Emily Culpepper: Nobody has quite said this, but we're still acting as if, were there simple sex selection technologies developed, it would be up to the conceiving parents or mother to use it. I don't have any faith that established medicine wouldn't market sex selection products. We have heard about DES being put into vitamins, without women knowing they were taking it. Sex selection medication could be developed and used on unknowing people. That's a spectre, especially in the so-called "undeveloped" countries (though I have a real problem with the terminology of undeveloped, primitive, etc.).

Ruth Hubbard: I want to reuse the word "eugenics." We have a history of it. This is not an isolated instance. If we are scared, we have reason to be scared. The eugenics movement *thrived* in the latter part of the nineteenth century. It thrived in the early part of the twentieth century. And it helped produce the immigration legislation that the United States operated under for thirty years and that was, in part, responsible for the effectiveness of Hitler's genocide in Europe. A lot of the people who wanted to emigrate to the United States to avoid that genocide came from the wrong "racial stock." That is, they were eastern Europeans, and US immigration laws had been formulated to exclude people born in eastern Europe. If eugenics died down in the 1930s, it did so partly because of horror at the German practices of race purification and partly because it didn't work. The techniques then available could not eliminate "undesirables," short of killing people. We now have a whole series of techniques that *will* do the job. Sex preselection is one of them; amniocentesis is another.

Ruth Nentwig: I'd just like to reinforce one thing. It is possible without technology to preselect the sex. There is an 89% success rate in choosing male or female with natural kinds of methods. It seems to me that we must work on increasing value and self-esteem among women. You can do it in your own home.

Becky Holmes: Shettles claims 85% success, but his studies are not double-blind. It may work for some people, but it doesn't work across the board. We do have to ask—if parents try a do-it-yourself technique and it fails—how they will behave toward that child of the "wrong" sex. Unperfected techniques bring a different series of problems with them.

Jill Wolhandler: I am concerned about the question of who would use the technology, and for whom. What Jan told us about who is funding this research is very significant. Population control groups want to keep down the numbers of certain populations, regardless of the cost to women or to the society. We've heard about sterilization abuse, we've heard about Depo-Provera, and I think that the implications of eugenics and population control should be very primary in our analysis of this field.

Manipulative Reproductive Technologies

Organized by
Betty B. Hoskins

Overview

Betty B. Hoskins

The final articles in this volume examine laboratory techniques and industrial technologies that are only now under development—egg banks, parthenogenesis, egg and cell fusion, in vitro fertilization and implantation, cloning, chimeras, and cell modification. We still have time to make conscious choices about these applications, in contrast to most of the other reproductive technologies we have discussed. *What techniques shall we use in studying reproduction and cell behavior? How shall we use technology to address the human condition?* The writers here first state the nature of the work being performed, then tease out some of the assumptions, the symbolisms and ideologies, the overt and covert conditionings, the axiomatic values of our society that underlie the work. We believe these lead to the present choices of funding, research, and application. In reaction, our writings and discussions raise both standard and nonstandard questions.

Rosalind Herlands reviews the biological and clinical state of the art, and shows that it is more advanced than has been generally recognized. She suggests a motivation: western scientific civilization usually acts upon its desire to know, to understand, and to take apart and put back together again.

Susan Anthony Salladay gives an ethical-social framework for asking questions. Our spectrum of control and choices exists in a context of implicit value judgments. Biological "truths" as well as social choices arise from a cultural milieu. Scientific perceptions change with time. Our present model of gene sequences portrays them as ticker tapes or computer bits; we no longer think of genes as pearls on a string or as poker-runs as we did in the 1940s and 50s. We no longer speak of the activist sperm awakening a quiescent egg. We conceive, so to speak, of fertilization as the fusion of two co-equal cells, initiating the development of an individual. And the social choices change; lobbying by infertile people and physicians has increased funding for microsurgery, cell manipulation, fertilization outside the maternal body, and cell transplantation. Previously, adoption and the acceptance of "fate" were the only recourse.

One technique is already in human use: in vitro fertilization and embryo transfer. Barbara Eck Menning and Ruth Hubbard argue for and against further development of these techniques. Does every woman have a right to bear a child? Can people choose for themselves when social dangers for others may be forecast?

With such divergent and deeply held convictions in our pluralistic society, what policy stance (if any) should the federal government take? How should such positions be reached? Robert Murray describes the deliberations that *did* lead to the policy recommendations to the secretary of HEW by the Ethics Advisory Board. Much of the ensuing discussion probes the roles of ethical discourse and political persuasion. In my view the usefulness of the former is dismissed prematurely; academic cautiousness is judged unsympathetically.

The requirement that prospective parents be married in order to participate in in vitro fertilization provoked considerable discussion. It highlights one of the patriarchal assumptions of our society: offspring are often viewed as property. The concept of legitimacy implies male-dominated and male-identified ownership.

Many of the debates at the conference reflect to me another patriarchal habit in our dualistic society: we women, too, are conditioned to make choices whether we need to or not. Pronouncements are made that it is "better" to speak from the head (citing documentable cases, valid statistics, verifiable assumptions) or from the heart and gut (stating a personal, experiential base of knowledge). Such unnecessary evaluations deny the integrity of the whole person. In another example of false dualism, immediate and future consequences are placed in opposition: worries are stated that while the futuristic topics are interesting, should we not choose to deal solely with present problems?

Despite our differences, a cluster of values emerges as important in women's consideration. They include: wholeness, oneness with nature, community responsibility for other humans (whether or not they be wanted, handicapped, female, less than perfect), responsibility for the earth, empowerment, affiliation, bonding, and network. We think and feel with the symbols of circles and cycles and cooperation. We move away from the predominant symbol of the ladder—of hierarchy; of quantitative rank-ordering of bad, good, and better than; of competition against others.

Our value perceptions at the conference have usually favored the social good. For instance, the risks to society in developing in vitro fertilization are seen as outweighing benefits to individual women or couples. Because of that calculus, it was argued that individuals ought to be denied the choice. Such a community focus may also be one-sided, in my estimation. It may too easily slight a woman's control of her own life and the essential confidentiality of her medical and social records.

A very important question raised by Dennis Livingston provokes no response: "How do you deal with patriarchal women?" Yet it is they (we)—and they were active in the conference—who pronounce judgments upon other women. They are forceful both "within the system" and within women's groups that purport to provide alternative, caring health and educational services. All of us have been reared in a culture that evaluates continually, hastily, often unnecessarily. This makes the struggle to establish affiliation and empowerment in a better world doubly hard.

A final section examines science fiction stories about alternative reproductive strategies. Livingston's remarks illustrate how science fiction supplies a vehicle other than the political process to project and choose among possible future developments in our society. He makes the startling point that no utopian societies have been exclusively male. Becky Logan stresses the dangers of eugenics and male-control. Is there a liberating alternative to the oppressive use of technology by oppressive societies?

Our society has an uneasy grasp of the specialness of life. Because life resources have been so abundant, we exploit and destroy them. Because development so ordinarily occurs with precision, we submerge our ability to wonder at the process that starts with a single cell and ends with a starfish, or fern, or person.

Human beings are no more special than, and just as fascinating as, all other life on this planet. But we regard human reproduction as trivial, as being something that women do, as requiring no brains; simultaneously, we declare pregnancy and birth to be processes requiring the guidance of experts. When we pierce through these polar contradictions, we better understand why there is an uneasy awe and jealousy of women's ability to create life:

research and development

the schedule
called
for me
to
create life

in
three days
just to
show
that we
could
do better.
—Philip Gordon[1]

Biological Manipulations for Producing and Nurturing Mammalian Embryos

Rosalind L. Herlands

One egg, one embryo, one adult-normality. But a bokanovskified egg will bud, will proliferate, will divide. From eight to ninety-six buds, and every bud will grow into a perfectly-formed embryo, and every embryo into a full-sized adult. Make ninety-six human beings grow where only one grew before. Progress.

A. Huxley[1]

Aldous Huxley's description of large-scale assembly-line production of humans in *Brave New World* represented replication of an individual embryo into multiple copies as a tremendous achievement in his grotesque "utopian" society. Just how close have today's scientific and technological advances brought us to achieving such asexual human reproduction and manipulation of human embryos outside the natural environment?

Most of the techniques Huxley described have not yet been (and may never be) realized for human embryos, principally for ethical considerations. However, variations of many of the techniques have been successfully employed to produce, manipulate, and nurture early embryos of many other mammals for use in basic and applied research. Although biologists have experimented with a variety of mammalian embryos (including mice, rats, guinea pigs, marsupials, cattle, sheep, horses, monkeys, and humans), most research has been conducted on mice and rabbits. Mice are favorite experimental subjects because they are easy to maintain in the laboratory, their genetics is better understood than that of many other mammals, and many genetic strains are available. Rabbits are also easy to maintain in the laboratory, and their eggs and embryos are relatively large; in fact, they were the first embryos to be produced and studied in vitro.

In this article, I will survey the various techniques biologists have developed to artificially produce and nurture mammalian embryos in vitro. I have divided these technical manipulations into seven broad categories: (1) obtaining embryos and use of foster mothers; (2) culture and storage of embryos; (3) in vitro fertilization; (4) parthenogenesis; (5) cloning; (6) chimera production; and (7) artificial placentae/ artificial wombs.

OBTAINING EGGS, EMBRYOS, AND SURROGATE MOTHERS

Any attempts to study egg (oocyte) maturation, fertilization, early development, implantation into the uterine wall, and subsequent organ formation rely entirely on the ability of the experimenter to grow oocytes and embryos in tissue and organ culture outside the female body. Up to now no mammalian embryo has developed entirely in culture; instead it must be inserted into a pregnant or pseudopregnant female which will carry the embryo to term. The successful collection of eggs and embryos at various stages and the use of surrogate or foster mothers has depended on our increasing understanding of the hormonal influences on egg maturation, on ovulation, and on the preparation (actually differentiation) of the uterine wall for implantation, and subsequent maturation of the developing embryo.

Large numbers of eggs (superovulation) or embryos at the exact same stage of development can be induced by administering precisely timed hormone injections, irrespective of the estrus (fertility) cycle in prepubertal females. If eggs are to be collected, hormone-primed females are not mated.[2] If early embryos are desired, mating and several days of development occur.

The procedures used for obtaining eggs and embryos of mice are similar to procedures used with other mammals.[3] Mice are especially handy; they have frequent fertile periods—every 30 days following puberty. Ovulation occurs one to five hours after mating. The presence of a hard horny mass, the vaginal plug, indicates that mating has occurred. Eggs and embryos are collected, usually after the donor female has been killed. Her oviducts and uterus are removed and the eggs or embryos are flushed out with an appropriate culture medium kept at 37°C and at the correct acidity. Under aseptic conditions, donor females of domestic animals such as cattle and horses are often not sacrificed and their embryos are instead removed surgically.[4] A similar series of hormone treatments in a human female, at the appropriate time in the menstrual cycle, leads to the ovulation of several oocytes.[5] The oocytes are then collected as they rupture from the ovaries, using a technique called laparoscopy. This technique entails making an incision in the woman's abdomen and inserting a laparoscope, a long metal tube containing a light and optical system to view the ovaries, and a micropipet to remove the oocytes.[6]

Once an embryo has reached the blastocyst stage, it must be returned to the uterus of a suitable female or foster mother if further development is to occur. This procedure is known as embryo transfer. The cells of the blastocyst have already begun to differentiate into two types: a layer of enveloping cells called the trophoblast that forms extraembryonic tissues, such as the fetal part of the placenta, and a tightly clustered group called the inner cell mass, which gives rise principally to the embryo. The embryo is thus ready at this stage to implant into the uterine wall.

Mouse embryos reach the blastocyst stage three days after fertilization and are usually then injected with a fine glass micropipet into the uterine wall of host females who are made pseudopregnant by mating them with a vasectomized male.[7] The host female is at a gestation stage similar to or 24 hours behind the stage of the transferred embryos.[8]

CULTURE AND STORAGE OF EMBRYOS

The ability to culture early mammalian embryos and even immature oocytes[9] has removed an earlier restriction on experimental studies. The introduction of antibiotics in the 1950s greatly increased the success of routine rabbit and mouse embryo culture,[10] building upon Brachet's pioneering studies in the 1910s. The successful culture of other mammalian embryos, including pig, rat, marsupials, humans, sheep, and cattle, up to the blastocyst or pre-implantation stage has also been achieved.

Many different culture systems for mouse embryos are used in different laboratories. Embryos are usually cultured in test tubes, in microdroplets of medium under mineral oil in a petri dish, or in special chambers in which a constant flow of gas is maintained. All media are basically physiological saline solutions plus energy sources (pyruvate, lactate, glucose) and the antibiotics penicillin and streptomycin.[11] These media can be chemically or biologically defined. The latter type includes some biological fluid, such as fetal calf serum or bovine albumin, and is usually more successful. However, a system that uses chemically defined media has the advantage of being reproducible and capable of being varied in quite controlled ways to study the nutritional requirements of different stage embryos or the effect of added molecules, such as hormones or teratogenic (defect-causing) agents, on development. Such tissue culture techniques have also allowed biologists to examine metabolic changes and to manipulate embryos in a variety of ways. Lin has injected or removed cytoplasm from mouse zygotes with micromanipulative techniques; the manipulated embryos can be transferred to oviducts or to the uterus of foster mothers.[12] Microinjection of macromolecules into embryos may provide a method for determining their effect on the differentiation of early mammalian embryonic cells.

In vitro development of post-implantation stages of mice, rats, and rabbits has also been achieved to a limited extent[13] allowing biologists to study early organ formation (embryos can develop with primitive beating hearts and primitive central nervous systems), the changing nutritional and environmental requirements, and differentiation of nutrient membranes. For example, Hsu found that post-implantation mouse embryos require human umbilical cord blood serum in the medium.[14] New found that older embryos grow better in an atmosphere of 60% oxygen.[15]

In 1971, a method for preserving viable pre-implantation stage mouse embryos in a frozen stage became available.[16] Since then, the procedure has been extended successfully to store embryos of rats, rabbits, sheep, goats, and cattle at –196° C, the temperature of liquid nitrogen.[17] Embryos can probably be stored in this way for decades. They must be thawed slowly and can then be transferred to foster mothers. This technique already is being used to transport embryos, particularly embryos for commerical animal husbandry.[18] It also has the potential for maintaining "egg banks" similar to established sperm banks. With the success of in vitro fertilization, selective embryo production based on the desired genetic makeup of the egg and the sperm could be achieved. Certainly the proponents of positive eugenics for humans would applaud this achievement.[19]

IN VITRO FERTILIZATION

Once the obstacles of obtaining eggs, culturing embryos, and then transferring early embryos back to a suitable uterus have been successfully overcome, external fertilization and the subsequent development to term of mammalian embryos becomes a relatively easy procedure. All that are needed are ripe eggs ready to be fertilized, sperm, a medium in which to mix the two, and a medium in which to support early embryonic development.[20] The sperm are put in a salt solution that mimics the environment of the female reproductive tract. In this solution, the sperm undergo chemical and ultrastructural changes that prepare them for fertilization. The activated sperm are placed in droplets of culture medium and inert oil. Then one ripe egg is pipeted into the droplet. Fertilization occurs within a few hours, and some hours later the developing embryo is transferred to a different culture solution.[21]

In vitro fertilization in mammals is an established technique. It was first achieved two decades ago in rabbits[22] and has since been adapted for use in animal husbandry and in humans.[23] Louise Joy Brown, born July, 1978, is the first human reported to have been conceived in culture and to develop successfully to term; to date, three other such babies have followed her. None of the subsequent techniques that I discuss in this paper has yet been realized for humans, but the kinds of scientific and ethical issues raised by in vitro fertilization forewarn us of the Pandora's box that may await us if and when these techniques become available for use on humans.

PARTHENOGENESIS

Parthenogenesis is the production of an embryo from an egg in the absence of any contribution from a sperm. Natural parthenogenesis occurs in some social insects. Males result from unfertilized, parthenogenetically activated eggs. There are also cases of spontaneous parthenogenesis in higher animals; for example, Stevens and Varnum[24] have found parthenogenetic embryos in the ovaries of strain LT mice and there are some species of lizards that can undergo parthenogenesis.[25] However, most parthenogenetic embryos, known as parthenogenotes or parthenotes, are produced artificially. The resulting embryos possess only maternal chromosomes, either one set or two.

The techniques used for artificial parthenogenesis mimic some aspect of fertilization that activates the egg to start division and development. Those techniques probably affect the cell membrane. Recently ovulated eggs of rabbits and mice have been stimulated within the oviduct of an anesthetized animal or isolated from the oviduct and stimulated in vitro.[26] The activating techniques are usually extreme conditions, such as heat shock (42–46° C), treatment with the enzyme hyaluronidase, electric shock, anesthetizing agents, and culture in medium lacking calcium and magnesium ions. "The art of activation lies in damaging the egg without killing it."[27]

Most parthenogenotes go through only one or two divisions.[28]

Most embryos with one chromosome set do not develop beyond the cleavage stage. However, Kaufman[29] has obtained complete development to the blastocyst stage in mice following activation in culture medium lacking calcium and magnesium, and many of the blastocysts implanted and developed within the uteri of foster mothers. Balakier and Tarkowski[30] reported that with heat shock in vitro followed by cytochalasin B treatment, diploid parthenogenetic mouse embryos developed to the blastocyst stage.

Scientists study parthenogenetic embryos to learn about: (1) natural activating mechanisms occurring during fertilization; (2) the point in mammalian development when active decoding of the embryo's genes occurs; (3) the precise role of the sperm in development; (4) the expression of genetic mutations during development; (5) chromosome mapping of biochemical mutants.

CLONING

Cloning is a type of developmental engineering in which one or more genetically identical copies are made of an organism. By its very definition, cloning is an asexual and duplicatory process; its results bypass the usual sexual reproduction involving merger of a sperm and egg to produce a unique individual. It occurs in plants and lower invertebrates more frequently than in vertebrates. The formation of twins from the same fertilized egg and the formation of buds in *Hydra* are natural methods of cloning in animals. Biologists have developed methods for creating clones in amphibian vertebrates, and have attempted to apply some of these methods to mammals. The various techniques usually involve embryonic cells subjected to nuclear transplantation, chemically induced self-replication, development from single blastomeres, or egg fusion.

Nuclear Transplantation

Briggs and King in 1952 pioneered this field in order to study whether a nucleus from a differentiated cell could support development of an undifferentiated egg.[31] They devised a way to transfer by microinjection an intact nucleus from a donor cell to a frog egg whose nucleus has been removed. Donor nuclei came from cells of different developmental stages of frog embryos; some of the embryos produced by this method developed into normal, functioning tadpoles. Subsequently, John Gurdon has shown that nuclei taken from differentiated cells, such as the tadpole intestine[32] or adult skin,[33] and transplanted into enucleated eggs of the African clawed toad,

Xenopus, could, in a few cases, also support full embryonic development.

Frog eggs are a thousand times larger in volume than mammalian eggs and so are much easier to micromanipulate. Nuclear transplantation has recently been attempted in rabbit eggs by Bromhall[34] using two methods: microinjection of radioactively labeled donor nuclei from early embryos into eggs and the virus-induced fusion of an egg and an early embryonic cell with an inactivated (Sendai) virus. In many cases, the recipient eggs cleaved normally, but only four embryos developing into morulae (18–26 cell stage) clearly resulted from nuclear transplantation. Fusion of adult and embryonic cells with one- and two-cell mouse embryos has been attempted by Graham;[35] like Bromhall, he had very limited success in achieving nuclear transfer by this method. No long-lived mammalian clones have yet been produced using this or any other method.

Chemically Induced Self-Replication

Sea urchin and frog studies have shown that cells need two sets of chromosomes for development beyond cleavage stages. When an organism with genetic information from only one parent is desired, research has been aimed at removing either sperm or egg nucleus from a newly fertilized egg before they fuse while still permitting the remaining (pro) nucleus to undergo chromosomal replication. Modlinski[36] has successfully removed one of the mouse pronuclei by microsurgery. Eggs developed up to the morula and occasionally to the blastocyst stage. Chromosomal analysis revealed that all such embryos had only one set of chromosomes. Peter Hoppe removed the sperm pronucleus from a newly fertilized mouse egg and treated the egg with cytochalasin B (which prevents cells from dividing, but allows the chromosomes to duplicate). Instead of receiving one half of its chromosomes from the father and one half from the mother, this genetically altered egg contains two identical sets of maternal chromosomes.

Development From Single Blastomeres

Individual cells from the early embryo, before cell differentiation has overtly occurred, can be separated, and their ability to develop normally can be determined. This approach has already been applied to rats, rabbits, and mice. Tarkowski[37] has isolated cells from mouse embryos at the two-cell stage; he utilizes two methods: (1) eliminating one cell (blastomere), either by microbeam irradiation or by puncture with a glass microneedle, and leaving the acellular zona pellucida membrane intact, or (2) isolating the two blastomeres from each other chemically after the outermost membrane (zona pellucida) has been removed. The single cells are then cultured in vitro to the blastocyst stage and transferred to foster mothers. The second method can theoretically be used on older embryos, but Tarkowski believes that the 8-cell stage in the mouse is the last one to possess cells capable of developing into a whole embryo. One may thus produce a mammalian clone by separating the blastomeres from 2-cell, 4-cell, or 8-cell embryos, culturing all the cells from the embryo and transferring the blastocysts to a foster mother.

Egg Fusion

Attempts to fuse two mouse oocytes, zygotes, or cells from a two-cell embryo together have met with partial success.[38] The outermost membrane (zona pellucida) is removed by enzymatic treatment. The denuded oocytes, zygotes, or cells are then fused together in vitro (by inactivated Sendai virus); the fusion products are cultured in a standard medium and, if appropriate, transferred to uteri of foster mothers. Graham found that a small percentage of fused zygotes or fused blastomeres could develop to the blastocyst stage, but that these embryos did not develop beyond initial implantation. He believes that the tetraploidy (four sets of chromosomes) of the embryos' cells may interfere with normal post-implantation development in some undefined way. This technique was the forerunner of the fusion technique used for nuclear transfer in rabbits by Bromhall. Soupart and his colleagues believe that oocyte fusion may represent a way to alter radically the sex ratio at conception and, hence, to provide a large number of female offspring as further research subjects.

CHIMERA PRODUCTION

A chimera is any animal or plant composed of two or more genetically different cell populations. Primary chimeras, in which the different cell populations constitute a single embryo from a very early stage of embryogenesis, are formed by aggregation or injection methods.

In the 1960s Tarkowski and Mintz aggregated mouse embryos at cleavage stages into a large clump that continued to develop to the morula or blastocyst stage. After mechanical or enzymatic removal of the egg membrane, the naked embryos are pushed together with glass needles, forceps, or hair loops, and cultured for 24 to 48 hours until aggregation is complete and a blastocyst is formed.[39] Aggregation is possible at any stage of cleavage, but the 8 to 12 cell stage has proved to be the most convenient. The best results are obtained when the fused embryos are at the same stage of development.[40] More than two embryos can be fused; Mintz has produced a giant blastocyst by aggregating 16 early embryos. She has suggested the term "allophenic" to describe progeny derived from embryo aggregation.

Gardner devised an alternative procedure by injecting cells or pieces of tissues into a mouse blastocyst cavity or into the inner cell mass.[41] The blastocyst stage seems to be more tolerant of in vitro manipulation than the earlier cleavage stages. Besides overcoming the experimental difficulty often encountered with production of aggregation chimeras, the technique of injection chimeras allows different combinations to be created. For example, interspecific hybrids of rat and mouse cells can be formed. Implantation will not occur unless the trophoblast is of the same species as the foster mother. Malignant cells can be injected into normal blastocysts, or mixtures of early cleavage stages can be injected into blastocysts to determine when cells specialize.

In both methods, the resultant chimeric embryos are transferred to foster mothers. Confirmation of chimera production depends on the use of specific permanent cell markers, which can be used to distinguish between the genetically different cell populations. Radioactive nuclear labeling, biochemical variations, chromosomal variations, and surface antigen differences have provided adequate cell markers.

Chimera production in mammals has illuminated a number of aspects of mammalian development. The extent to which the inner cell mass contributes to the embryo and to extra-embryonic tissues has been clarified by this procedure.[42] Chimeras composed of chromosomally male and female cells have shed light on the mechanisms of sex determination in mammals. Chimeras also may be used to indicate the main focus of activity of a mutant gene.[43] In adult mice derived from chimeras, all tissues examined have been composed of cells from the different cell population sources, indicating that cells of mammalian morulae migrate. In addition, the basic mechanisms underlying the highly malignant state of teratocarcinomas are being studied by injecting embryonal carcinoma cells into normal blastocysts.[44]

ARTIFICIAL PLACENTAE/ARTIFICIAL WOMBS

Although there has been some limited success in culturing mouse and rabbit embryos beyond the implantation stage, there exist no baby hatcheries of the kind described in *Brave New World.* The placenta formed from both fetal and maternal tissues provides the vital link allowing viviparous development in mammals. Research in this area has taken two directions: (1) studying in vitro implantation of mouse and rabbit blastocysts to gain an understanding of the factors that are involved in the initial development of the placenta and (2) duplicating the environment of the uterus and functions of the placenta in an attempt to save premature human babies.

Glenister and Sherman have followed the implantation of mouse blastocysts into monolayers of uterine cells in organ culture.[45] Glenister has also cultured post-implantation rabbit embryos with their developing placentae for up to 48 hours. These studies permit the researchers to study the effects of hormones and oxygen levels on the implantation process. Kirby[46] has transplanted mouse blastocysts to extrauterine sites as a way to study implantation production of placenta hormones, control of trophoblast differentiation and its invasiveness into the maternal tissue, and the general immunological problems of pregnancy. In addition, Bergstrom[47] has experimentally delayed implantation in the mouse by removal of the ovaries; this technique offers another method to study the hormonal regulation of implantation.

Attempts to mimic the uterine environment of a pregnant mammal and the functions of a fully formed placenta have been limited. Zapol *et al.*[48] tried to construct an artificial placenta and womb for premature lamb fetuses; the fetuses survived for about 55 hours before they underwent cardiac arrest. This extrauterine support system was developed to study physiological and biochemical variables of an isolated, late-term fetus. At Stanford University, scientists have developed an artificial womb or fetal incubator.[49] Into it, oxygen and nutrients are carried under pressure; young human fetuses, products of spontaneous abortion, have been kept alive for up to 48 hours. Not only would artificial wombs and placentae provide extensive knowledge into post-implantation development and physiology that might aid in saving fetuses, they might also provide the means to increase the survival of premature 20–28 week-old fetuses who can usually live only up to five days outside the uterus.[50] Advantages and disadvantages can both be projected.

To summarize: I have outlined a number of techniques that biologists have devised to produce mammalian embryos artificially and to nurture mammalian embryos in vitro. The research utilizing these techniques has been principally aimed at facilitating our basic understanding of mammalian embryogenesis and other developmental phenomena. The therapeutic uses of these techniques were not always immediately evident. The state of the art in this field is quite advanced—to such an extent, in fact, that biologists and society at large must be aware of its inherent dangers as well as its great benefits if we wish to avoid the human production scenarios depicted in *Brave New World.*

Ethics and Reproductive Technology

Susan Anthony Salladay

In educator Lawrence Kohlberg's model of stages of moral development, those who reach the most advanced stage achieve "harmony" between the various dimensions of personal experience, group identity, and general principles.[1]

In debates about the moral acceptability of manipulative reproductive technologies, such harmony is yet to be satisfactorily achieved. Situations such as the recent DHEW Ethics Advisory board hearings about the morality of in vitro fertilization (IVF) or the "Ethical Issues in Reproductive Technology: Analysis by Women" Workshop may serve as examples of potentials for a "trap milieu" in which the exploitation of controversy increases to a point where problems come to seem overwhelmingly complex, and moral decision-making is stalemated or compromised by policy or economic concerns. In such situations there is a rise in individuals' feelings of frustration and powerlessness that leads either to a decrease in personal commitment to the difficult decision-making process (and a corresponding decrease in group creativity) or to a "counter-activism" that is retaliatory, but usually short-lived or misdirected. This sort of "trap milieu"[2] is an ideal precondition to the spread of an undesirable moral fatalism.

To thwart the trap milieu that destroys creative moral decision-making, it is necessary to employ techniques that facilitate group communication and personal honesty. As the morality of manipulative reproductive technologies is evaluated, it is essential that those concerned with the deliberations make clear their own "gut level" feelings and intuitions about reproductive technologies and about technology in general, its values, promises, and liabilities. This must involve a value-clarification process that will, most likely, place individuals in one of four categories. Concerning technology generally, we may believe:

1. That it can be tamed, managed, or controlled successfully.
2. That society must co-exist with it in a delicate balance.
3. That it must be repudiated completely.

4. That it must be exploited to the fullest extent while still possible (in this view technology becomes like an addiction, hence a further understanding of the term "technological fix").

It is possible that an individual may admit to a "public" feeling about the value of technology for society, holding (for example) to category two while, in the moral debate, actually argue from a "private" feeling based on personal experience (category three, for example). It is helpful to remember that one's stance on technology does represent a (conscious or semiconscious) choice. Choice is the key term because our beliefs about values do very frequently become self-fulfilling prophecies, a strange recurring phenomenon that we call history.

What are the major issues, problems, and concerns involved in the moral decision-making process now taking place in relation to the various new reproductive technologies such as IVF, sex-preselection, and cloning? Why are these issues and problems *moral* concerns? What is "morality" and how is it studied? Let's work backwards on these questions. Ethics concerns itself (broadly speaking) with human morality, that is, judgments about goodness and rightness as opposed to badness or wrongness. Ethicists study the various moral traditions and beliefs of societies and observe the actions, policies, and rules of behavior connected with these. In its descriptive function, ethics notes contrasts, contradictions, and conflicts between individuals and between cultural systems. In its prescriptive function, ethics evaluates moral systems and behaviors against one another by metaethical standards in our attempts to solve moral dilemmas with justice and equity.

Two important criteria are usually involved in evaluating any system of morality: its universality and its force. A morally valid judgment or sanction must be widely and fairly applicable and not represent the special interest of a small, privileged, or controlling group to the detriment of other groups' interests. At the same time moral judgments must apply to situations realistically. They should be accepted and promulgated by personal conscience and general will rather than by coercion or prejudice.

Debates about the morality of manipulative reproductive technologies raise issues concerning (1) the approach to decision-making; (2) the terminology of decision-making; and (3) the social implications of decision-making. Group 1 concerns the grounds for moral determinations, the nature of moral authority, and whether particular authorities are asserted to be absolute or not absolute. Group 2 relates to the meaning and application of terms used in making key value judgments. Group 3 includes questions about the assumed effects or results of research in various forms of reproductive technology upon human endeavors and institutions, and biological evolution, e.g., patterns of sexual reproduction, sex roles and family structures, traditional moralities, and the distribution of genetic traits within gene pools. All three of these groups of questions interact simultaneously with three dimensions of deliberation: (1) personal conscience and private experience, (2) group awareness and the extent of common corporate identity and/or commitment, and (3) general humanistic ideals, universal goals, rules, and norms.

CHOOSING THE APPROACH TO MUTUAL DECISION-MAKING

Let us first consider the approach to moral decision-making and how this involves questions about moral authority. Two different methods or "world-view" orientations lie behind any moral judgment. A judgment may arise from either an *a priori* or an *a posteriori* orientation. No individual uses one method exclusively. The tendency to prefer one or the other method lies deep within the individual psyche and depends upon the sense of trust, view of human "nature," level of moral development, and ability to tolerate open-ended, ambiguous, or "disorderly" situations.

An *a priori* approach usually involves a notion of universal principle or absolute authority. Right or wrong is determined by reference to this principle or authority and the determination is often thought to be "final" in the sense that a particular change in circumstances will not alter the principle or the determination. The principle or authority does not admit of exceptions, thus: murder is always wrong. The absolute authority may be God, the Good, a policy, or an "ism"; it may have a "name and face" or it may be highly abstract. Nonetheless, it assumes a *priority* over all other principles, standards, and circumstances in the moral decision-making process.

An *a posteriori* approach uses guidelines other than "absolute" authority in solving moral dilemmas, and solutions thus reached may be considered "working" or temporary solutions. This notion of a "working" solution suggests that the pragmatic (that which is "workable") might be one such guideline in the *a posteriori* determination of rightness or wrongness. Workability is sometimes determined by balancing needs and desires, or by balancing the desirable consequences of an action against the undesirable ones. When such a judgment is required "before the fact" in order to proceed with or to stop actions, it becomes a risk-benefit analysis.

Moral dilemmas may arise when *a priori* and *a posteriori* positions conflict. For example, one might ask whether IVF is, in principle, *always* wrong or whether such technology will *always* be misused and, if so, how is this position proved true without exception? Or is it the case that IVF cannot be judged at all in a generalized sense or with absolute authority, but only in a relative sense, perhaps on a case-by-case basis or only by those choosing the process as therapeutic treatment? Is IVF's rightness or wrongness to be weighed in terms of its workability: whether it produces individually satisfying consequences with minimal risk? Are we able to make either a *strictly a priori* or *strictly a posteriori* judgment about IVF? How essential is it to know all the consequences and their magnitude in order to determine the morality of this or any use of technology? It is doubtful that such knowledge is possible.

This debate between an *a priori* and an *a posteriori* approach often translates into conflict between a "sanctity-of-life" ethic and a "quality-of-life" ethic. The principles frequently appealed to as being absolutely determinative in an *a priori* system are those having to do with divine commandments or natural law, principles held to be inviolable by any particular circumstance or need. "Thou shalt not kill" is one such priority commandment over which, according to a sanctity-of-life ethic, no other concern can claim superiority. A quality-of-life ethic, by contrast, is more relativistic. All principles may admit of certain limitations, and not all would be equally applicable in every situation, depending on particular circumstances. Regarding this contrast between absolute and relative applications of moral principle, theologian Daniel Maguire writes:

> To say that something is morally right or wrong in all possible circumstances implies a divine knowledge of all possible circumstances and their moral meaning. To say that something is universally good or bad is non-sense for it is to say that something is *really* good or bad apart from the *reality-constituting* circumstances.[3]

Yet from their various positions, each side finds compromise difficult. For the absolutists a particular (perhaps divine) principle is at stake. For the relativist or the pragmatist, human responsibility and individual freedom are on the line. As ethicist Joseph Fletcher says:

> Moral judgments differ. Some people fear new and unexplored risks. They prefer to forget the risk-benefit calculations; they like to stay on the safe side. Others distrust any enlargement of potential powers that might give some advantages over others. This is the rock-bottom issue and the definitive question: are we to

> reason from general propositions and universals to normative decisions, or are we to reason from empirical data, variable situations, and human values to normative decisions?[4]

A moral dilemma is best defined as a forced choice between two equally unappealing (or appealing) alternatives. The relentlessness of technology appears to be the main coercive factor forcing choices in the area of reproductive technology. Even supposing it were possible to do so, is it morally incumbent upon us to halt all forms of research in reproductive technology? And for how long? Or would such action constitute irrevocable shortsightedness? The eventual recommendations of the DHEW Ethics Advisory Board—to continue federally funded research and create structures to monitor the ongoing consequences and set guidelines—represent an *a posteriori* approach to the morality of IVF. However, apparently as an appeasement gesture to intense pressure from religionists arguing the *a priori* approach (that IVF is against divine or natural law), the Board recommended: "that embryo transfer be attempted only with gametes obtained from lawfully married couples."[5] Such an *a priori* principle, sanctioning the heterosexual, two-parent family as the only right or "legitimate" context in which IVF births may occur, represents extreme prejudice against all women (but particularly against single and lesbian women) and also against infertile men.[6] That there was such a Board and that such a decision was reached has not, of itself, resolved more fundamental questions about the nature of moral decision-making and moral authority.

THE TERMINOLOGY OF DECISION-MAKING

In considering IVF we find traditional problems of terminology and value-clarification. The distress and inability to communicate and resolve such differences as those that plagued the "pro-life vs pro-choice" debates on the morality of abortion reappear in the arena of reproductive technology. Supporters of the patriarchal family and its heterosexual system of division of labor, being challenged, feel obliged to retaliate. The terminology questions reflect this challenge. They are primarily centered around a preoccupation with "defining the nature of human": is humanness something given at conception or inherent in the event of conception, or is humanness something that develops? Is the product that results from the joining of nuclear contents in ovum and sperm "human?" Does the blastula or product of conception have "human rights"? As philosopher/poet Adrienne Rich comments:

> . . . these forms of debate are framed in terms of . . . an ethic and a social conscience which is male-defined. The questions raised thereby (At what point is a fertilized egg a person? When does the soul start to exist?) are inevitably male questions, posed in a world-view and an ethical system which has persistently denied moral and ethical value to women, viewing us as marginal, dubious, or dangerous, and in need of special controls.[7]

Indeed, one woman defines this as the essence of patriarchal chivalry: "In the system of chivalry, men protect women against men . . . it is an age-old protection racket. . ."[8] The sorts of concerns that are evidenced by questions about the human rights of the blastula or about the "unnaturalness" of reproductive technologies are "control questions" that stem from a world-view that sees women and children (even unborn or newly conceived) as vulnerable to men and their "rapist" tendencies and technologies. But these very control questions perpetuate the need for the patriarchal protection racket instead of exposing it.

In addition to these terminology controls, our system of logic and our language create an "either/or" sort of dualism that makes questions like "is the embryo a person or not" seem sensible. We feel that we must "choose one of the above." But such determinations inevitably involve a compartmentalizing and limiting of thought that may actually restrict ethical insights. The term "natural," for example, is often taken as a standard by which moral rightness can be judged. Are reproductive technologies "natural," we ask, assuming that either they are or they are not. Those who purport the "unnaturalness" of IVF or cloning, for example, rely upon a tradition of heterosexual intercourse within marriage as a definition of "natural." On the other hand, those who purport that IVF and cloning are indeed "natural" may choose as a standard of defense the observation that it is in man's nature to manipulate, restructure, and control his environment and his own evolution. Now what does a concerned, thoughtful *woman* do when faced with this "either/or" sort of logic? Perhaps to escape this verbal dilemma of equivocation, we must expose it for what it is: whether you take the "either" or the "or" side, "natural" really means "what is in the best interest of those in control."

THE SOCIAL IMPLICATIONS OF DECISION-MAKING

These are perhaps the most difficult questions because they present problems not only to the individual in terms of judgments and conscience, but also to society in the necessary formation of public policy. Questions in this group include those about the known and imagined risks of reproductive technologies, and about the desirability of such technological expertise and its potential for altering established social value systems. Will developments in reproductive technologies cause the elimination of pregnancy? Or will pregnancy become a class-related function? Will protective legislation be required to determine the inheritance status of clones? Will reproductive technologies prove to be a means of pollution whereby deleterious genes continue to contaminate gene pools? Or perhaps these technologies will mean the subtle beginning of a millennium of eugenics for the 21st century.

Will reproductive technologies eventually eliminate any significant division of labor and inequality between male and female in the family structure (or eliminate the traditional heterosexual, two-parent family altogether)? Will further research in the area of artificial contraceptives and placentas end sex-role stereotyping and discrimination or will it serve to enhance patriarchal ideologies by actually placing increasing powers (of gestation, birthing, and/or asexual self-reproduction) in the exclusive hands of male technocrats?

Here it can be counter-argued that if technologies such as IVF are already available and the risks appear to be minimal, do we not have a moral obligation to offer treatment to whose who choose it without indulging in futuristic speculation and science-fiction predictions? How can such obscure prognostications but frustrate and anger an infertile woman who has come to her own personally significant choice to have a child by IVF before her reproductive period in life is ended?

It is at this point that one frequently meets with the dreaded "slippery-slope" or "wedge" (i.e., foot-in-the-door, camel's-nose-in-the-tent) argument, especially when people attempt to speculate about the value of remote vs immediate consequences. It is often assumed that if we do "A" now, it will inevitably lead straight to "B." Thus, if we approve "A-type" actions or policies, we are implicitly sanctioning their "B-type" counterparts down the road. Although it is true that moral insight requires a thoughtful examination of known and potential consequences, it also requires that we step back from moral fatalism to discern acutely *real differences* between doing A and doing B. If we assume an automatic cause-and-effect relation between A and B, we may harmfully obscure real causes, thus helping to bring about the B we had hoped to prevent.

How does this apply to a discussion of the morality of reproductive technologies? Fatalism develops from the double-binds that have so long limited and crippled women's judgments and life-choices. One woman portrays the extremes of this trap and the terrible expense it entails for women:

> From an early age we are alienated from ourselves as sexual beings by a male society's ambivalent definition of our sexuality: we are

> sexy but we are pure; we are insatiable but we are frigid. . . . Caught between the demands of a male-dominated society and the demands of our own self-determination, we survive by fully accepting the masochistic symbol-world given to us by male society at the expense of our own experience.[9]

In discussing reproduction, technology, and morality, we feel acutely the many dimensions of this bind: gestation and birthing (at least at present) are exclusively, as physical processes, the power of women; women's bodies are essential for reproduction; the supervision of and technological expertise necessary to supervise these processes presently is controlled by men; women are valued and approved in today's society as mothers, through successful child rearing and domestic service; child rearing and domestic service are disvalued in this society as marginally important and deprecated as "women's work." Clearly women are in a "no win" situation, whether they rush to glorify and render exclusive their reproductive situation or to repudiate it altogether yet go on having babies!

Such a situation will continue to bind women as long as we accept, literalize, and limit women's total scope of creativity to one dimension: the uterine.

Response

Theresa Mayrand

In our consideration of in vitro fertilization (IVF) I wish to question our increasing dependency on technology, the application of informed consent, and current research priorities. Then, I wish to focus on our need to assess the values that underlie our decision-making, to supplement a concern for rights with an assumption of responsibility and to look at the long-range effects of adopting manipulative reproductive technologies.

As we move into IVF, we of necessity become more dependent on technology. We remove the control of reproduction to some extent from the woman herself, and open ourselves more to control and possible abuse by that technology. This issue has surfaced and resurfaced in this book. On the other hand, as Barbara Menning points out, infertile women ask for this technology to enable them to gain control of a natural process that they do not have. Hence—our dilemma. Although we are aware of the abuse that reproductive technology has heaped upon women in the past, we are also aware of the potential promise IVF holds for some infertile women.

Although women requesting this procedure will give consent, many people question whether women were adequately informed by Edwards and Steptoe, especially in the early stages of their work, about the low success rate of fertilization and full-term pregnancy. Did they make it clear to these women that they were, and at this point still are, participating in an experiment? According to Grobstein in a June 1979, *Scientific American* article,[1] Steptoe admitted that, although 79 women entered treatment since he began his clinical trials, only two actually gave birth. Of the 79, 68 underwent laparoscopies and 44 yielded usable eggs at a correct stage of maturity. There were 32 successful cases of fertilization and cleavage. Four women actually did become pregnant; two miscarried and two gave birth. In fairness we must ask how this compares with in vivo reproduction. Grobstein states that of 100 human eggs exposed to sperm in vivo, an average of 84 are fertilized, 69 implant, 42 survive the first week, 37 survive to the sixth week of pregnancy and 31 actually reach full-term birth.

Regarding maternal health, were the risks adequately assessed and described for repeated laparoscopies, and for the hormone administration needed to cause superovulation?

What about possible risk to the offspring? Besides considering the known, but supposedly low, risks of amniocentesis, is in vitro fertilization a proven safe process in terms of effects on the fetus? Edwards and Steptoe of course do believe that there has been adequate animal testing; Mastroianni from the University of Pennsylvania School of Medicine does not: "Most investigators" he says, "presently hold that in vitro fertilization is important solely for biological experimentation," and that ovum transfer "involves risks of a different order of magnitude," risks that must be "scrutinized with great care."[2] He feels that there has not been statistically valid proof of normal offspring in animal work. Although the Brown baby from England appears to be normal, will this be borne out in later life and will this be true of most in vitro children? Is compensation for research-related injury provided for, and by whom?

Another question involves priority of research funding. If our goal is indeed to help the woman who is infertile because of blocked oviducts, is it better to work toward perfecting methods to correct blocked oviducts or to develop in vitro techniques? Of course many who advocate funding of in vitro research have goals other than helping the infertile woman, and these goals too deserve careful evaluation.

In my own view, three concerns stand out. First, I feel that we have to carefully assess the values that underlie our decision-making in this area. We can easily get lost in our technological advances. I agree with Susan Peterson that we usually treat our moral problems merely as technical problems. We seem to step to the tune of "progress", and "progress for the sake of progress." We must question this mentality and the attitude that if we can do it, we will do it. Together we must look deeply at our basic values. If we value individuality, individual freedom, and dignity, and believe that each one of us has a right to a unique, unprecedented, unrepeatable existence, this will no doubt influence our decision on cloning. Do we value each person as a person *or* for her productivity, her IQ, and her "perfection"? Our answer to this question will influence our decisions regarding the handicapped neonate, eugenic sperm banks and donors, mandatory screening and coercive sterilization, and the use of in vitro fertilization with ectogenesis. Whether or not it is in fact possible to reproduce the "ideal" person, one motive behind ectogenesis is that it would enable us more easily to manipulate the genes during gestation to create the kind of person that we want. The values we hold will influence our decisions. It is vital that we examine and assess these values!

Secondly, and I say this in response to an attitude that I sense is present to some extent at this conference, it is important that we not get lost in just demanding rights. Our justifiable anger and our zeal in trying to achieve our previously denied respect and rights can sometimes blind us to the rights of others. I think that we have to move from a rights orientation to a responsibility orientation. While we are responsible for our lives and our happiness, we are also responsible for our fellow women, men, children, and even our children's children, our earth, and our universe, as Katsi Cook so eloquently said.

Finally, I emphasize that we must look at the long-range effects of adopting these reproductive technologies. Although I don't think we can adopt the morally fatalistic or "slippery slope" mentality that Susan Salladay described, I do think that everything we have said in this book speaks to the fact that we cannot be careful enough. What do we do? Do we create a moratorium? That response is not always possible, nor always good; but we do have to proceed with great vision and great care. The real question is: how do we perfect our vision? How do we give ourselves enough time to adequately discern these long-range effects?

In conclusion,we have many questions to answer and values to assess, but I am not pessimistic. I do believe in a Creator that in some way set forth this universe; but I also believe that *we* are called to be co-creators, and by that I mean we are to be instruments in transforming human life in the direction of wholeness and fulfillment. I believe that this requires that we be deeply and ethically absorbed in the profound meanings of what we are doing, and that we cultivate a spirit of contemplation—a contemplation that will put us truly in tune with our bodies and ourselves, our people and our universe.

Manipulative Reproductive Technologies Discussion

Part I

Moderated by Betty B. Hoskins

Claudia Card: Rosalind, you mentioned very quickly in talking about culture and storage of embryos that usually the female, except in humans, is sacrificed. Could you elaborate on that and explain why? That shocked me when you said it casually.

Rosalind Herlands: I didn't mean to be casual about it. I assume it's easier to keep a large stock of mice around, and just to do a cervical dislocation instead of performing sterile surgery and storing the mice. Some experimenters claim to get 75–80 eggs out of one female mouse.

Betty Hoskins: When we talk in lab jargon about "sacrifice" and "cervical dislocation," that distances us from our procedures. I think we usually have a different sense, perhaps *too* different a sense, of the lab animal and the human person. One of the reasons for the increasing use of tissue culture in biomedical research has been internal distress at the use of animals, even animals bred for study, and there has been a search for other sources of living forms to use in getting the information we want and need. But we do use up other living forms in order to get knowledge for our benefit, use, and curiosity.

Emily Culpepper: What are the implications of the massive use of experimental animals in all kinds of so-called "advanced specialized technologies?" What are the profound effects of removing ourselves, as a species, in our view of the world—of the cosmos, if you will—and distancing ourselves to the extent that we condone the torture of animals? And I'm not off into some naively sentimentalized view, but, besides my concern about what it is like to inflict this kind of pain, I wonder what it means about the mind set of the person and the profession that can do this, and how that carries over in ways that are not quantifiably measurable.

Susan Peterson: I don't think technical language does defuse the emotionally charged realities of medical practice. For instance, when I ask nursing students about the psychological protection afforded by technical language they say it doesn't work anyway. This may be because if you begin to use neutral word B instead of loaded word A, after a dozen times, all the meaning, impact, and emotion in word A just gets transferred over to word B anyway.

Elizabeth Kutter: I began working with bacterial viruses partly because of philosophical problems involving experimentation with animals. Now I've just spent the last five months at the University of California at Davis learning about nutrition, working with trace minerals and fetal development. They're doing important work with rats showing, for example, that a lack of zinc very early in pregnancy creates serious fetal abnormalities that persist.

This forced me to consider again the issues raised by animal experimentation. I think we need to focus on developing an atmosphere in which we first ask: Is the experimental question important enough and approachable enough at this point to justify using animals for it—and secondly, are the experiments being conducted humanely. I would answer "yes" to both questions at the lab I've just worked in, and yet I still couldn't do it. But raising these issues, for those of us who are in environments where animals are used, is extremely important.

Carol Korenbrot: Those of use who do study animals—and I study their behavior and their hormones—have other serious questions. There's a real problem when you're studying hormones in animals that are kept in confining environments. For instance, they're either put into solitary confinement or segregated according to sex even when they're not homosexual; they're made to live in crowded conditions; the food isn't what they normally eat and may have cockroaches in it. Those are not tortures, but what is the value of research in hormones if you change all their living conditions and their food?

Caroline Whitbeck: Let's consider the more general question of why some reproductive technologies are discussed (and funded) while others are ignored by our society in general. Cloning, for instance, gets a lot of attention. It is the final realization of a very old and popular masculine myth or theory of reproduction. You find this theory presented in Aristotle, and it recurs with variations throughout Western European thought. The theory is that the male provides the form (the genetic material), but the female provides no form (no genetic material) but only matter for the fetus. I call it the flower-pot theory of generation: the man provides the seed and the woman provides the dirt. In contrast to cloning, innovative uses of artificial insemination (insemination by donor), are rarely discussed (or funded). Now, this is a technology that *works,* and rather easily for human beings. (It may just take a few tries.) When I have raised the subject of the widespread use of donor insemination, that is, its use in cases other than male infertility, somebody usually gasps, "You're talking about the breakdown of society." But, of course, there were lots of societies that hadn't discovered paternity. If this technology were in widespread use, women would have the control of reproduction, but that seems only fair if we are to continue to bear the great majority of the responsibility for both child rearing and child bearing.

Barbara Menning: Artificial insemination by donor is a current, accepted technology. About ten to twenty thousand children are born of it every year, and heaven knows how many thousand children exist already. It is a kind of counseling I do daily in my work with infertility, although not everyone agrees with it. Perhaps that would be an even more valid case study—as an existing technology—than in vitro. The problems of artificial insemination are legal and social as well as technical; they deal with issues of male parent identification, and ownership of offspring of the male donor and surrogate father.

Janet Farrell Smith: The term 'artificial insemination' implies that the male is the active principle, the agent, while the female is the passive object upon which the act of insemination occurs. The term recalls the ancient Aristotelian biology of male principle giving "form" to the material supplied by the female. 'Artificial insemination' is artificial only because the male agent is not engaged in the act. But this account leaves out the female entirely, especially the fact that the natural process of conception occurs in the woman's body. What is 'artificial' about that? 'Artificial insemination' reflects a patriarchal, male-centered mode of thinking which in turn points to the fact that certain technologies are male controlled.

Diana Axelsen: Through the use of "surrogate mothers," an infertile woman who wants to raise her husband's biological child can do so without technology. Even with the consent of all three persons, and apart from issues regarding financial arrangements, such cases raise serious ethical issues about the nature of relationships, sexuality, and parenting. The *psychological* dynamics involved in deciding the preferred sex of a child, or in placing so much value on connections between biological parenthood and long-range nurturing, need to be examined more fully.

Sheryl Ruzek: I'm particularly perturbed at the comment that perhaps ethics is lodged in the unconscious. It seems to me that whether people decide *a priori* or *a posteriori* depends on where one is in a society and the historical context. Any ethical discussion must look at who has the power to impose their ethical view.

Susan Salladay: My point was not to equate ethics with the unconscious, but to remind us that moral decision-making includes unconscious dimensions that need to be looked at.

Ruth Hubbard: I think power and our unconscious are not separate. That's what "internalizing the oppressor" is about. Power determines what our unconscious tells us about the nature of reality. And as women who have internalized some, or even perhaps all, aspects of the oppressor, we are trying to become conscious of that fact. Obviously a great deal of that bringing into consciousness requires that we interpret the power relationships that have determined what we can and cannot do.

Karen Lebacqz: The elements of our own particular world view come to us from a number of different places. One of them is our position in the social structure, and in that we have to include such things as socioeconomic class and particular training. For example, those who are trained in our culture to be professionals usually have learned to adopt a quasi-scientific (if not scientific) world view. Though we are struggling to find alternative criteria for the validity of data, or the validity of knowledge, most of us here still seem to operate out of a basically scientific world view. We expect things to be presented to us in a verifiable form before we accept them as reality. That perception automatically suggests a link not only with our professional training, but also with the broader social and cultural values of our society. Ultimately what we need is an analysis of the shape of the age that gives us our cultural values, our professional training systems, and our very upbringing. For example, there's no one in this room who didn't have a mother at some time, and our mothers and that generation were different from us. Such forces influence what I call a person's basic perspective—or bias, or loyalty, or cathexis, if you will—out of which we analyze data, make our interpretations, decide which facts are morally relevant and which facts are not morally relevant. Looking at the exact same situation, we come out with radically different policy proposals and interpretations. Because all those things are in our subconscious, part of the task of ethics is to bring those things out. This is what we have been saying to each other: "Here are the values that we think have formed dominant interpretations in our society. Here are some alternative interpretations that come out of our own life histories, out of our own training, out of our own perspectives as women who have been involved in the Women's Movement." We have to bring out things that have been in an unreflective mode in order to engage in a dialog with each other.

Judy Norsigian: Our moral deliberations are connected with our ultimate actions—the policy recommendations we make, the things we do in our lives. And it's very clear to me that our moral deliberations are only a small part. At this conference I have heard women in academic settings who are extraordinarily threatened right now, who, when they speak what they really believe, will get fired. Clearly it's not going to be primarily their moral deliberations that determine what they say and do in their settings. I'm not blaming anyone for that. I'm saying this with sympathy. It doesn't matter what we believe in and what we think is ethical if, in the end, we're too afraid to do something about making what's ethical a reality because we'll lose our jobs.

I keep coming back to wanting to struggle more and more with settings like this, something very difficult when we're coming from different places. We need to begin in dialogs among ourselves. When we find positions we can agree upon, we need to find ways of taking political action and supporting one another so that if somebody acts as she believes and gets fired, the community will support her.

Judy Luce: I don't have as much concern about whether I or people I know are going to be afraid to take a stand as I do that no one's going to ask me what I think is right about what's happening. No one ever asked any of us whether it was right for Depo-Provera to be exported and used on Third World women. I feel that much energy and time can be put into making sure we make the pristine, pure ethical decision for ourselves, but that no one cares at all about what *we* think is ethical.

The Case Against In Vitro Fertilization And Implantation

Ruth Hubbard

One reason we must talk about in vitro fertilization is that it is a reality now. Two or three babies who were conceived in vitro and reimplanted into their mothers' uteruses have been born. As a society, we therefore must decide how we feel about this new technology and what should be done about it. In fact, a first decision has been made by the HEW Ethics Review Board; Robert Murray will later describe that decision and how it was made. I think that the decisions we come to in this instance and the mechanisms we develop in order to reach them are likely to have a bearing on future decisions and future processes of decision-making as other kinds of biotechnologies are contemplated or developed.

My personal history will help you to understand where I come from. I have never taken the "pill" or worn an IUD, though I've been heterosexually active from age eighteen through menopause. During my pregnancies, which predated the thalidomide disaster, I did not take any medicines or vitamins or other supplements beyond a regular balanced diet, except for a very rare aspirin for a headache. (What's worse for the baby, the headache or the aspirin?). Now, I did those things not because I am blessed with Cassandra's kind of foreknowledge, but because as a woman and as a biologist I have always had the utmost respect for the enormous intricacies of the workings of organisms. And I also have always had very little respect for the physical models we devise in order to try to understand and explain how biological organisms work. That is not to say that I do not use those models but rather that I know the models are vastly oversimplified. And therefore, when it comes to thinking about how a complex organism works, be it a person in her or his own life, or more especially a pregnant woman carrying a fetus, I have always felt that one ought to interfere as little as possible, and only when it is absolutely necessary in order to avoid severe pain or death. After all, embryonic development is the most complicated of biological processes, one in which an infinite number of reactions are taking place in intricate interrelationships, where timing and all kinds of factors in the chemical environment are fantastically important and split seconds or tiny changes in concentration can make a difference. So, coming from this perspective I frankly view with incredulity and horror the notion that one can "simply" remove an egg from a woman's ovary, put it in a culture medium in a dish, fertilize it, and let it go through the first few divisions, and then "simply" pick it up and re-insert it in a uterus that is at the proper stage of preparedness, and have it implant and go through development, without these many manipulations having some effect on the process of development. I cannot believe that there is no effect. This is an act of faith, or lack of faith, on my part, but I believe there must be an effect or, more likely, effects. How or when the effect will express itself is another question, or whether it will be overt and noticed.

Unfortunately, I see no way of answering these questions until there exists a statistically significant number of in vitro people so that one can look at their health patterns, and until they have been around for a long enough time (perhaps lived out their lives), so that one can compare their health and disease patterns to other people's. I see no way around the fact that every in vitro fertilization and implant, and every person who results from it, is an experiment and a different experiment: both the women who bear these babies and the babies-on-into-adults themselves are guinea pigs. Therefore I see the disasters that have resulted from the use of thalidomide, the pill, the Dalkon shield, DES, Depo-Provera—all disasters we have spoken about here, and all surely lesser interventions into normal physiological processes than in vitro fertilization and implantation—as probably rather minor compared to what we may be in for as a result of this new technology.

Now, having said this I must ask whether there are considerations that outweigh the terror I feel in looking at the future of this experiment. An issue that has been mentioned here is the notion that every woman has a right to bear a child. In fact, earlier Martha Mathis raised this question: does she have the right to a baby of the correct sex? There is an undercurrent in our society that implies that this is so, that these *are* "rights," or at least should be.

I first heard the expression that every woman has a "right" to have her own baby from Barbara Menning at the first of the occasions at which we both spoke. I had never thought of it that way until then. It had never occurred to me that every woman has a right to bear a baby any more than that every woman has a "right" to a 34 inch bustline or a 24 inch waist. I am not trying to trivialize the issue, but I had never thought of circumstances or events that have a strong biological component (as well as, of course, environmental ones) as describable in terms of "rights." So I have tried to think in what way it makes sense to say that every woman has a right to bear a child.[1] There is indeed a sense in which this is true, and that is that a great many, most, all women in this society grow up paying their dues. As girls and women, we are taught from earliest childhood that we cannot or may not do any number of things that we would like to do, be it play baseball, climb a tree, be king of the mountain, or whatever. Later, perhaps, our parents tell us that they cannot afford to send us to the same schools as our brothers, that we cannot study the same things, get the same kinds of jobs or promotions. And we are led to understand and accept that the reason for all this is because our rewards are different: we will grow up to marry and be mothers, to have children of our own. It seems to me that it is only in this context—of women paying their dues—that not being able to bear a child is in fact a real denial, a bargain unfulfilled.

Only in this sense can I understand the "right" to bear a child; but also in this sense the claim that in vitro fertilization is a way of fulfilling this right, is a reinforcement of the status quo. So, acknowledging the genuine hardships and sufferings of women who want children and cannot bear them, I question whether there is not some better way to help than to lead them down the garden path of in vitro fertilization, which I believe to be a path to disaster. Some strong, deep, feminist, consciousness raising might end up being far more therapeutic in the long run than broadening the scope of the technological fix. When I think of what coming to understand the force of my own internalized socialization did for me—and past age forty-five—I have the greatest respect for the changes in self-perception that become possible in the right social circumstances. (How to become able to act on those insights brings up a whole set of other questions, perhaps to be discussed at some future conference.)

Let's talk a little about reinforcing the status quo: Having thought these thoughts, to me the blatant proof that this technology will not liberate women by offering them new options—and a decision that appalls me—is that the recommendations from the Ethics Review Board to the Secretary of HEW include that this procedure can only be used for a couple within the legal state of matrimony. And the first clinic in this country that is opening in Virginia lists as its first qualification that to be a candidate for in vitro fertilization, a woman must be married and want a child as part of that marriage. Now, if this is a technology to liberate women and put them in possession of a natural right, then what does the holy state of matrimony have to do with it? To have this technology immediately coupled with patriarchal definitions of where and when and how childbearing must be carried out gives the show away.

This brings me to my next point. Besides being worried about the health risks, I am also very concerned because this is an extremely complicated technology that involves many steps. It therefore is hard to demystify and requires highly skilled professionals. There is no way to put this technology into the control of the women who are going to be exposed to it, or of their support systems. It really locks women and their babies into the high-technology medical system: it requires that the women and their babies be monitored from before conception through birth, and probably that the children be surveyed through life. I have read that Drs. Steptoe and Edwards, the men who produced two of the in vitro babies—and it isn't clear whether they are the doctors' babies or the families', certainly in terms of the publicity they have generated—made each woman promise to have an abortion if the doctors felt it should be done. (Though I am dedicated to a woman's right to choose, I am not for giving that right over to doctors or scientists.) For these women and their babies, the process of gestation was monitored all along the way. But we have already seen in this conference that all the technologies used to monitor pregnancy themselves involve hazards. Therefore, what I am saying is that these women from the start become locked into subservience to the professional establishment in a way that I find impossible to interpret as an increase in reproductive freedom, rights, or choices.

The final issue—and a major one—is that this is an expensive technology that requires highly skilled professionals and costly equipment. We must remember that we are talking about it in a context in which, as we have heard, poor women with minimal access to minimal health care are being sterilized or otherwise coerced into *not* having babies they want and can have, while women who can pay are encouraged to participate in the expensive and risky technology of in vitro fertilization.

In Defense of In Vitro Fertilization

Barbara Menning

It is important to understand the magnitude of the problem of infertility. It is estimated that 10 million Americans are currently infertile. Of that number, one third have problems related to the woman and one third of those are problems relating to the Fallopian tubes. The Fallopian tubes of the woman might be described as the most vulnerable point in her reproductive system. Even the slightest inflammation or infection in this area may result in partial or complete blockage owing to scarring and adhesions, or may cause damage to the cilia that transport the ovum or to the biochemical secretions so vital to fertilization. Although modern surgical techniques and microsurgery have improved the success of surgical repair of the Fallopian tubes, this is still successful only 30% of the time. This means, of the 1 million women who have serious tubal disease, 700,000 cannot be helped to become pregnant by *this* means, at this time. I will first comment on in vitro fertilization (IVF), in terms of who decides, screening of candidates, risk, and the issue of technological remedies for technologically related infertility. I will then discuss the general matter of infertility in more personal terms.

I am tired of hearing that the technology of in vitro fertilization should not be researched and developed as a safe alternative for infertile women. It is invariably stated by women and men who have achieved their families, or celibate clergy for whom it is not an issue. At the Ethics Advisory Board hearings it was amazing how many "right to lifers" and other witnesses stood up and gave among their credentials the number of children they had borne, as if to add credibility to their testimony. In my opinion, and in the opinion of other infertile women, the fact that they had achieved their families *disqualified* them from any understanding of the pain of childlessness. Pro-choice advocates are inconsistent if they are willing to apply technology for contraception and for abortion, but not for procreation. It smacks of eugenics to suggest that "not all people were meant to bear children" or that infertility is Nature's Way of selecting people out of the genetic pool.

On the matter of *informed consent,* couples desiring in vitro fertilization are going to be screened so rigorously that there is no danger of inappropriate application of this technology. If anything, the screening is highly restrictive. At the Norfolk, Va., clinic that began accepting IVF candidates in early 1980, the following are requirements: maternal age under 35 years, excellent fertility and general health, except for a hopeless tubal situation; a couple must be married to each other, and must be able to pay $3000 out-of-pocket expenses for the procedure.

With respect to *risk*, I am satisfied that in vitro puts the recipient couple no more at risk for the usual maternity risks than the average population. We have discussed risks in depth at this conference and have accepted the following as facts of life: 15% of all pregnancies will end in miscarriage; 3% of all pregnancies will result in perinatal death; and 5% of liveborn children will have a congenital defect. There is no reason to expect the in vitro conception to escape these risk factors. One thing is sure: the couples who are infertile owing to hopeless tubal damage run a 100% risk of remaining childless if they are not allowed access to in vitro fertilization as a technology. It has been said here repeatedly, "Let those who will incur the risk make the decisions about the technology." I repeat that mandate for you now. Let those of us who are infertile decide whether we are willing to subject ourselves to the instrumentation and intervention necessary to unite ovum and sperm and reimplant the conceptus in our bodies. Let *us* make informed consent, since we will incur the risks.

I think technology owes infertile couples this option known as in vitro fertilization, since they have often been victims of other technologies: the Dalkon Shield; sepsis after abortion; coerced sterilization; salpingitis or pelvic inflammatory disease following use of any IUD. We can add to the growing list of man-made causes of infertility: DES, Depo-Provera, and exposure to chemical toxins and nuclear radiation.

Now, I will turn my attention to infertility in general. It hurts to be infertile, to make the conscious and informed choice to have children and then to be denied. As I listened to the midwives discussing their birth histories and the birthings they have attended, I felt an old familiar ache reawaken in me. I have been a midwife too—for two years in the Peace Corps, in Afghanistan. Unfortunately, the birthings there were not usually peaceful and beautiful; the women were too young, were malnourished, and had no prenatal education. They entered their labors in terror of dying, a terror based on reality. I have taught maternity nursing in America. Each time I saw a birth or conducted a birth, I did so thinking, "One day this will happen for me." It was never a question of *whether*, just *when*.

When I was married at 27 I tried almost immediately to achieve a pregnancy. What followed were four years so filled with medical and surgical mayhem that they are remembered mercifully blurred. I will not recount the particular details of my infertility struggle—just a brief summary of events: I underwent a year of testing biopsies, uterotubograms, post-coitals; my husband also had repeated tests. We had a programmed sex life keyed to a basal temperature chart. At the end of that year an acute abdominal episode, improperly handled, cost me the ovary and tube on the right side. After recovery from surgery, on to a new doctor—more tests, more programmed sex life—everything was just fine, "relax." Relaxing did no good. On to a new doctor. Discovery of a cyst on the left ovary—resection by surgery. Six months later, success. Pregnancy—followed by miscarriage at 13 weeks. On to another doctor—an activist. "We'll have you pregnant again in no time!" Emergency admission to the hospital after an acute reaction to the fertility pills he prescribed. My cycles ceased. The best efforts of men and their medicine could not coax another cycle forth. At 31 I experienced menopause owing to the surgical and medical assault on my ovaries.

If it is painful to hear these things, then I am getting my message across. This experience *changed* me. It radicalized me. For a while I felt very much a victim. I became a whole person again when I realized I had to stop feeling like a victim. I had to stop reacting to my own pain and sorrow and start a purposeful course of action to help others.

I founded an organization called RESOLVE from my kitchen table in 1973. Our purpose is to offer counseling, advocacy, and support to infertile people. We believe the best consumer is an informed consumer, so we publish a bimonthly Newsletter and many fact sheets on aspects of infertility. We survey doctors who claim to be "infertility specialists" every year and publish our list of recommended specialists in a state-by-state Directory. Last year only 260 doctors in the country met our criteria for inclusion in the Directory. Most important, RESOLVE gives infertile people a way to find each other so they can share feelings and experience. Since infertility is so *invisible,* most infertile couples believe themselves to be "all alone" and cannot identify the 10 million others who are all around them. Our support groups for women and couples are a way people can validate each others' feelings and problem-solve their way to solutions. Defining technology as "application of knowledge to solve problems," this is *our* technology—software, not hardware.

From these humble beginnings, we have grown to a national organization with a membership of over 3000 couples and chapters in 30 cities. Recently, we received half of a $100,000 grant from DHEW to collaborate with a model infertility clinic and do trainings in the New England area. This award was one of only four made in the country. HEW has defined infertility as a family planning problem only since 1976, and in 1980 the $1 million it funded to infertility services represented less than 1% of the 147 million dollar family planning budget. Clearly, if 15% of the population is infertile, more equitable funding must be given to infertility services in the future.

The infertile person needs advocacy for a number of reasons. Gynecology is still predominately male and the infertile woman is often brutalized by a patronizing and patriarchal system. The terminology of infertility is revealing: blighted ovum, incompetent cervix, infantile uterus, habitual aborter—and that most outrageous of all infertility conditions, *hostile cervical mucus.*

The infertile person may become vulnerable to exploitation through her very desperation to achieve pregnancy. I am *not* overly concerned about exploitation with in vitro fertilization, as I have expressed. But I am concerned about a lot of real and present risks that the infertile woman may be unwittingly subjected to:

1. The infertile woman who achieves pregnancy is always termed "high risk." She is carrying what doctors love to call a precious pregnancy. She is at risk for close monitoring via ultrasound and all the new birth technology and monitoring. We estimate the C-section rate of infertile women to be almost double that of the national average—about 40%.

2. Many believe that infertile women are at risk for not bonding with their babies, whether conceived after great effort or adopted after great effort. It has something to do with unrealistic expectations of what that child can and will possibly do for them. There has been a push at RESOLVE for post partum and post adoption women's groups to share these concerns.

3. Infertile women are at risk for health problems secondary to their cause of infertility: in DES exposure, the risk of cancer follows; Depo-Provera exposure brings the possible risk of immunologic impairment. In endometriosis is the risk of hysterectomy, and in case of surgical menopause the risk of estrogen replacement therapy exists.

4. Finally—and this may be most important—there is the unmeasurable risk of impairment in something I call the "quality of life." Personal self-esteem and joy may be hopelessly compromised by a diagnosis of infertility. Who knows what destructive palliatives, such as alcohol and drugs, are used to ease the daily despair of childlessness? Who knows the divorce rates, the suicide rates, the rate of mental

breakdown for infertile women? I await these figures with a sure dread that they are worse than any of us imagine.

Katsi Cook mentioned the native American woman as being the miner's canary. Do you all understand that metaphor? I will take her metaphor one step further. I think the reproductive organs are the miner's canary of the human species. When our miscarriage rate approaches 40% in some areas near illegal chemical waste dumps and nuclear reactors; when our children are born defective not in the 5% range, but in the range of 25% where agent orange has been sprayed; when our infertility rate approaches 20% in the 1980s—then I think we as a species are in deep trouble.

On a more optimistic note, women ought to share with each other their strategies for success in their personal and professional lives, and I have three to share:

1. When I felt I was a "victim" I was by definition vulnerable and controlled. By being in a *reaction* mentality, I was like the knee jerk reflexively following the hammer. Society is full of hammers—it can leave any one of us twitching reflexively for the rest of our lives. Instead I suggest that a person ought to set a course of purposeful action—carve out a territory and work hard. Refuse to be sidetracked or attenuated by reflex reaction to unrelated issues: confine your area of effort to a manageable size. I am taking care of infertility issues the best I can so you won't *have* to.

2. As for power, I used to believe that men had it all and, of course, they *did*, since I ascribed it to them. I no longer believe that. In my area of expertise I believe that *I* have the power to make change. Since I believe it, it has become true. You have it too, and together we can work wonders with our collective power.

3. Finally, we women are the caretakers and nurturers of this Good Earth and of its women and children. We must be *vigilant*. We must pay attention, listen carefully and overlook nothing. I will close with a favorite quotation from Adrienne Rich:

This eye
is not for weeping
its vision
must be unblurred
though tears are on my face
its intent is clarity
it must forget
nothing.

"From the Prison House," *Diving into the Wreck,* 1973, W. W. Norton & Co., Inc., New York.

In Vitro Fertilization and Embryo Transfer

The Process of Making Public Policy

Robert F. Murray, Jr.

INTRODUCTION

The public policy generated with respect to research and application of in vitro fertilization and embryo transfer in the United States grew out of the interaction of several elements. A major contributor to the process was the Ethics Advisory Board to the Secretary of the Department of Health, Education and Welfare (HEW). This body of eleven men and two women sought to consider the broad range of opinion and fact that existed on the topic and, using the perspective and background of its members, to arrive at recommendations for the implementation of this new reproductive technology. My objective is to present briefly the elements of the procedure used and some of the rationales for the recommendations and conclusions finally made by this board, of which I am a member.

BACKGROUND

The Ethics Advisory Board was established to advise the Secretary of HEW with respect to the ethics of current and proposed departmental research and other activities including missions, programs, agency assignments, or procedures that are reviewed, supported, conducted, sponsored, monitored, or regulated by the department, or which may involve the department directly or indirectly. In addition, the Board may initiate inquiries, hold hearings, conduct public meetings or symposia, or deploy other means for developing an appropriate recommendation to the Secretary.

The Board spent its first two meetings reviewing the range of ethical dilemmas that presented themselves to the various agencies of the Department of Health, Education, and Welfare. During this period, the announcement by Dr. Edwards and Mr. Steptoe in England of the imminent birth of Baby Louise Brown, conceived by in vitro fertilization and embryo transfer, hit the public press and media. The birth of the baby on July 25, 1978, led to a flurry of discussion in various governmental agencies and the Houses of Congress. At the same time, attention was focused on an application for research that involved in vitro fertilization without embryo transfer that had been submitted by Dr. Pierre Soupart three years earlier,[1] and had been waiting for the establishment of an Ethics Advisory Board to review its ethical acceptability.[2] HEW Secretary Califano directed the Board to consider the questions that "reached to our most profound moral and ethical beliefs," including (1) whether techniques of in vitro fertilization and transplantation of the embryo might damage the fetus and lead to abnormal children; (2) whether this research might lead to selective breeding and attempts to control the genetic makeup of offspring; (3) or, whether rich men might pay poor women to carry their children, leading to the use of "surrogate parents"; (4) whether the researchers or the supporters of these researchers might be legally liable for defects produced in a child conceived in the course of such research. The Secretary also directed the Board to emphasize public participation in the decision-making process by holding public hearings in each of the ten HEW regions to stimulate a national debate on the subject.

The Ethics Advisory Board was already considering an impressive array of ethical problems that existed in HEW. Were it not for the Secretary's memo and the Board's desire to be of assistance to the Secretary, it probably would not have chosen this issue as the first on its agenda. Nevertheless, it proceeded to tackle this problem, beginning with hearings in September of 1978 and continuing through to its final approval of the report and recommendations and conclusions in March of 1979.

COMPOSITION OF THE BOARD

The same information assessed by a group of individuals with drastically differing outlooks and philosophies from those reflected on the Board would possibly have yielded significantly different conclusions and recommendations. The Board, throughout these deliberations, consisted of 13 members: 11 male and two female.[3] Had this reproductive issue been in mind at the time of its development, additional female members might well have been appointed to the Board. Thus one serious criticism of the Board's perspective was focused on the fact there there were really too few female members if one considered the nature of the problem that the Board was addressing. The issue of appropriate sexual representation on policymaking boards is, of course, one that is extremely controversial and one that I will not attempt to address further here. The members of the Board consist of theologians, lawyers, physicians (of which there are seven), and a philosopher. One of the female members of the Board is an ethicist and the other has a degree in law, but is currently not practicing. Only one of the physicians involved could be considered a practicing physician; the others are from academic institutions.

GATHERING INFORMATION AND OPINION

At monthly meetings the Board heard expert witnesses representing both sides of the issues dealing with the state of the art of in vitro fertilization and embryo transfer, the ethical issues involved that grow out of the application of this technology in research and practice, and the public policy issues that would arise from the approval of research by DHEW and the support of research by this department.[4]

Another critical element in the process of evaluating the relative significance of these issues is the selection of the "experts" who testify. I believe that the points of view presented to the Board were relatively well balanced. All hearings were public. As time went on, greater and greater interest developed so that, toward the end of the hearings and deliberations of the Board, newspapers, magazines, radio, and television were heavily represented. All members of the Board were interviewed numerous times; most tried not to give definitive opinions.

In addition to hearings from expert witnesses, the Board received more than 2000 pieces of written comments from the public. Most of the Board members attempted to review a representative sample of it. Staff members reviewed all of this correspondence and reported on especially salient or imaginative comments or criticisms. One hundred seventy-nine (179) individuals presented oral testimony in hearings in Bethesda, Maryland; Boston, Seattle, San Francisco, Atlanta, Kansas City, Detroit, Philadelphia, Denver, Dallas, and New York City. Eighteen people submitted formal written testimony in lieu of oral presentations. An attempt was made to have at least one Board member present at every public hearing so that they might be able to question the witnesses in order to be certain that the points that each witness was making were clear on the record. There was a clear difference in the positions of the witnesses from various regions of the country on these issues. For example, in the Northeastern part of the country, witnesses tended to favor going ahead with research into in vitro fertilization as well as in vitro fertilization with embryo transfer. On the other hand, in the Midwest and Southwest, witnesses tended to oppose the further development of both technologies. Of course, the witnesses who presented testimony at these hearings might not be representative of the attitudes among *all* the people in that region.

Both the Gallup and Harris survey organizations conducted polls in which they sampled the opinion of the American public, especially American women. In the Gallup survey, 60% of men and women were in favor of using the technique and those who clearly understood the technique were more likely to approve it (75%) than those who did not understand it. Most women in the Harris survey wanted this technique prohibited until testing had established that it is safe; they also opposed federal funding of such research. However, eighty-five percent of the women in the Harris poll felt that the procedure should be available for couples who were otherwise unable to have children. Both polls indicated that from 53 to 58 percent of women of childbearing age might consider using in vitro fertilization, if necessary. On the other hand, most women surveyed in the Harris poll said that they would prefer adoption to in vitro fertilization if they were unable to have children. Only a small percentage, about 25%, wanted in vitro fertilization to be used immediately before further testing had established its safety.

The Board found significant differences of opinion among the scientific community. Some reputable researchers recommended that further research be conducted immediately. Furthermore, the very high frequency of chromosome and other birth defects that normally occur during the process of fertilization and in early embryonic development suggests that embryos damaged by this procedure would probably not survive throughout pregnancy, but would be spontaneously aborted. It was also clear that there was a paucity of legal opinion on the status of the human embryo and that eventually court action would have to determine its "human" status.

DELIBERATIONS AND CONCLUSIONS

There was a clear difference of opinion among Board members with respect to some of the issues that were discussed. Initially it appeared that there might have to be two or even three minority reports prepared because of these differences in opinion. However, as Board members began to consider the implications of various actions or inactions, there evolved a broad consensus that enabled it to submit to the Secretary a single report. In the full report submitted to the Secretary, the Board found four critical issues that strongly influenced the conclusions and recommendations it reached. These were: (1) the moral status of the embryo, (2) the safety and efficacy of the procedures, (3) the potential long-range adverse effects of such research, and (4) the appropriateness of support by DHEW.

Conclusion 1: The Department should consider support of carefully designed research involving in vitro fertilization and embryo transfer in animals, including nonhuman primates, in order to obtain a better understanding of the process of fertilization, implantation, and embryo development, to assess the risks to both mother and offspring associated with such procedures, and to improve the efficacy (efficiency) of the procedure.

Conclusion 2: The Ethics Advisory Board found it acceptable from an ethical standpoint to undertake research involving human in vitro fertilization and embryo transfer provided that: (A) If the research involved human in vitro fertilization without embryo transfer, the following conditions are satisfied: (1) The research complies with all research provisions of the regulations governing research with human subjects (45 CFR 46). (2) The research is designed primarily: (a) to establish the efficacy of embryo transfer, and (b) to obtain important scientific information toward the end not reasonably obtainable by other means. (3) Human gametes used in such research will be obtained exclusively from persons who have been informed of the nature and purpose of the research in which such materials will be used and have specifically consented to such use. (4) No embryos will be sustained in vitro beyond the stage normally associated with the completion of implantation (14 days after fertilization). (5) All interested parties and the general public will be advised if evidence begins to show that the procedure entails risks of abnormal offspring higher than those associated with natural human reproduction. (B) In addition, if the research involves embryo transfer following human in vitro fertilization, embryo transfer will be attempted only with embryos formed from gametes obtained from lawfully married couples.

Conclusion 3: The Board found it ethically acceptable for the Department to support or conduct research involving human in vitro fertilization and embryo transfer provided that the applicable conditions are met. However, the Board decided not to address the question of the level of funding, if any, that such research might be given.

Conclusion 4: The National Institutes of Child Health and Human Development (NICHD) and other appropriate agencies should work with professional societies, foreign governments, and international organizations to collect, analyze, and disseminate information derived from research, in both animals and humans, and from clinical experience throughout the world, involving in vitro fertilization and embryo transfer.

Conclusion 5: The Secretary should encourage the development of a uniform or model law to clarify the legal status of children born as a result of in vitro fertilization and embryo transfer. To the extent that funds may be necessary to develop such legislation, the department should consider providing appropriate support.

The Ethics Advisory Board is only, as its name indicates, advisory to the Secretary of HEW. Only actions taken by the Secretary can determine whether or not the outcome of the work of this Board will become public policy. In the final analysis, the reaction of the public-at-large should finally determine whether these policies are acceptable and are in the best interest of American citizens, especially women who wish to have children.

The Board did not resolve all the issues that were raised in its deliberations, nor did it expect to. Many of these issues will require further research and discussion, as well as further consideration by members of the public before they can have any kind of meaningful resolution. The fact that there has been no further success with this new technology in the past several months suggests that a great deal more understanding of the details of the reproductive process is needed before we will be able to say that in vitro fertilization with embryo transfer is a safe, reliable and acceptable reproductive technique.

Manipulative Reproductive Technologies Discussion

Part II

Moderated by Betty B. Hoskins

Sandra Sewell: Is the method of in vitro fertilization used in this country? I ask that because with this method and without enough data compiled, how will you deal with parents who end up with "imperfect" babies? If you counsel people for this process, is it your responsibility to deal with its possible failure?

Barbara Menning: RESOLVE does not offer medical services. RESOLVE is a counseling, referral, and support mechanism only. I don't expect to do a lot of in vitro counseling in the next five years. But I will deal with that as I dealt with any other issue surrounding choices of adoption, donor insemination, childfree living, in vitro—four legitimate choices. The responsibility rests with the couple to make a decision they can live with. I acquaint them with risks and benefits. I am an information source only. I do not impart values.

Sandra Sewell: But, when people are advocating these technological methods to have children, how do you deal with parents not coming out with a "perfect" baby?

Barbara Menning: I would handle that in the same way as I would with any couple who have a child that isn't perfect. They would have an option to come for counseling or we would refer them to an appropriate resource. The people who usually do this kind of counseling are the medical providers, whether you like it or not.

Carol Korenbrot: In adding another technique for gaining fertility, mightn't you be raising more false hopes and perhaps hurting as many people as are helped? The IVF technique is not very successful yet—the percentages of success are still very low; improved technology may raise that percentage somewhat, but the technique is never going to be perfect. It could result in some defective children, or fail completely to provide children for some people.

Barbara Menning: I guess we're just asking for the right to add it to our "cafeteria of choices." That phrase has been used for contraceptives. I think IVF should be among the choices available for procreation.

Emily Culpepper: I'm concerned that the statement "every woman has the right to a child" blurs the distinction between one's desire to parent or mother and one's desire to bear a child—I'd like to stress the alternatives such as adoption. Justifying in vitro fertilization and all of the possible abuses that go along with it in order to focus on having the biological route to motherhood does not add up for me. I don't for a moment take away from the pain of not having that experience of birthing, but that's not the same, you know, as not being able to mother and to raise and rear a child. I feel that's a really important distinction.

Barbara Menning: Among the people I counsel, and myself, there is a real pain in not being able to bear a child when you wish. Most of what I grieved was the loss of the ability to have a pregnancy experience. I have a parenting experience, a beautiful one. I have three beautiful children. I have found another way to have my family. Not everyone goes on to adopt a family; not everyone wishes to. As you know, it's very difficult to adopt.

Emily Culpepper: Right. And not everyone feels that they can bond with the child if they did not give birth to it. But I don't think I'm comfortable with statements that say we all have a right to certain things that are within one way of stating our biological capabilities. Does everyone have a right to a certain IQ? Or, can we justify rigid, forced training programs to produce certain sorts of athletic children? That sounds like fetishization of specifically biological traits such as reproducing against which I weigh all the accompanying abuses of risks of IVF. A pregnancy experience may not happen, but mothering and parenthood can happen.

Robert Murray: The legal analyses presented to us [the Advisory Board] stated that strong support might be developed for a constitutional right to reproduce by means of in vitro fertilization. That is to say, we often justify rights from the so-called natural rights standpoint, but from a legal standpoint a strong argument could be made for the constitutional right to procreate.

Elaine Locke: I'd like to make one distinction without attempting to define "rights." I think intuitively you might agree with me that there's a difference between the right to have or bear a child and the right to *want* to bear a child. Ruth Hubbard's ascription of a motivation to women who want to have a child, suggesting that it's a payoff for the insult of being a girl, is probably not accurate. Men who want to have a biological child certainly don't have that same reason. Finally, I'm a little concerned about the idea that consciousness raising is a better remedy than trying to find a way to have a child. I think women who have expected to become pregnant and do not usually consider their motives for having a child at great length. By comparison people who become pregnant much more quickly may not have considered their motives for wanting a child.

Tabitha Powledge: The Ethics Board sidestepped the issue of funding level. Was that part of a compromise solution?

Robert Murray: Yes, that was definitely a compromise. Some people felt that it would be unethical to approve research on this technique without funding. Other people felt that we could say to the Secretary, "We think that this research is ethically acceptable, but that it shouldn't be funded, because, on an ethical basis, we feel that its priority in terms of the general welfare is so low that HEW's money should not be used for this." There were others who felt we were not in any position to set priorities for HEW.

Tabitha Powledge: That means that a number of members of the Board didn't see allocation of scarce resources as an ethical issue.

Robert Murray: Some of them didn't and they were very persuasive.

Janice Raymond: Could you clarify either my interpretation of the Board's logic, or the Board's logic itself on limiting such research, in humans, to married couples? Would you say that members of the Board thought that in vitro fertilization was an unnatural process to begin with? Did the stipulation of including it within the constraint of marriage make it more natural? Or was that a compromise measure?

Robert Murray: The two were quite separate issues. People critical of the technology, including clergy, deemed it unnatural. The Board's reason for restricting the technology to married couples was based on legal criteria. Since there are legal ambiguities about the status of children so conceived and born, those children would be classified as legally "illegitimate" if born outside of marriage; therefore, the technique should be restricted to married couples.

Caroline Whitbeck: What is supposed to be the value in knowing paternity? We get strong *prima facie* evidence for paternity with legitimacy. Rousseau wrote that it is absolutely essential to ensure that the husband's paternity is assured. He argued that it would be the worst fraud if a man financially supported children who were not "his own." This obsession with paternity invariably leads to a double standard of sexual behavior and punishment of the children who are labeled "illegitimate." Historically, this concern with paternity and legitimacy has been extremely destructive. Although I've argued that male infants particularly should have at least some of their nurturing from a male, we see that paternity in this culture has *nothing at all* to do with providing nurturance for an infant. What then is the advantage of a system that safeguards paternity? Why should the state have an interest in reducing illegitimacy?

Susan Salladay: What in the Board's eyes makes a child legitimate? Did the Board see that, in accepting a particular definition of legitimacy and in sanctioning this particular social policy, they were in fact defining a certain kind of morality for our pluralistic society?

Robert Murray: The Board did not wrestle with the concept of legitimacy or illegitimacy. There is a legal definition of legitimacy or illegitimacy. We had nothing to say about that definition or its status. The Board listened to public testimony at 10 sites, read letters, and heard legal analysis in order to recommend policy. Acting within the context of our society, the Board said the government has an interest in fostering marriage and in discouraging illegitimacy however defined.

Susan Salladay: Did the Board question the concept of legitimacy it reinforced or advocated?

Robert Murray: I believe that concept is a fiction. There's no such thing. The word has no meaning. Every child is legitimate. But our society recognizes a legal definition and the Board, in the process of making public policy, had to recognize that definition. If any Board members were asked if they believe that children should be considered illegitimate, they would probably say no. But our society says, yes. And we have to operate in the context of our society *now*. If we took it on ourselves to say that we should try to change society we should resign from the Board.

Ruth Hubbard: In the process of trying to set up an ethical or quasi-ethical situation about a new procedure for which new definitions have to be made (and I think that's the context we're wrestling with), if we're talking about in vitro fertilization, why do we have to do it in the context of the holy bond of matrimony?

Judy Norsigian: What might have happened if members of the Board had said that they would not mention anything about marriage because they felt it was inappropriate?

Robert Murray: The committee recommended that a model law be developed. In that context the legal concept of illegitimacy would have to be addressed. But our legal system deals with the old by establishing new precedents. If you're suggesting that we change our whole legal system that's quite another issue. I'm saying that we as a Board are there to provide the Secretary with policies that he can use. And he has to operate within the legal framework of our society.

Julie Melrose: Something happened here a little while ago that was passed over as a small incident, but I feel that it touched on a central issue in the making of public policy concerning women.

Right after Barbara Menning's presentation, Robert Murray commented that he wasn't going to pull at anyone's heart-strings. I assume that was a reference to Barbara's presentation, which included some very painful details of her life. Although I don't agree with everything Barbara said, I believe it takes real courage—particularly in a setting like this—for a woman to speak openly about her life and what is done to women in this society by the medical establishment. Time and time again, women who dare to tell the truth about their lives are accused of telling sob-stories, but are never really heard. I'm very uncomfortable with the idea of a man who would reduce a woman's act of truth-telling to "pulling at heart-strings" being in a position to make public policy that affects the lives of individual women.

Robert Murray: I didn't mean it that way; I'm sorry that you misinterpreted what I said. I think that Barbara understood that my remarks were not intended to criticize her presentation or to put her down. I merely intended to point out that my presentation of public policy would be rather dull, dry, or even boring in contrast to Barbara's poignant and very moving talk based on her painful personal experience. I have the greatest respect for Barbara, what she is doing, and what she stands for.

Elizabeth Kutter: What is the make-up of the Board in terms of women?

Robert Murray: Two women: the ethicist Sissela Bok and a lawyer, Agnes Williams. That's two out of fourteen. Now the Board can go up to twenty members, and I have a strong feeling that some of the additional members will be women. The problem is not the number of women, but who *are* the women and what are *their* attitudes. None of the people on the Board could be classified as anywhere near grass-roots, in terms of their current status, although some of us had come from there, and still maintain ties there.

Barbara Menning: Are there any infertile people on the Advisory Board?

Robert Murray: No.

Barbara Menning: Why not?

Robert Murray: Certain classes of professionals were supposed to be represented on the Board. Infertile couples were not listed as one of them. We heard this issue among others to be considered, and it was not one we would have selected.

Gena Corea: The HEW Ethics Advisory Board is almost entirely composed of clergymen, physicians, and lawyers. When I saw that, I recalled that priests, doctors, and lawyers are what 19th century popular health activists had called The Devil's Trinity. The activists understood that by mystifying religion, healing, and the law, professionals made it difficult for common people to control their lives.

I think it is the Trinity of Satan that is involved here in this decision on in vitro fertilization—a decision that will so greatly affect women. With only two exceptions, the priests, doctors, and lawyers on the Ethics Advisory Board are men. These men, however unconsciously, will serve the interests of their own gender caste. The two token women were not included on the grounds that they are women and that women have a right to decide how their lives are lived. Being a woman is not enough. Just being a woman doesn't make you an expert on the moral aspects of your own procreative life. The two women needed male professional credentials in order to claim any right at all to help make these decisions. One woman was a lawyer; the other, an ethicist.

Another point: I value the contributions made by some of the professional ethicists here. At the same time, I cannot tell you how weird I find the notion that we should extract "ethics" from daily living and make a profession out of it. Ethical decision-making should be part of all our lives—not a function reserved for professionals. And I don't like the idea that the decisions of professional ethicists may be seen to have more validity than the decisions of ordinary people. Ethical decisions—like the supposedly disinterested "truths" promulgated by the Devil's Trinity—are often related to what sexual, racial, or class caste you belong to. Since those who have the readiest access to professional training tend to be white, middle or upperclass men, they end up giving ethical seals of approval to what others of their gender, race, and class decide, in their own best interests, to do.

The Biology of Utopia

Science Fiction Perspectives on Ectogenesis

Dennis Livingston

Science fiction is an important source for probing the interactions of science, technology, and society.[1] First, it is a laboratory of the imagination, offering the author a framework for carrying out a series of thought-experiments on the consequences of current or foreseeable trends and events. Science fiction does not so much make predictions as ask "what if" something should come to pass, with a range of answers bound only by the author's literary skill, imagination, and assumptions about human nature and social evolution. Though not usually written for didactic purposes, science fiction stories may be powerful heuristic models. As entertainment, they induce an empathetic response in readers provoked to consider the array of options open to humanity reflected in the plots of particularly compelling tales.

Second, many science fiction stories, though ostensibly set in the future or on other planets, are commentaries on our own society. With such tools as satire and metaphor to distance the reader from her own time and place, science fiction holds a mirror up to the present, reflecting in distorted or exaggerated form familiar human foibles. As with all good literature, the best science fiction provides us with new perceptions or questions to ask about the conventional wisdom.

Science fiction taps and gives modern expression to certain mythic themes that fuel the collective subconscious of human cultures. These include the origin of life and the universe, the just ordering of society, and the quest for knowledge about the meaning of life. Particularly prominent in science fiction are explorations of our hopes and fears about the Promethean forces unleashed by science and technology.

Finally, science fiction has a presumptive impact on the society from which it emerges. That is, science fiction *matters.* Most directly, it has influenced the career choices and aspirations of many individuals, including some of the most important innovators of this century. The options it helps clarify about social and technological futures may influence the boundaries of public debate on where we are or should be going as a society.

Each of these facets of science fiction is relevant to examining the topic of concern here, the implications of ectogenesis. Ectogenesis comprises the fertilization of an egg, nurturance of the zygote, and carrying of the fetus to term entirely by artificial means. Variations on this theme include implantation of an embryo back into the womb of the natural or a surrogate mother, or even a nonhuman mammal; manipulation of the genetic material of the zygote; and cloning or parthenogenesis.[2]

Science fiction, of course, has warned of the unanticipated outcome of biological experiments, ever since Doctor Frankenstein's man of parts wandered from the laboratory into a hostile world. Perhaps the recent spate of films on the havoc wrecked by devilish offspring (*Demon Seed, The Omen, Prophecy*) carry some symbolic message on the dangers of tampering with nature for fun and profit, but the message has not been developed with great sophistication. For this analysis, I have selected stories only for the acuteness of the comments they make on ectogenesis in the biomedical revolution. In particular, they address three overlapping questions: Why undertake ectogenesis in the first place? Can it be used by the state for purposes of social control? What impact might it have on women's role in society? Perhaps the most fascinating suggestion is that clones, possessing identical genetic heritages, could be used to carry out field tests in telepathy and other psychic research (as happens in Cowper's *Clone*[3]).

Stories that play on the theme of reproduction through cloning of particularly significant individuals illustrate other forces that might promote ectogenic research. The criteria of significance obviously varies according to whomever is in charge of the process. Thus, in what might be called the Daddy Warbucks hypothesis, a person of means decides that if he can't take it with him, he can at least leave it all to himself. David Rorvik's *In His Image*[4] features, according to the paperback jacket, "'Max'—worldly, self-educated, aging millionaire who was determined to have a direct male descendent—but could find no woman fit to be the mother." He then finances the development of his clone by the scientist "Darwin," who places the zygote in "'Sparrow'—the gentle 17-year old native virgin who . . . would come to mean more to Max than he ever dreamed possible."

More ominously, 93 little Hitlers are placed in different families around the world by an unrepentant Nazi doctor in Levin's *The Boys From Brazil*[5] in the hope that one or more of them will turn out to be chips off the old block. Similarly, in LeGuin's 'Nine Lives"[6] a dead, multitalented genius is the source of a "ten-clone," a set of males and females sent as a team of planetary engineers to a distant world. The major advantage of this group of bisexual clones over "singletons" is their ability to function as an efficient, self-sufficient group, each of whose members has total peer support from the others and knowledge of each others' abilities. On a more speculative note, clones might be used to replenish the planetary gene pool or increase the population following some global catastrophe[7].

The role of an authoritative group—usually the state—in setting the rules for the use of reproductive technology is more explicit in plots that deal with eugenics. Negative eugenics is already with us in the form of prenatal genetic screening and counseling. A step beyond this would be governmentally mandated screening and appropriate corrective measures enforced by a public agency in order to improve the quality of the population by eliminating hereditary defects or carrying out such genetic repair as science makes feasible.

The coercive potential in the nonvoluntary application of negative eugenics is often stressed in stories that link such procedures with governmental licensing of the right to reproduce. Even more controversial in this context is positive eugenics, attempts to improve the genetic quality of the race by enhancing particular physical and mental abilities supposedly dependent on one's genes. Thus, in *The Eyes of Heisenberg*[8] Frank Herbert's "submolecular engineers" in the far future engage in gene shaping within the zygote, following in vitro fertilization. Their purpose is to work for the creation of "optimen," the immortal elite who run the society. A contraceptive gas enables these rulers to allow the breeding of only those couples that they choose. The English author John Brunner has treated this concept with telling effect in several of his novels.[9] In *The Shockwave Rider,* the US government secretly engages in genetic research, callously creating and destroying embryos and deformed children developed in experiments to enhance intelligence. The same purpose is given to an Asian country in *Stand on Zanzibar*; its efforts threaten to set off a "genetic race" among countries skeptical of its claims of success, but wary of conceding it a lead in the creation of a possible superrace. This book is also one of the few to acknowledge that genetic manipulation is available to many countries outside the West and could become one more source of contention in an already overburdened international system.

But is it possible to promote specific human qualities, in contrast to inhibiting disease or deformities, by genetic engineering, inside or outside the womb? Could the state, or any other group, create human beings behaviorally matched to fit its own perceived needs, thereby maintaining control over the population to a degree unknown in history? The fear that this might someday be the case has provided a pervasive theme in science fiction, at least since the Director of the Central London Hatchery and Conditioning Center took a class of schoolboys on a tour through his facilities in the opening scenes of Huxley's *Brave New World.*[10] In this classic model of better living through chemistry, the individual is literally designed to fit pre-established occupational categories. Both the heredity and physical environment of embryos are controlled, by adjusting oxygen content, temperature, and the like, to meet the intelligence and skill requirements of the job castes. The Director notes that after they leave the Social Predestination Room, "We decant our babies as socialized human beings."

This vision is part of the larger tradition of dystopian (anti-utopian) fiction in which technology is used by the totalitarian state to subject the individual to the whim of a ruling class in which he or she has no role. As one scholar has put it, it is the "synthesization of experience" that this situation represents that so awakens our apprehensions. The variety and plurality of human experience that mold personalities are to be suppressed in the name of efficiency and order by ensuring the conformity of every individual to an artificially constructed prenatal and social environment. History ends in the test tube.[11]

Thus, society will be perfected by controlling the process of personality formation and, thereby, abolishing the individual's capacity to choose—or, more subtly, by manipulating the illusion of the capacity to choose. However, in contrast to the brutal police state techniques of Orwell's *1984,* the scenario of *Brave New World* and its imitators stresses the fact that people will be happy in their chosen slots and perfectly tailored for those slots. It is guaranteed, to the benefit of both individual and society. As the Hatchery Director says:

> "Bokanovsky's Process [a type of cloning] is one of the major instruments of social stability! . . . Ninety-six identical twins working ninety-six identical machines!" The voice was almost tremulous with enthusiasm. "You really know where you are. For the first time in history." He quoted the planetary motto. "Community, Identity, Stability." . . . "The principle of mass production at last applied to biology."[10]

Several decades later, a character in *The Boys From Brazil* echoes this sentiment with regard to cloning:[5]

> What planned society could resist the idea? Multiply your superior citizens and prohibit the inferior ones from reproducing. Think of the savings in medical care and education! And the improved quality of the population in two or three generations.

But why would the state want to go through the expense of genetic engineering at all when the same ends can be accomplished through various techniques of behavioral modification after birth? This is the case in Skinner's *Walden Two,* in which, as in *Brave New World,* citizens will be happy, and useless emotions are eliminated through behavioral science alone. Sparta did perfectly well millenia ago in molding its warrior caste without benefit of the higher biology, and children were raised by the state to ensure good citizenship in Plato's *Republic.* To put it another way, if clones from a desirable type are to receive the optimal environment and training to realize their full potential, why cannot similar conditions be provided to other sectors of the population?

On a mythic level, ectogenesis and cloning represent the fear that technology will be misused if it is placed under the direction of institutions that are themselves unjust, hierarchical, and oppressive. Such institutions tend to use the available tools for enhancing their own power and perpetuating their vested interests. Reproductive technologies simply give them the ultimate means of treating citizens as interchangeable parts, manufactured in the service of the state, and disposable according to shifts in the master plan. Many, of course, would feel that we have already reached this condition, so that biomedical horror stories symbolize or extrapolate from existing governmental surveillance, advertising, CIA drug experiments, and so forth.

But this implies one further point about social control. Is such technology inherently dangerous? Or is it conceivable that reproductive technologies could be used for liberatory, choice-enhancing goals if the institutional context were radically different from that depicted in most science fiction? This is the challenge presented by Piercy's *Woman on the Edge of Time,*[12] the only novel I know of that discusses ectogenesis in a positive vein.

The key difference is a revolutionary alteration in the political structure of the US (and most of the rest of the world) in the direction of decentralization. The small community is the basic unit of this brave new world, featuring consensual decision-making, a flow of representation from the grassroots upward to regional and global planning councils for decisions of more than local importance, and a sophisticated communications system that links everyone to each other and to computerized data banks. Communities seek to realize such goals as preservation of the environment, production to fulfill basic needs, resource recycling, enhancement of cultural diversity, apprentice-based education, and development of self-reliant working/living collectives.

In this context, communities, presumably on the basis of local choice, may use ectogenesis for negative eugenics and in order to mix racial genes throughout the population. The result is a society without racism, in which each community has a consciously chosen ethnic "flavor" (black, Jewish, etc.) that has no relation to the genetic or cultural heritage of its members. This is plurality with a vengeance. Piercy's society also faces the issue of using its"brooders" for positive eugenics. Here, the point is strongly made that such a decision will only be taken after careful and deliberate thrashing out at all levels of governance by all who wish to take part, and not imposed by centralized authorities on the basis of their own presumed wisdom. Such a process for the direction of science and technology is inevitably slow, but that is its strength. A truly democratic environment does not ensure that wise policy will result, but it roots the ultimate locus of choice on those who will be affected by the consequences—in this case, everyone.

The third general theme raised by science fiction is changes in women's roles and, consequently, in the shape of society itself, under the impact of reproductive technologies. One obvious impact would be to relieve natural mothers of months of pregnancy, placing the job of incubation on artificial devices or surrogate mothers. The literature has not given great attention to this issue, or for that matter, to the whole experience of having and raising children: "Most sf, when it bothers to deal with childbirth at all, sees it either as only a regrettable necessity or the most important thing a woman can do."[13] A third perspective may not be much more helpful, though it is often encountered. This is the view of male futurist and nonfiction author F. M. Esfandiary that pregnancy is inconvenient and primitive, as well as antisocial. The decision to have children should be "an event which cannot be left to the whims of individuals. It is an event in which everyone must be involved."[14]

However, Adrienne Rich provides an important corrective by noting that whether or not pregnancy is in fact drudge labor, to be given up when technology makes this feasible, depends on the "political and emotional setting" in which birth takes place. It is "patriarchal childbirth" and "institutionalized motherhood" that make pregnancy an alienating, technocratic, power-depriving experience for many women.[13] If the birth process were humane, Rich argues, ectogenesis might compete on equal grounds, instead of by default, as one of several alternatives open to women who wished to choose the method of nurturing and/or creating their fetuses.

In any case, a recent wave of feminist utopian fiction has looked in some detail at the profound connections between reproductive modes, family systems, and gender-based social roles. It is, of course, conceivable that progress toward an androgynous society, in which roles are filled according to ability, may be made without the technological fix of ectogenesis. However, precisely because ectogenesis seems more likely to lead in the opposite direction, some feminists are alarmed. There is the possibility that reproductive technologies will take their place in society as it is, becoming the ultimate example of man's (i.e., male) domination over nature. Woman's body would become the field site for experiments in genetic engineering—the Vietnam of ectogenesis—while, to mix metaphors, Frankenstein's monster creeps back into the laboratory to ask the boys from Harvard to create for him a bride.

However, stories that do postulate social change as the route to androgyny invariably stress a variety of communal alternatives to the nuclear family. This is the case in LeGuin's *The Dispossessed*[15] and McIntyre's *Dreamsnake*[16], where it is not technology that frees women for full participation in society—or for making the choice to participate. Rather this freedom develops from an intertwined nexus of values, child rearing arrangements, and social institutions. Although the means for child raising may vary, such visions have in common the elimination of any expectation that the natural mother must be solely responsible for the rearing and early education of her offspring. This task is usually shared within an extended family, undertaken communally, or taken on by self-selected members of the community.

To be sure, this was the system for child rearing, after decanting, in *Brave New World,* a reminder that there is no one institutional or technological panacea for human liberation. It is the decision-making context that counts. In Huxley's book, choices are in the hands of the world government leaders and experts from the College of Emotional Engineering. In the recent utopias, localized collectives, operating by town meeting democracy, are in charge.

Ectogenesis, however, does play a role in some of these works. If reproductive technologies potentially contribute to the triumph of patriarchy, there is no inherent reason why they should not have the opposite result. They extend the function of contraceptives and abortion to give women complete control over their biological destiny, and therefore freedom of role choice, *if* women are able to participate in guiding the uses of these techniques. Thus, it is possible that male genetic researchers will one day be seen as traitors to their gender.

Woman on the Edge of Time employs ectogenesis to show how to break the bond between gender and social roles, on the one hand, and end the predominance of the traditional nuclear family, on the other. Piercy presents the provocative view that, far from shunning artificial reproduction as a male power ploy, women in the future welcome it for its political implications. It symbolizes the giving up of power over others, to which men contribute by relinquishing a dominating role over the direction of society. For the same reason, the women also accept hormonal treatment for men who wish to breastfeed children taken into their families.

> When we were breaking all the old hierarchies . . . [we had to give up] . . . the only power we ever had, in return for no more power for anyone. The original reproduction: the power to give birth. 'Cause as long as we were biologically enchained, we'd never be equal. And males never would be humanized to be loving and tender. So we all became mothers. Every child has three. To break the nuclear bonding.[12]

The careful balances at work here are made clear by glimpses in the novel of a high technology, patriarchal enclave that has survived our time to fight the decentralized communities in a war of annihilation. The male rulers of the former use biology to create a force of deadly androids and to engineer their women for sexual pleasure, a chilling merger of Pentagon and Playboy.

If one believes that women will never be free as long as men are in the way, ectogenesis provides the final solution through various forms of parthenogenesis. In Gilman's recently discovered utopia, *Herland*,[17] women reproduce by sheer act of will. The genetically altered women of Charnas' *Motherlines*[18] are able to mate with their genetically altered stallions, giving new meaning to the love of a young girl for her horse. And in Russ' *The Female Man*[19] the women of Whileaway give birth to offspring drawn from merging the ova of the parents. These all-female societies are lesbian civilizations in the broadest sense. The women are not only sexually self-sufficient, but are depicted as fully capable of constructing a total society that, in all cases, is more satisfying than what we enjoy at present.

Whether a female society is used as a satirical foil for commentary on the present, as a serious prediction, or as a metaphor to inspire current social change, the full flowering of women's capabilities and a supportive value system are based in such visions on liberating women from any dependence on men for reproduction. Incidentally, the men in these socieities have either all died off from disease or war, or the women have withdrawn to separate parts of this or other worlds, leaving the male-dominated civilization to its own devices. Curiously, I know of no attempt to portray a society of men going it alone, let alone a male world that might be devoted in its way to humanistic relationships and institutions. Nor is it clear why an all female society would not have its share of Hitlers, large and small, unless one assumes that the absence of men automatically deprives the women of access to oppressive role models.

In conclusion, these stories highlight several important public policy and interpersonal issues that society presently faces regarding technology in general, even if ectogenesis itself is not a likely prospect for the near future and even if the impact of genotype on behavior is often fudged.

(1) The impact of reproductive technologies on society will depend heavily on what individuals and groups are in charge of the policy process that controls advances in and applications of such techniques. The impact of ectogenesis, for example, need not be automatically pro- or anti-feminist.

(2) However, in the absence of change toward a society based on ecological values, human dignity, and localized decision-making, reproductive technologies are likely to find use as toys of the rich and powerful, as research tools of scientists whose experiments may give rise to inhumane or disastrous consequences, and eventually, as part of the arsenal of means by which governments control citizen behavior and compete for power with each other.

Ectogenesis and Ideology

Rebecca L. Logan

When I look at the future scenarios that Dennis Livingston has presented, I find that most of them, with the exception of the societies depicted by Marge Piercy and the lesbian feminists, are based upon two ideological assumptions. I would like to look at these assumptions and explore their implications for women.

The first assumption is biological determinism: the notion that "biology is destiny." This is especially obvious in the cloning stories, where exact duplicates of selected individuals are sought; ectogenesis, too, is usually performed to produce desired genetic traits. The characteristic most commonly desired is intelligence, sometimes defined as high IQ and sometimes as an ability to synthesize information. In a story entitled "The Last Woman," intelligence is combined with the elimination of emotion.[1] The researcher in *Clone* produces four men with eidetic memories who function together as a group mind.[2] Clones in these scenarios are always produced from men.

The other ideological assumption is population control, the notion that social problems and scarcity of resources are caused by an overabundance of people—a concept that ignores social structure, power, and the unequal distribution of wealth. Population control and biological determinism come together in the ideology of eugenics, where the quality as well as the quantity of people is controlled. A common scenario features a world in which all people are sterilized, ectogenetic reproduction makes use of frozen sperm and egg banks, and decisions about who to reproduce are made by an "objective" scientific elite. The goal in some of these societies is to create a race of "supermen"; in others, such as *Brave New World,* a permanent genetic caste system is created. Some of these societies seek to solve the problem of racism by eliminating nonwhite races or by mixing genes to create one racial type.

I am not concerned here with the technological feasibility of these scenarios, nor with the correctness of the assumptions of biological determinism or population control/eugenics. Instead, I see them as ideologies, as belief systems or world views. If one views the world through this particular set of ideological lenses, what are the likely consequences?

Historically, biological determinism has functioned to justify the oppression of immigrants, blacks, women, and the poor, all perceived to be biologically inferior to white men. In the nineteenth century, women were considered to be low on the evolutionary scale, dominated by their reproductive organs, and possessing deficient brains.[3] Black men were considered intellectually equivalent to women, children, and senile whites.[4] Today, biological determinism supports the argument that IQ is genetically determined by race. It is also the basis of sociobiology, which justifies patriarchy as the inevitable result of innate male–female differences.

The history of eugenics reveals the same pattern. In the early part of this century, American eugenicists advocated larger families for the "fit," that is, white upper-class yankees, and birth control and sterilization for the "unfit"—immigrants, nonwhites, and the poor. Restrictive immigration policies were established. Twenty thousand prisoners, mentally ill, and mentally retarded people were legally sterilized between 1928 and 1935, followed by another 38,000 between 1935 and 1956.[5] Today, the population controllers, many of whom are eugenicists, focus their attention on poor and third-world people, now considered "surplus" rather than "unfit."

Thus, historically, these ideologies have functioned to perpetuate and rationalize the oppression of the powerless—women, blacks, other people of color, immigrants, the poor, the institutionalized.

Today, adherents of these beliefs claim the future of the human race requires rational planning, that it is too important and too delicate to be left to the whims and self-interest of individuals. They raise fears about resource scarcity and deterioration of the gene pool. Drastic measures are advocated—for example, if third-world people selfishly continue to have babies, they must be prevented from doing so. Reproduction is the key to controlling population size and quality. And ectogenesis offers, for the first time, effective means to control reproduction.

Efforts to control reproduction up to now have had disastrous consequences for women. Coercive population control methods are common; women's bodies have also been used to test contraceptive and sterilization procedures. Those that have been developed, especially the pill and the IUD, are distributed widely, despite the physical and emotional damage they cause.

But, one could ask, won't ectogenesis and cloning change that by removing reproduction from the bodies of women? David Rorvik's book, *In His Image,* suggests otherwise.[6] His cloning experiments are carried out in a third-world hospital where women are paid for their eggs, which are chemically stimulated to maturity and then removed during sterilization operations. Embryos are transplanted into the wombs of women without their knowledge or consent. Some of the women become pregnant for short periods of time, but are not told. A surrogate mother eventually gives birth to the cloned boy.

In fact, the development of new reproductive technologies does require experimental research on women. Eggs must be surgically removed from women's bodies. Embryos must be transplanted into women's wombs. It is interesting that "surrogate mothers" are cited as a means to relieve women of the burden of childbirth, since "surrogate mothers" are women. And, in the tradition of wet nurses, they are likely to be poor and nonwhite women.

I would like to close by suggesting that reproductive technologies are controlled by the same people—the same multinational corporations, the same medical establishment, and the same patriarchal values—who brought us DES and thalidomide, who encourage sterilization while denying abortion, who perform thousands of unnecessary hysterectomies, and who are poisoning our air, water, land, and bodies. Their control of reproductive technology is not likely to benefit women.

Manipulative Reproductive Technologies Discussion

Part III

Moderated by Betty B. Hoskins

Betty Hoskins: As a woman and an embryologist I think that one of the hardest things for us to grapple with, to contemplate clearly, is the extraordinariness of the reproduction of life. Whether it be human life, or plant or animal life, the process that starts with an egg and a sperm and ends with a person, or a fern, or a clam—occurring almost every time with precision and accuracy—is extraordinarily unlikely. It's like telling a fantasy, a myth, to teach embryology. Since it's very hard to cope with the sense of awe and with the sense of the creative power women have, curiosity and the attempt to take life apart and understand it result. It's hard to choose what kind of research is appropriate in order to gain the knowledge and understanding we in the Western scientific world want.

Janet Farrell Smith: It is important to look beneath the surface of talk about rights to the psychological needs and social structure which might stimulate that kind of talk. In US society, especially in white middle class communities, children are very much privatized or isolated from adult society in large public schools. If we took a cross-cultural perspective, we might find that in other societies adults relate more easily and naturally to children. In Tahiti, for example, an adult who wants to be a parent finds it natural and easy to bond with a child. Social parenthood does not depend so exclusively on biological parenthood. The strong needs expressed by women at this conference to bear and have children should be affirmed. At the same time as we sympathize with these needs, we should be aware that the technology of in vitro fertilization is an inadequate solution to the complex psychological and social need and capacity for bearing children.

At the Genetics and Law Conference in Boston in May, 1979, (sponsored by the American Society for Law and Medicine) a presentation on In Vitro Fertilization included actual photographs of the fertilized ovum projected on a screen 12 feet high. The photographs of the 2-celled to 8-celled stage were dramatic and awesome, like the first photographs of the moon or Mars. I was struck by the fact that the speaker mentioned the slides came from Chile, a country in which thousands of people have disappeared under military rule. The political background of the biological research was not discussed. The experience was for me a vivid metaphor for the power of the state which stands behind the biological power we now have.

Karen Lebacqz: Marge Piercy's *Woman on the Edge of Time* presents a picture of an alternative and at least quasi-utopian society in which (1) women have given up their right to biological reproduction, and (2) mothering or parenting has been broken down and reconstituted. She presents both of these changes as necessary to a society that wishes to empower people rather than to have power over others. Piercy is pushing us to ask the question of what it is that we must give up if we really want empowerment and other feminist values we have talked about at this conference. She suggests that we may have to give up the ultimate power, because really our biological reproduction may be in some sense the ultimate in power (not to say that it's the only power that women have, should have, can have, and so on). Is that the price of a utopian society in which one shares power and empowerment?

Becky Logan: I think Piercy is very naive. She didn't really think through the effects of ectogenetic technology. Development of that technology would require a lot of experimentation on women's bodies. Secondly, what kind of children would be produced in test tubes or outside the body? There is a deep emotional and physical relationship between a mother and a child. Women have real power in childbirth, although it is a power that has been significantly controlled by men in this society. But I think that the notion of giving it up in that kind of technological way is just not desirable.

Ruth Hubbard: We shouldn't forget Shulamith Firestone. Piercy told a mythic story around a theme that Firestone elaborated earlier—a theme that I think is a mistake. But it has to be part of the record of feminist thought that these women believed that we may need to develop external, technological reproduction in order to achieve a more just society. Obviously I think that the technological fix that gets into both of these stories misses the point.

Judy Luce: I object to the concept that women have power to give up in any real sense. You can only talk about giving up something that you've had, and, although having babies is a capacity women have, I'm not sure it's a power in any political sense.

Betty Hoskins: I see it as an extraordinary creative power. We are using the word "power" in several different ways.

Susan Peterson: Power as control or domination is indeed a masculine definition of power, and in this sense women do not have that power to give up. But there is a more creative and fulfilling kind of power that women do have. We must make this distinction between the two meanings of power.

Tabitha Powledge: No one picked up on Martha Mathis' point during the sex preselection discussion: these technologies are mostly used by the white upper middle classes. They are just not addressing some of the serious problems that a great number of other women have. I would like to ask whether these discussions (intellectually intriguing as I have found all of them) are perhaps not distracting us from a problem we haven't solved: we still need a good contraceptive.

Betty Hoskins: This session started with the premise that there are certainly pressing present problems. The topic of manipulative reproductive technologies gives examples of technologies that are still being developed. I'm very sensitive to the criticism that scientists have never been able to look ahead and see what they were heading society into, that they have used their self-interest to pursue the fascinating study of development and have not seen risks, benefits, consequences. Here we have a prospective chance. These manipulative studies *are* going on; these applications *are* contemplated; they are fascinating; they do receive some funding; they have implications we can try to foresee. Please consider putting your attention to *both* present and imminent technologies that have social and ethical implications. I do take the poem I began with seriously: it is a formidable power to be able to create life. It is more than "interesting" to contemplate creating life in the laboratory.

Jill Wolhandler: Although scientists have been accused of not thinking out the implications in advance of their research, individual scientists don't have that much control over what research is done. A value system determines what will be funded or given credibility. The high technology research we've been talking about is a priority; food for pregnant women is not. I can't ever get those things out of my mind in all of these discussions; sometimes it has been hard to sit here and listen to some very interesting and important things because these other realities are so close. And it's also very hard to hear so much emphasis on creating biological motherhood for women who don't have that option, without first stopping sterilization abuse and abusive medical experimentation on women.

Helen Holmes: Possibly as women we have a special connection with the future—through our children, our children's children, and so on. Possibly we are able to predict and suggest actions to prevent future problems, instead of having to wait 20 years to see the cancers develop. The victims of this technology again may be the poor and the people of color.

Joyce Berkman: It might help us to speculate on historical situations that might spur government policy to encourage in vitro fertilization. I can think of some rather scary situations in the future where for some reason or another (e.g., war, pollution, nuclear plant leakage) 75% of the female population becomes sterile and the government becomes very concerned about future offspring. Under those circumstances I wouldn't be surprised if large numbers of men and women in this country conclude we have no other choice, given a population crisis, than to accept this super technology. This is no abstract discussion.

Susan Bell: I've been struck by parallels between the histories of in vitro fertilization and DES. In each there were women who wanted to bear children and couldn't, and who were desperate to bear them. Yet, by looking only at this desire, we obscure what else is influencing the production of technology to aid childbearing in these two cases. It is developed to promote childbirth in white and/or middle class or rich women. Simultaneously, other technologies are developed to prevent childbirth in third world and/or poor women. Additionally, some women are sterilized before they can work in certain industrial situations. Maybe we should keep this political undercurrent in our minds when we evaluate IVF.

Adele Laslie: On the issue of informed consent Barbara Menning seemed to say "Look, we're informed, we're consenting, and we want it. Who are you to say we shouldn't buy into the system? We're ready for that." Barbara's recital of the things she went through reminded me of the case of a black woman, in Barker-Benfield's book,[1] a woman who as a slave underwent some 30 operations without anesthesia until J. Marian Sims perfected the silver suture. It was said, yes, she was a slave who was owned, but she had faith in her doctor and said, "Try it again, I don't want this urinary incontinence. It's an awful thing to be leaking urine all the time." Other women thought the same thing. There were lots of other cases of women who came begging for operations. In that kind of situation, the issue is not just what the couple wants or the woman wants, no matter how informed she feels about what the risks are. It's experimental and there's another decision to be made concerning the responsibility of researchers and doctors. A national task force should make that decision.

Diana Axelsen: It's good that we're using analogies and looking to history, as well as to the future, to deal with these issues. However, the analogies need to be examined carefully. In the case of the slave women, they had only the "choice" of staying in the field or accepting Sims' experimental surgery. IVF involves women with access to a variety of medical and social options; we aren't talking about slaves. But I agree that the history of reproductive technology does involve massive societal manipulation of individual women.

How much risk are we entitled to take in using experimental reproductive technologies? It may be all right to be a "guinea pig parent," but what about the *children* born as a result of experimental technologies? It's one thing to say 'I'll be an experimental subject," but it's different to say, "I'll bring an experimental entity into the world and hope that it turns out all right."

Barbara Menning: I didn't say, because I thought it was obvious, that I am a consumer advocate. No one is more caring and is more protective of infertile people who are greatly exploited than I am. I have been exploited myself; I know what it feels like. If I thought that there was an increased risk that they would have a congenitally damaged child I would never advocate "in vitro." Further research is needed. I'd be the last person to see people who've gone through a lot of pain go through additional pain. I just say let's make it available as a choice. And I would imagine that many people would choose not to have in vitro. If I qualified for in vitro I would choose not to have it. I've had enough instrumentation on my body.

Elizabeth Kutter: First, the number of infertile women to whom this technology may apply, a million women, is far more than the number potentially affected by most of the other diseases we're trying to treat with large amounts of tax dollars.

Second, I think we can't make the argument that a woman can't take a risk on herself of having some small chance of having a defective child. We don't tell a woman with genetic risk of even 1 in 2 or 1 in 4 she can't have a child. On the other hand, the more I think about it the more I am opposed to this technology now for a rather different reason. Ruth Hubbard alluded to the question of genetic engineering. I think it's far closer than most of us realize. At the last recombinant DNA Committee meeting we approved experiments that involved moving the genes for monkey hemoglobin into a teratocarcinoma cell, then putting that cell into an early blastula stage mouse embryo and letting it develop into a mouse. So mice will be formed that carry functional monkey genes. There's reason to do that, to understand how genes are controlled. We said such work cannot be done on human beings. But there is going to be a lot of pressure to use that kind of technology for genetic engineering on the human gene pool. There will be experiments on curing diseases like sickle cell anemia; the key animal experiments are there now. But I see the one crucial step for development of the broad technology being re-implantation of the ova that have grown for a short period in a test tube. This seems to me to be the one step in the social acceptance of the technology and also in the technology itself at which we can draw the line. We used the word moratorium before.

Perhaps we can make all people aware from the beginning that there is a possibility that they won't be fertile; helping them to deal with the problems in other ways may in fact be the most desirable solution, at least at this time.

Reflections

Uncovering Patriarchal Agendas and Exploring Woman-Oriented Values*

Emily Erwin Culpepper

A hallmark of the feminist movement (and feminist scholarship as part of that movement) is the radical rethinking we bring to our lives and the world women face. The feminist movement is not just one of "personal growth" unconnected with social realities. We are concerned to create whole and healthy lives for ourselves and to aid this process for all women. This inextricably involves us in assessing society as we find it. It means seeing many hard and frightening conditions that are the current situation of our sex. It means channeling for change the exhilaration welling up from deep sources of primal self-knowledge and love.

From just such a specifically personal and globally expansive grounding, the best strong-minded feminist analysis develops. Already in the current wave of feminism, there are key insights and methods of thinking that we find especially helpful to bring to bear on issues of concern to us. Here I discuss what several of these methods uncover when we look at ethical issues involved in human reproduction technologies.

First, I want to focus on the portion of the conference title that said, "Analysis by Women." This is not a mere de facto, circumstantial occurrence. Nor do we regard ourselves as doing one-half of a complete analysis. To think, to discuss, to argue, and to agree in a

*The EIRTAW Workshop Advisory Committee chose five Workshop participants to appear in a symposium at the January, 1980, Annual Meeting of the American Association for the Advancement of Science (AAAS) in San Francisco. Avery and Cowan from Volume I (Birth Control and Controlling Birth), and Steinbacher and Hubbard from the present volume were asked to adapt their papers for a larger audience. Emily Culpepper was then invited to synthesize the four papers and to develop an ethical analysis. A revised version of her talk follows.

space that is female created and controlled has a primary positive value for us. Reflection and action in space that is ours is different, more open and strong than if we limit ourselves to a traditional, male-defined orientation for our work. Let me be clear. This is not a separation out of weakness—it is a tough and determined clearing out of free space, free from the dilutions and distortions of standard intellectual and social frameworks that are heavily skewed toward the "interests" of men. To be even more clear: feminists do not naively believe that such all-female thinking will somehow be magically pure or perfect or unified. We *do* know from our experience that we will be working from more solid ground, the better to draw out our own differences, find our own mistakes and right directions, confront and change the dangerous status quo. Energized by our woman-oriented experience, we may still choose to join coalition efforts. Once this is no longer a necessity, but one choice to share ourselves, to make alliances, coalitions are, in fact, all the more effective.Although some feminists make coalitions and others do not, or do so rarely, we all share a deeper, common woman-identification.

I am stressing this feature of our work—that we are consciously and strategically women working with women—because it qualitatively affects the process and results of what we do. For women to choose each other, we are breaking vast taboos internally and institutionally, going against male authority, moving out from under male control. We are women who desire to know our own minds and to have minds of our own. In so doing, we become especially better equipped to envision our values, to draw distinctions, to make moral judgments—which is, after all, what the enterprise of ethics is about. When we are first true to our Selves as women, the truer our ethics can be.

Another primary feature of feminist method is the recognition that *the personal is political* (and vice versa). Including information that is traditionally considered private or personal, rather than public and supposedly more detached or objective, is an intentional intellectual and emotional decision. This inclusion is not for purposes of adding color or being anecdotal, nor does it mean being less than rigorous in our philosophical, theoretical thinking. It springs, in fact, from a rigorous honesty—including as primary data in our considerations our own experiences and attitudes. Thus, we see for ourselves, and make available for others to see, how these inform, obscure, inspire, and otherwise affect our thought. Including the personal breaks conventional academic distinctions. Women recognize that these function to divide us from important sources of knowing. This does not mean that we jump to making claims of absolute truth based on our individual herstory. We are adding, rather, a rich and fermenting source of further information—just the information that has been so often ignored, distorted, erased, or belittled when applying the criteria that usually count in patriarchal scholarship.

I want to accent the diversity that this opens up for us. Contrary to the androcentric attitude that women's personal concerns are all alike—an undifferentiated mush—we are each quite dramatically different. Our oppression does not manifest itself in our lives in the same ways; the paths of our lives do not always lead through the same terrain. In our united commitment to improve the situation of "our kind," we encourage the exploration of our uniqueness, the uncovering of our complex diversity.

Sharing this real presence of our selves in our reflections and seeking such sharing from other women—especially those we know or imagine to have different experiences, opinions, and needs than our own—grounds us in a solid, "real life" orientation to our work and theorizing. Now, what better safeguard can one build into the sensitive undertaking of ethical reflection and action? How better to guard against the notorious pitfall of mere armchair ethics! Feminists are committed to practical, flesh and blood, active, livable ethics. One important motivating force of this commitment is our knowledge that remote ethical abstractions—developed and enforced by men in the male institutions of religion and government—have had disastrously harmful effects on women.

A further asset to ethics that comes from including the personal is that we are therefore more likely to discover and to appreciate the subtleties of experience—the nuances and ramifications of issues and how they are lived. We gain greater inclusion of those features of experience that are not quantifiable, not so easily and tidily weighed in the balance. Thus attuned to more of the fabric of experience when we assess whether actions and approaches are right or wrong, beneficial or harmful, life affirming or death dealing, we realize that ethical decisions are not so easily fitted into the dualisms on which patriarchal models are typically built.

From our discussions here I want to recount a few examples of personal information being part of our thought process. In moderating the panel on Sex Preselection, I volunteered my own status as a first-born daughter. I stated that this has highlighted for me over the years the fact that such a status runs contrary to the patriarchally preferred, depicted, and rewarded norm (though fortunately not contrary to my family's values). I brought up my direct experience in this role as one source of my information and also as a condition that prompted me to notice and retain other information (including psychological and sociological studies) that I ran across about first-born daughters and sex selection preferences. Further, my status produces a valid vested interest that I have in assessing sex selection technology and its possible implications. These facts do not determine, limit, or blind my thought—especially if I place them out in the open for all to assess. In fact, openly expressed and examined, they are less likely to do so, less likely to remain submerged and function as an unconscious bias. Two examples I can give of this latter phenomenon concern abortion. Some people who know or fear that they were unwanted children oppose women's right to choose abortion because they fear that they would not have been born if their mothers had had this free choice. Or again, I know a male ethicist, who has testified in legislative hearings against women's right to legal abortion, who does not publicly acknowledge that his interests as an adoptive father inform and affect his arguments and feelings.

In the Workshop, my reference to my own first-born daughter status sparked one woman to ask our entire gathering about this. We learned that we had a majority of first-born daughters in our group. We recognized that this added a specific dimension to the matrix of our considerations. On this same note, Martha Mathis reminded us that the daughter-preference often expressed by Black women presents a different model within American society. As another conference example, Ruth Hubbard (in her paper opposing in vitro fertilization) spoke of the personal and professional experiences that inform her perspective and her appreciation of the biological and ethical issues involved. Barbara Menning, who was on the panel with Ruth in June, acknowledged her own role as an activist proponent of this technique and, further, her wish that she could have made use of it herself. In these books are further rich, moving, and thought-provoking examples.

I want to move on now to another principle of feminist ethical analysis and its specific relation to the issues concerning our conference. Feminist method is inevitably and invaluably *interdisciplinary* or, even more fully, transdisciplinary. This means we see and examine together information usually kept separate by traditional divisions of knowledge. In this connection, I want particularly to refer you to Mary Daly's work and especially to her recent book, *Gyn/Ecology: The Metaethics of Radical Feminism*. She is a primary incitrix (a female who incites) of my own thought. Her work especially develops and exemplifies how feminist thought weaves together threads of connectedness, finding meaning past the fragmentations of overly disciplined disciplines. The feminist inclusion of the personal as political is already one instance of how women reclaim the relatedness and relevance of wisdom that is hidden by standards that sever and segregate knowledge into pieces. Further examples abound.

Belita Cowan's paper on government funded contraceptive research places side by side the fact that women—and particularly Black and Third World women—are overwhelmingly the objects of this research, although the researchers, policymakers, vendors, and doctors controlling it are predominately male and white. Thus, the ethical considerations here do not remain on the level of looking at how the subjects of the experiments and procedures are affected. Cowan goes on to the ethical issues now evident in such a great power imbalance.

Byllye Avery, in her consideration of birthplace contrasts, not only compares women's experiences in hospitals and birthing centers, but also holds up as relevant and revealing the fact that these are very disproportionately available options, since 98% of US births take place in hospitals. Further, Avery adds to our assessment of the situation the disturbing harassment and legal suppression of midwifery. Feminists learn that our enemies often name themselves by the way their actions in one area belie their words in another. The issues become even clearer when we view the above in light of the long history of persecution and murder of midwives and witchhealers in many diverse patriarchal cultures. Thus, while Avery logically starts with the experiences of the woman giving birth, her ethical reflections proceed to take in a larger picture.

As we pay attention to placing diverse information side by side, we also look at facts in *contexts* that are often ignored. Many at the conference brought up the financial vested interests of men in medicine, research, academia, government, and industry. It significantly adds to our assessments to realize that medicine in this country is business for profit. It functions more to perpetuate and further itself than to promote well-being. Judy Norsigian and Norma Swenson spoke of the reality that patient warning labels on drugs are written more with an eye to protect legally the manufacturers than to inform genuinely and fully the patient (or even the doctor, for that matter). Thus, the phenomenon of patient package inserts can and is being subverted from its original intent and, in fact, functions to provide a false sense of security while protecting male power and privilege. Helen Rodriguez brought to bear on our discussion the drug company bribes to foreign countries to gain markets for drugs (often drugs not approved for use in the US) and experimental populations. One documented case is Upjohn admitting $4.7 million in bribes to

Latin American countries. Women are saying it is important to place what these companies have to offer and what they say in the context of such economic realities.

Here is a different sort of example of establishing a woman-oriented context for our deliberations. Feminists see the connections between the apparently dissimilar techniques of in vitro fertilization (which allows some women to become pregnant) and forced sterilization (which keeps other women from becoming pregnant) because we see a common theme here: male efforts to control and manipulate female reproductive abilities. Further, these examples above all point up another facet of a feminist approach, which I also consider a genuine principle of analysis: we bring a healthy, questioning *suspicion* to assessing the products of powerful patriarchal institutions. We refer to the horrifying track record of women's experiences with DES, thalidomide, the birth control pill, and the IUD (to name a few blatant, known examples) in our consideration of new proposals from the same sources. Ruth Hubbard aptly calls this an issue of belief, of trust. It is an active, informed distrust (and not a rigid cynical retreat) that feminists utilize as a valuable principle to apply when considering arguments and practices of doctors, drug companies, government officials, and researchers. We know it is valid to ask whether the men who brought us thalidomide, and who want to bring us cloning, are using the desperation of infertile women to justify in vitro experiments. Although these men claim that cloning and total laboratory reproduction of humans are not on their agenda, we see consistent themes of deceit and destruction emerging as we put our diverse sources of information together. We know that it is important for us to put the pieces together, for rarely are members of the medical establishment unsophisticated enough to admit directly their true intentions.

One who did was a physician instrumental in the case of Durga Argowald, the "in vitro baby" born in India. He said on a recent television network news special, "The Baby Makers," "We are not really worried about abnormalities. This pregnancy is so valuable we would rather have an abnormal baby than no baby." His "we" is no doubt the "royal male medical we." I seriously doubt that the parents felt this way. I also seriously doubt that the only value to which he had reference was the solution to a few women's infertility. This quote is a classic example of how doctors appropriate ethical judgments to themselves. (I found an interesting reflection of this in the Webster's Dictionary definition of "ethical." A secondary meaning states that an 'ethical drug" is one that is "restricted to sale only on a doctor's prescription.") I want also to note briefly here the enormous ego involvement in these technologies that the men developing and using them have. These techniques function as male extensions of themselves, an observation that leads feminists also to consider them as sophisticated [sic] forms of rape, battering, and mutilation of women. In sum, feminists find it important and valid to look not only at direct, explicit effects of ideas and actions, but also at connections, themes, and patterns that we find applicable in contexts we consider appropriate.

Another, less obvious at first, method of proceeding is that feminists look for the astounding *absences* of information and concern that further alert us to additional dimensions of a situation. Belita Cowan names the absence of concern in the government birth control studies with safer, less drastic barrier methods; the omission of programs that include a self-knowledge approach for women; and the lack of male agitation for male birth control. As a Lesbian, I notice the lack of concern for Lesbian mothers, the silence regarding parthenogenesis (we know they are working on it), the minimal funding for laywomen's health projects and clinics. Many women at the conference spoke of whole neglected populations of women—such as Chicana, Native American, and Asian women. Their interests either are not considered at all or are paternalistically assumed to be understood and included or overridden by the policymakers who also prevent these women from speaking for themselves.

These absences are visible to us. Roberta Steinbacher stressed the visibility to feminists of the glaring gap between the work on sex selection techniques and any comparable attention to the behavioral, social, and ethical results of such technologies. Janice Raymond cited the absence of concern with the ways in which many of these technologies tie people into long term dependency on doctors and the traditional medical establishment. Gena Corea saw significance in the omission of serious attention to the long term effects of drugs, surgery, and hormones (as evidenced by the lack of real follow-up studies). We all noticed the absence of attention to the whole person and a distorting, fetishizing focus on body parts and specific bodily processes. All these absences are real and present dangers for women. Attention to their inclusion constitutes part of a feminist method.

Another area where feminists are developing our analysis is in examining the *language* we use and that we hear from others. The very naming of issues can play a great role in how these issues are perceived and analyzed. Passive acceptance of traditional words can lull us into false descriptions that skew us away from naming the real issues and being able to work effectively on answers and theories that are pro-woman. In my remarks, I usually find it more appropriate to speak of women as "we," for example. This is not because I presume to speak for all women, but because I find I think more accurately and caringly when I do not speak as if women were a separate group from myself. Many feminists find this significantly alters the character of discussion and presents issues in new ways. Equally important, those opposed to the well-being of women often utilize language that blurs distinctions and conceals information and consequences. "Acceptable risk" can translate in medical jargon to mean number of deaths. "Side effects" can turn out to mean serious and lasting illness. "People in primitive countries" and "the uneducated," and so on frequently function to imply less decision-making capacity by individuals directly affected by the technologies and to legitimate their exclusion. As Sandra Serrano Sewell said, "informed consent" may mean that a consent form in English gets read to a primarily Spanish-speaking woman with no attention to her genuine comprehension. Other status quo language unintentionally reveals aspects of the situation. People receiving medication are "target populations." Babies are pseudo-generically "he" when infants' risks are contrasted to mothers' risks. This is loaded language in a culture where "he" is assumed and enforced to be more valued than "she." In vitro proponents often speak of "the right to motherhood," blurring the crucial distinctions between child-bearing and child-rearing.

Another key linguistic issue confronted at the conference is the pseudo-liberal use of the term "choice," which can actually function to justify developing and administering dangerous drugs and procedures. A feminist approach involves us in seeking out who is offering the choices, how fair or biased are the options, how does the recipient come to the situation, and so on. Further, feminists do not back away from making new words, creating new speech that will better convey our information and intentions. As feminists, we continue to become more alert to the ways our language informs thought. This is not a simplistic attention to semantics, but a concern with the reality-making power that words have. Certainly in the development of ethics, accurate and careful language is essential.

Finally, a feminist method does not only criticize. Even though here we had the starting point of examining existing technologies, we were actively concerned not just to react. This involves us in offering *alternative suggestions* and theories. It means taking the risk of having a point of view, of constructing working hypotheses and acting on them. It means planning, getting funding for, and staffing alternative birth centers as well as criticizing traditional hospital experiences—and knowing that both actions are valid and indeed essential. It means testifying at government hearings. It means organizing where we live and work. Throughout our work, women here put forth positive suggestions of actions, theories, principles.

A feminist method means, then, that we do not wait until some perfect, ideal imagined state of affairs is established before trying out alternatives. This necessitates, as Simone de Beauvoir said in *The Ethics of Ambiguity,* "taking the risk of creating an original solution." We are fashioning an ethic of respect for the diversity of responsible decisions that women reach on many of these issues, rather than constructing false absolutes. We realize that this commits us to challenge actively, support, and discuss these different decisions, so that we do not slide into an "anything goes" attitude.

Not holding back from challenging all assumptions, including our own, also leads us to take seriously previously devalued perspectives, respecting what these might have to offer—especially if they too have been the objects of attack by those we have found to be dangerous. One example is feminist interest in the traditions of the witch-healers, of psychic and spiritual powers for healing, of herbal remedies and the natural, wholistic health movement. Another specific example is the Native American Indian prophecy shared with us by Katsi Cook. Long ago, tribal seers predicted that one day the white man would go to the moon and that this would interfere with the abilities of women to bear children. Non-Indian feminists hear this story with open ears and open minds. We too in our way see disturbingly direct connections here. The invasive, colonizing male mentality that wants to possess the moon is only another face of the same male dominating drive to possess female bodies and reproductive abilities.

Feminists know that, as we ponder connecting such disparate sources of knowledge and what their similarities might mean, we risk ridicule as being crazy, romantic, silly, not serious. But we know that we are serious. We know the scope of the change we need is as large as reimagining the very nature of reality. We are not, however, deadly serious—a revealing phrase that indicates the ultimate orientation to death in established values. We are serious in a living way—we are vitally serious and proud to be so.

And now I have come full circle (another familiar pattern which feminists find our independent thinking often takes, rather than conventional linear models). My full circle brings me back to one of my original points: the value of including the personal and recognizing this as political. I want to make a final remark on my own process in deciding what to include in this paper. From my perspective as a radical feminist and Lesbian, I have tried to honor the obligation I felt to include not only my own thoughts but to represent something of all the women at the conference. I have made it a point to include references to the dynamics and opinions at the conference and especially to cite women from underrepresented groups.

I want to close with some warning words from WARN (the Women of All Red Nations): "Truth, and the communication of that truth is a basic survival tactic." Our gynergy is great, yet the situation of women is extreme. Ethics is one implement with which women can fashion a different world and a larger truth. If this paper, then, is true to my purpose, it will take some of you beyond it—to further reflection and action of your own—as women moving independently and variously together for the survival and liberation of our kind.

Appendix

Resolutions

OVERVIEW

Throughout the Workshop discussants lamented that, although it was stimulating to discuss these issues, this conference was likely to turn out like any other, in that there would be no differences in health policy after everyone had gone home. The inequities would not be rectified. The value system beneath the status quo would remain unchanged. Our official purpose did not include setting up an action agenda. But a surge of participant activism urged that we make specific policy recommendations while we were together, in the form of resolutions. These were created before the final session and brought to a vote on the last day.

Resolutions were written by Workshop panels and by special interest groups that formed during an additional mid-workshop plenary session. They were compiled by Gena Corea and Judy Norsigian. At the voting session, a copy was distributed to every three participants. With Sheryl Ruzek as moderator, the two compilers read the resolutions. For lack of time no discussion could be permitted. Many persons then expressed their misgivings about the lack of a chance to give calm and thoughtful consideration to each issue. It was moved, seconded, and passed:

> That the *general* resolutions dealing with further conferences and funding of information activities passed by this body, and the resolutions dealing with the new Presidential Commission [on ethics in medical research], be considered as officially passed by this body and be transmitted to NSF and other appropriate agencies; further that the Advisory Committee supplemented by volunteers review and refine (i.e., make minor grammatical changes and eliminate duplication of) all other submitted resolutions and submit them to all attendees for mail vote.

GENERAL RESOLUTIONS

1. All health-related conferences supported with public funds should include women of diverse social, ethnic, racial, and class backgrounds, including persons with disabilities, in the planning and design of those conferences as well as such women as participants.

2. NSF and other public agencies should expand the number of conferences of this sort—women's analysis of critical social and scientific issues—which include both professional and lay representatives.
3. In order to allow for participation of women and consumers as witnesses before Congressional and regulatory agency hearings and proceedings, there must be a broader definition of "expert witness," availability of travel funds, and adequate lead time or notice.
4. In recognition of the key role of networks, and to help facilitate communication among women on health and ethical issues, groups such as the National Women's Health Network and the Women and Health Roundtable should continue to expand their information and clearinghouse functions to help serve community and professional needs, especially with regard to resources and expertise-sharing.
5. Recognizing that one factor contributing to medical research abuses is the system of values used in selecting medical students, we recommend that the admissions committees of community medical schools (since they receive public funds) be required to include professional women and nonprofessional community representatives, particularly women and minorities.
6. That all publicly funded conferences on ethical issues, science, and technology be required to incorporate analysis by women in the content and structure of the program.
7. That all federal agency or intra-agency policy-making bodies that determine policies affecting reproduction must have a majority of women members.
8. Because there is a dearth of community forums in which to discuss issues surrounding women, technology, and society, NSF and other agencies should fund more small regional workshops based on the needs of the community as expressed by community members and developed by community organizations in conjunction with professional consultation.
9. To potential sponsors: A followup conference should be held on ethical issues in parenting. The conference would consider such issues as: mothering (parenting) a child with a handicap; feminist perspectives on mothering; the revolution of rising expectations and the desire for "perfect" children; the impact of population control on modes of parenting; changes in societal values and their impact on norms for parenting, etc.
10. We urge the establishment of better working relationships between academic/professional women and nonprofessional community activists, in part through workshops and conferences designed for sharing perspectives, needs, skills, etc.
11. That NSF and HEW develop mechanisms for the implementation of the recommendations passed at this conference and that

the US Congress appropriate funds for the above implementation.

12. We urge President Carter, in choosing members for the newly forming President's Commission for the Study of Ethical Problems in Medicine and Biomedical and Behavioral Research, to include at least 50% women, and to include at least one participant from an EVIST [Ethics and Values in Science and Technology Program of the National Science Foundation] project as well as lay representation.*
13. Because women have had so little voice in determining research priorities and conducting research in the area of human reproduction, this conference recommends that the following decision-making bodies be composed of at least 50% women, including some lay women:
    (1) All government committees and bodies that determine research priorities in human reproduction.
    (2) All government peer review committees that determine funding for research proposals in the area of human reproduction.
    (3) All Institutional Review Boards.
    (4) All editorial committees that review submissions to publications concerned with reproduction.
14. This conference urges NSF as well as other private and public funding sources to sponsor forums for laywomen and professional women researchers to come together for the following purposes:
    (1) To develop models for research in human reproduction to be designed and conducted jointly by professional researchers and laypersons.
    (2) To develop strategies for obtaining funding for such research.

MAIL BALLOTING

The rest of the resolutions were submitted to attendees on a mail ballot of 67 resolutions. They are grouped below by the level of support in voting: (1) those receiving support of more than 90% of those voting; (2) those supported by at least three-quarters, but less than 90%; and (3) those that gained a majority, but less than three-quarters support.

The results of the voting on these resolutions are notable for a number of reasons. First, a great number of policy issues emerged, and, in the voting, many of these policy resolutions gained very wide support. Second, that level of support is significant because of the diversity of participants, and because

*As of June, 1980, there are ten commissioners. Four of these are women, with PhDs respectively in psychology, sociology, economics, and research science, each with experience in bioethics.

they gave such support despite concern, during our voting session and later on the ballots, about the specific wording of the resolutions. On the one hand, a number of voters felt that the resolutions were too idealistic or impractical; on the other hand, some felt that they did not go nearly far enough.

Third, since voters could and often did abstain, the proportion of votes that are not affirmative includes those from participants who would have accepted a resolution with the omission or addition of a word or phrase.

Finally, although the voting procedure inevitably limited opportunities to discuss the motions, the mail ballot allowed generous amounts of time for people to deliberate before voting, away from any of the immediate impact and sense of urgency which they may have felt during the conference itself.

The extent of positive support is therefore impressive evidence of widespread consensus, despite reservations, on a number of very important policy issues. Furthermore, those issues receiving less strong support lay the groundwork for further discussion among women to explore other possibilities and to develop policy goals.

Resolutions Receiving 90% or More Affirmative Votes

More data should be gathered on procedures that are often performed unnecessarily, including: hysterectomy; oopherectomy; tubal ligation; cesarean section; dilation and curettage (D&C); breast and uterine biopsies; episiotomies; and radical (Halsted) mastectomy. Data should determine:

(a) When, on whom, and how often they are currently being performed.
(b) Their effectiveness in the treatment and prevention of the conditions for which they are utilized.
(c) Their long term effects and sequellae.

Alternatives to the above procedures should be investigated.

Because Medicaid cutbacks for abortion services represent unconscionable discrimination against poor women, we support the restoration of Medicaid coverage for abortion services.

We recommend that neonatal and maternal morbidity should be used as official standards of the United States health care system, in addition to the traditional standards of mortality.

We recommend that basic preventive care should be provided to all women, with a focus on eliminating poverty and its effects. Nutrition is particularly important.

Background: Because most of the technologies, procedures, and drugs discussed have not been fully evaluated as to their safety and usefulness,

We recommend that patients be told of the experimental nature of these procedures and drugs.

We recommend that pregnant women and their advocates be given information about the effects of all drugs, hospital, and instrumental technology procedures—including physician office procedures and prescription drugs—likely to be "offered" them during pregnancy, labor, and delivery. ("Advocates" refers to appropriate advocates, not those with vested interests.) Such women must be allowed to participate in deciding whether to consume drugs or to be exposed to such procedures.

We recommend that electronic fetal monitoring should not be used routinely in childbirth.

Resolved, that the possibility of having a healthy child should be extended equally to women of all economic and ethnic groups through protection from environmental harm and provision of basic care to all.

Resolutions Receiving 75-89% Affirmative Votes

Resolved, that medical schools should be encouraged to devise courses or electives on the humanitarian issues in medicine.

Resolved, that medical schools be encouraged to act in a more humane manner in dealing with patients—particularly poor patients—for teaching purposes.

Background: Major provisions of the sterilization regulations issued by the US Department of Health, Education, and Welfare (HEW), include: a 30-day waiting period between consent and operation with waivers for early delivery and emergency abdominal surgery; that consent not be obtained during labor, abortion, or while a person is under the influence of drugs or alcohol; a continued moratorium on sterilizations of people under 21, in penal institutions, or adjudicated incompetent.

In recognition of widespread sterilization abuse problems, we support the HEW sterilization regulations and call for their strict monitoring and enforcement.

We support the recent establishment by the National Women's Health Network of a voluntary Depo-Provera registry.

Resolved, that we oppose the provision of the proposed Drug Regulation Reform Act of 1979, which allows the export of drugs judged too unsafe for use in the United States.

Women should be able to share the information obtained [when data are gathered on gynecological surgery]. Means of facilitating the sharing of this information through local women's health groups should be funded.

We urge government funding, on a pilot project basis, of women-controlled health centers and other women's health projects such as self-help groups.

In recognition that isolated services offered as part of population control programs can interfere with the reproductive freedom of women, we recommend that all foreign aid programs offering contraceptive services should, whenever possible, offer such services within the context of broad health services.

Resolved, that Diethylstilbestrol (DES) be banned for use as a food additive and as a drug.

Resolved, that federal legislation be enacted requiring hospitals, physicians, and clinics to review their records and notify persons exposed to DES.

Because birth is a normal process, we recommend that the mother should have ultimate responsibility and power of decision over attendant, place, and method of birth.

To make wise decisions, women need sound information. Therefore, we recommend that women should have access to information about all aspects of reproduction. Such information should be provided by other women through women's networks or health centers to be established in each community with the help of public funds. Such funding should not necessarily be contingent upon involvement with conventional professional practitioners. Information on drugs and instrumental technologies is particularly important. Whenever possible, women should have the alternative of health care by women.

Background: Where the cause of the death or deformity of a child is unknown, the woman is frequently blamed in spite of her effort to make responsible choices for herself and her child.

We recommend that adverse outcomes should not be attributed to the behavior of a mother who has done what she considers best for the child.

We condemn the current attacks on midwives and on homebirth, especially the assertions of spokesmen for the American College of Obstetricians and Gynecologists (ACOG) that homebirth is a form of child abuse.

We recommend that the need for more information on the benefits, risks, and costs of both existing and new medical technology be recognized.

We further recommend that new mechanisms be developed for controlling the use and overuse of medical technology.

Background: The proponents of medical technology have career, emotional, and financial investments in the development and use of medical technology that fosters these abuses.

We recommend that these relationships should be public knowledge.

We recommend that midwifery training programs should be established in each state. Non-nurse midwifery programs should be recognized.

We further recommend that hospitals and physicians recognize their moral obligation to provide backup to midwives and others doing out-of-hospital deliveries in case of complications.

We recommend that high risk scales be critically re-evaluated, with an aim of drastically limiting the number of women classified as high risk.

We recommend that hospitals receiving funds from HEW should be required to obtain informed consent for all procedures, especially experimentation with any drug or device not approved by the Food and Drug Administration (FDA) as safe and effective for labor and delivery. Strong financial sanctions should be applied against hospitals not complying. The form used should be a standard one drawn up by a national commission of women under the aegis of the HEW. The mother must be given a copy of this signed form.

We recommend that all mothers must be given copies of their medical records covering pregnancy (from the health care provider) and childbirth records, as well as the infant's records, upon leaving the hospital—if necessary, without charge or change. No bills for hospital care should be tendered or paid until the medical record transfer is made.

Background: Federal dollars for research and health care services related to women's reproductive life are allocated through a process that is controlled by men.

We recommend that such processes should be controlled by women in a majority, with full participation by laywomen, and with proportional representation by women from all socioeconomic, racial, age, linguistic, and geographical groups.

Resolved, that women should have ultimate responsibility for decisions about their bodies and their unborn children.

Resolved, that we affirm the fact that women have unique perspectives to communicate to other women.

Resolved, that funding priorities be given to proven technologies that are easy to apply and that result in the greatest benefit to poor women of all communities, rather than to elaborate and expensive technologies that benefit only a few.

Background: Nondrug products are those products in common use, such as spray-on insecticides, cosmetics, laundry products, diesel, gasoline, and items emitting microwaves or other radiation.

Resolved, that nondrug products, such as the above listed, should be examined by the appropriate regulatory agencies for effects on reproduction.

Because women's reproductive health, our children's health, and all life on earth are threatened by herbicides, pesticides, and dangerous chemicals in their production, distribution, and disposal, we call for protection from them.

Because cultures and technologies other than those emerging from western industrialized nations have been undervalued by so many, we urge renewed recognition and appreciation of these other cultures and technologies.

We recommend that public policy reflect an awareness of the need to go *beyond* "informed consent" in cases where people are under extraordinary stress, as when a woman is in labor or when parents are faced with decisions about care for a newborn who is seriously ill or has severe birth defects. In such cases, health care workers need to promote the parents' ability to make decisions with which the parents can live. We recommend, for example, that educational curricula for health care workers be revised to place greater emphasis on the skills necessary to fulfill these moral requirements.

We recommend that the costs for special medical, rehabilitative, and social services [for babies with birth defects] be a community responsibility.

We recommend that further steps be taken (a) to increase community acceptance of physical differences in children, and (b) to achieve a more realistic appreciation of the prevalence of birth defects. We oppose the view that children are *products* that need to be *perfected.*

The *moral* situation regarding children and those (most often women) who care for them is *not* a function of marital status itself. Therefore, we recommend that policies regarding reproduction contain no provisions which discriminate on the basis of marital status.

Resolutions Receiving 50-74% Approval

Resolved, that medical schools, in selecting candidates for admission, choose humanities students who have taken required science courses rather than just students who have majored in the sciences.

Resolved, that appropriate hospital services be decentralized and offered in the community.

Resolved, that the aforementioned decentralization begin in hospitals serving low income patients.

Resolved, that an in-hospital or community group review the function of each hospital department as it relates to patients in order to humanize policies.

Resolved, that patient education be incorporated as a separate hospital department or service.

Resolved, that community education be directed towards the appropriate selection of health resources for specific problems.

Resolved, that future conferences similar to this provide ample space and opportunity for community residents to observe conference deliberations.

Resolved, that we solicit more funds for a conferences or conferences specifically focused on the political, social, and economic consequences of reproductive technology, as discussed here, and on ways of implementing recommended changes. The responsibility and authority for planning such conferences should be given to panels of the present participants.

We call for the establishment of registries similar to the Depo-Provera one for: sonograms, prenatal X-rays, and estrogen replacement therapy.

Based on the fact that dogs and monkeys appear to have developed cancers of their reproductive systems while receiving Depo-Provera, be it resolved that we oppose the use of this drug as a contraceptive for women until and unless convincing new evidence is gathered to show either that these animal data are wrong or that Depo-Provera does not cause cancer in humans.

Mechanisms should be developed to control the utilization of surgical procedures for which there is already evidence of misuse.

Independent patient advocates and mandatory second opinion programs should be available for all potential surgery patients.

We call for both public and private funding of research designed and conducted jointly by laypersons and professional/academic researchers.

Because the potential hazards of in vitro fertilization, including its application to human genetic engineering, surpass the benefits it may offer to women who are unable to bear children, we recommend a halt to the development of the technology of in vitro fertilization.

Resolved, that federal legislation be enacted to benefit those who suffered harm from DES exposure as a drug, as a food additive, or in the workplace.

Background: Available evidence suggests that carefully screened pregnant women have no more maternal or infant mortality or morbidity when delivered at home by skillful midwives than when delivered in hospitals by skillful obstetricians. Therefore,

We recommend that the persecution of midwives and of women and couples seeking out-of-hospital deliveries should cease. Midwives should be allowed freedom to practice independently.

We further recommend that the use of electronic fetal monitoring should be limited to major medical centers where careful evaluation can be carried out of its use in high risk pregnant women with full informed consent.

Background: Despite existing government mechanisms for protecting the public, women and their infants continue to be exposed to unsafe and unevaluated instrumental technologies, drugs and other substances prenatally, perinatally and postnatally. The importance of protecting our future generations requires unusual action. As a first step,

We recommend that the Food and Drug Administration establish a permanent committee to deal with these issues. The members of the committee should be a majority of nonphysician women representatives of users of services by race, social class, etc. Any physician members should be chosen by the nonphysician women. The staff for this committee should be, to the extent possible, made up of women.

Background: At present, "safe tolerance levels" as exist for chemicals, radiation, and microwaves do not consider the fetus, and frequently become excuses for occupational discrimination against women.

Resolved, that the Occupational Safety and Health Administration should require one low Safe Tolerance Level for all: fetuses, women, and men.

Because women's reproductive health, our children's health, and all life on earth are threatened by the nuclear industry at each stage—exploration, mining, weapons production, power plants, waste disposal, and experimentation—we call for an end to all activities promoting the development of nuclear arms and nuclear energy.

Resolved, that a federal agency (*not* NICHD) be empowered to add a study section for funding research and related activities on behavior teratology and developmental toxicology, that the staff be female, that the majority of study section members be female, and that the others be selected by the women in the study section.

We recommend that the stigma attached to the mothers [of children with birth defects] be investigated and changed.

The American Medical Association, local medical societies, and The American College of Obstetricians and Gynecologists should bar their members from the nontherapeutic use of medical technology in the determination or selection of the sex of a child-to-be.

We recommend that all policy in the area of human reproduction be written to recognize that the disabled have a right to exercise the full range of reproductive and social choices.

Notes and References

REPRODUCTIVE TECHNOLOGIES, Helen B. Holmes

1. Raymond, J., "Response," elsewhere in this volume.
2. Pearse, W. H., quoted in *Ob. Gyn. News* **19,** 1, 33 (1977).
3. Swallow, H., "Midwives in Many Settings," in *Birth Control and Controlling Birth,* Holmes, H. B., B. B. Hoskins, and M. Gross, eds., Humana, Clifton, New Jersey, 1980, p. 250.
4. Luce, J., "Ethical Issues Relating to Childbirth as Experienced by the Birthing Woman and Midwife," in *Birth Control and Controlling Birth,* Holmes, H. B., B. B. Hoskins, and M. Gross, eds., Humana, Clifton, New Jersey, 1980, p. 242.
5. Ampola, M., "Prenatal Diagnosis," elsewhere in this volume.
6. Carlton, W., "Perfectability and the Neonate,'" page 129.
7. Cook, K., "A Native American Response," in *Birth Control and Controlling Birth,* Holmes, H. B., B. B. Hoskins, and M. Gross, eds., Humana, Clifton, New Jersey, 1980, p. 256.

OVERVIEW, Anne J. Davis

1. Herbst, A. L., H. Ulfedler, and D. C. Poskanzer, Adenocarcinoma of the Vagina: Association of Maternal Stilbestrol Therapy with Tumor Appearance in Young Women, *N. Engl. J. Med.* **284,** 878 (1971).
2. Bibbo, M., W. M. Haenszel, G. L. Wied, M. Hubby, and A. L. Herbst, A Twenty-Five-Year Follow-Up Study of Women Exposed to Diethylstilbestrol During Pregnancy, *N. Engl. J. Med.* **298,** 763 (1978).
3. Gill, W. B., G. F. B. Schumacher, and M. Bibbo, Structural and Functional Abnormalities in the Sex Organs of Male Offspring of Mothers Treated with Diethylstilbestrol (DES), *J. Rep. Med.* **16,** 147 (1976).
4. Dieckmann, W. J., M. E. Davis, L. M. Rynkiewicz, and R. E. Pottinger, Does the Administration of Diethylstilbestrol during Pregnancy Have Therapeutic Value?, *Am. J. Obstet. Gyn.* **66,** 1062 (1953).
5. Ferguson, J. H., Effect of Stilbestrol on Pregnancy Compared to the Effect of a Placebo, *Am. J. Obstet. Gyn.* **65,** 592 (1953).

THE DES CONTROVERSY, Susan E. Bell

1. Noller, K. L., and C. R. Fish, "Diethylstilbestrol Usage: Its Interesting Past, Important Present, and Questionable Future," *Medical Clinics of North America* **58**(4), 795 (1974).
2. DES Task Force, *DES Task Force Summary Report,* U.S. Department of Health, Education and Welfare, DHEW Publication No. (NIH) 79-1688, September 21, 1978. Also, Wellenbach, B. L., M.D., Philadelphia Pa., personal communication, April 13, 1979.
3. Brackbill, Y., and H. W. Berendes, "Dangers of Diethylstilbestrol: Review of a 1953 Paper," *Lancet,* **2,** 520 (September 9, 1978). Also, O. and G. Smith, personal communication, April 9, 1979.
4. Ethical drug manufacturers were generally family-owned producers of drugs, the "elite" of drug producers at that time, who produced for physicians and not the public. They shunned association with patent or proprietary manufacturers, presenting an image of being against patenting, advertising, and competing for prices. The ethical manufacturers purported to produce uniform, quality products, seeing themselves as a kind of gentleman's club. (Measday, W. S., "The Pharmaceutical Industry," in *The Structure of American Industry.* Adams, W., ed., Macmillan Co, N.Y., 1977, 5th ed.: 250–284.)
5. Barker-Benfield, G. J., "A Historical Perspective on Women's Health Care—Female Circumcision," *Women and Health,* **1,**(1), 13–15, 18–20 (January/February 1976). Also, Dodds, E. C., "The Practical Outcome of Recent Research on Hormones," *Lancet* **227** (December 8), 1318–1320 (1934). And Hall, D. L., "Biology, Sex Hormones, and Sexism in the 1920s" *Phil. Forum* **5**(1-2), 81–97 (Fall-Winter 1973–1974).
6. The quote is from E. C. Dodds, p. 1318. It is interesting to note that Dodds, loyal to his peers, lays blame for the "rubbish" on the public and business. My impression is that physicians and scientists added to the "rubbish." In addition, Barbara Ehrenreich and Deirdre English have explored the issue of the relationship between medicine and sexism in *Complaints and Disorders: The Sexual Politics of Sickness.* The Feminist Press, New York, 1973. I would like to point out that today there is a continued belief in the power of hormones—albeit more refined. See the following for a discussion of this: Gordon, L., *Woman's Body, Woman's Right,* Grossman, N.Y., 1976; Rich, A., *Of Woman Born: Motherhood As Experience and Institution,* Norton, N.Y., 1976; Seaman, B., and G. Seaman, *Women and the Crisis in Sex Hormones,* The Book Press, Brattleboro, Vt. (1977).
7. Paul Ehrlich's theory of substitutability and charmed bullets, and his research into chemical dyes, formed the background for this research.
8. Dodds, E. C., "Synthetic Estrogens," *British Med. Bull.* **11,** 131–134 (1955).
9. Theoretical and applied research (and trial and error), in laboratories at Oxford and London, as well as in Germany, led to this discovery. E. C.

Dodds, of the Courtauld Institute in London, and Robert Robinson, of an Oxford laboratory, are credited with having synthesized DES. Both men were knighted in later years for other research. (Dodds, E. C., L. Goldberg, W. Lawson, and R. Robinson, "Oestrogenic Activity of Certain Synthetic Compounds," *Nature* **141,** 247–248, (1938). (Golberg's name was misspelled in this communication and was corrected in the subsequent communications from the Courtauld Institute.) Also, in England, DES research received funds from the British government primarily. However, some of the researchers were supported by drug houses. For instance, Muriel Boycott had been a research fellow of the British Drug House since October 1937. In the United States DES research was funded primarily by the drug industry and by private foundation grants. (See also, Shyrock, R. H., *American Medical Research Past and Present,* The Commonwealth Fund, N.Y., 1947).

10. Golberg, L., oral deposition taken April 25, 1976 in *Barros v. E. R. Squibb & Sons, Inc.,* No. 75-1226 U.S. District Court, Eastern District of Pennsylvania.

11. Bishop, P. M. F., M. Boycott, and S. Zuckerman, "The Oestrogenic Properties of 'Stilbestrol' (Diethylstilboestrol)," *Lancet* **236** 5–11, (1939). Also, Winterton, W. R., and T. N. MacGregor, "Clinical Observations with Stilboestrol (Diethylstilboestrol)," *British Med. J.* **1,** 10–12, January 7, 1939.

12. Letter, Sir Henry Dale to Merck and Company, May 6, 1939.

13. See for instance, Ehrenreich, B., and D. English, *Witches, Midwives and Nurses,* Glass Mountain Pamphlets, N.Y., 1972. Also, Dubos, R., *Mirage of Health,* Harper, N.Y., 1979. Ehrenreich and English, Dubos, and others have documented this faith in potions, drugs and interventions generally in the western "organized" medical community from its origins to the present.

14. Noller and Fish, *op. cit.;* E. C. Dodds, 1955.

15. Federal Food, Drug, and Cosmetic Act. 52 STAT. 1040–1059.

16. New Drug Application #1643 filed with the FDA September 14, 1939.

17. See, for example, the following: Lacassagne, A., "Apparition d'adenocarcinomies mammaires chez des souris males traitees par une substance oestrogene synthetique," *Compt. rend. Soc. biol.* **129,** 641–643 (1938) *CA* **33,** 1392; Varangot, J., "Clinical Use of Stilbestrol," *Lancet* **236,** 296 (1939).

18. Letter, FDA to Sharp and Dohme, August 29, 1939.

19. Letter, FDA to Merck and Company, September 21, 1939; letter, ADMA to Abbott Industries, December 27, 1938; letter, ADMA to Parke-Davis, October 16, 1939; letter, ADMA to Parke-Davis, November 9, 1939.

20. Letter, physician to Sharp and Dohme, October 7, 1940.

21. Trip Report, January 30, 1941 by D. C. Hines of Eli Lilly (unpublished); letter, D. C. Hines to E. Gifford Upjohn, February 3, 1941.

22. The FDA had, in another case, requested that four companies file a joint application to streamline the approval process. Klumpp, T. G., oral deposition taken January 23, 1979 in *Payton et al. v. Abbott Labs et al.* No. 76-1514-S U.S. District Court, District of Massachusetts.

23. Letter, D. C. Hines to FDA, April 23, 1941. *Meeting Regarding Stilbestrol in New York City, March 24, 1941 and Washington D. C. March 25, 1941* by D. C. Hines (dated March 28, 1941 and unpublished).

24. Hines, Meeting Regarding Stilbestrol. . . .; *Memorandum of Interview* signed by T. Klumpp, R. P. Herwick, H. F. Kennedy (dated March 25, 1941 and unpublished).

25. The companies were: Abbott Laboratories, Armour Laboratories, Ayerst, McKenna & Harrison, George A. Breon & Co., Inc., Charles E. Frosst & Co., Eli Lilly & Co., Merck & Co., Inc., Sharp and Dohme, Inc., E. R. Squibb & Sons, The Upjohn Co., Winthrop Chemical Co., Inc., John Wyeth & Brother, Inc.

26. They reorganized what they had previously collected and undertook as little new testing as possible, having appointed a Small Committee to organize the data collection, to devise a questionnaire to distribute to physicians who had been researching DES, and to have ongoing meetings with FDA officials.

27. By the end of May, company officials were told informally that the FDA would probably have a positive response to their applications (internal memo, Upjohn, author unknown, May 27, 1941).

28. Of the twelve companies that originally filed the joint application, as of 1973, ten were among the 25 largest multinational pharmaceutical companies (cf., James, B. G., *The Future of the Multinational Pharmaceutical Industry to 1990,* Wiley, N.Y., 1977.)

ASSESSMENT OF RISKS FROM DES, Barbara C. Tilley

1. Noller, K. L., and C. R. Fish, "Diethylstilbestrol Usage: Its Interesting Past, Important Present, and Questionable Future," *Medical Clinics of North America* **58** (4), 795 (1974).

2. Chalmers, T. C., "The Impact of Controlled Trials on the Practice of Medicine," *Mount Sinai. J. Med.* **41**(6), 753–759. (1974).

3. Dieckmann, W. J., M. E. Davis, L. M. Rynkiewiez, and R. D. Pottinger, "Does the Administration of Diethylstilbestrol During Pregnancy Have Therapeutic Value?", *Am. J. Obstet. Gynecol.* **66,** 1062–1081 (1953).

4. Herbst, A. L., H. Ulfelder, D. C. Poskanzer, "Adenocarcinoma of the Vagina: Association of Maternal Stilbestrol Therapy with Tumor Appearance in Young Women", *N. Engl. J. Med.* **284,** 878–881 (1971).

5. Heinonen, O. P., "Diethylstilbestrol in Pregnancy: Frequency of Exposure and Usage Patterns," *Cancer* **31,** 573–577 (1973).

6. Labarthe, D., E. Adam, K. Noller, et al., "Design and Preliminary Observations of National Cooperative Diethylstilbestrol Adenosis (DESAD) Project," *Obstet. Gynecol.* **51**(4), 453–458 (1978).

7. O'Brien, P. C., K. Noller, S. J. Robboy, et al., "Vaginal Epithelial

Changes in Young Women Enrolled in the National Cooperative Diethylstilbestrol Adenosis (DESAD) Project," *Obstet. Gynecol.* **53**(3), 300–308 (1979).

8. Bibbo, M., W. M. Haenszel, G. L. Wied, et al., "A Twenty-Five-Year Follow-Up Study of Women Exposed to Diethylstilbestrol During Pregnancy," *N. Engl. J. Med.* **298,** 763–767 (1978).

9. Brian, D., B. C. Tilley, D. R. Labarthe, et al., "Breast Cancer in DES-Exposed Mothers: Lack of an Association," *Mayo Clin. Prac.* **55,** 89–93 (1980).

10. Bibbo, M., M. A. Nageeb, I. Baccarini, et al., "Follow-Up Study of Male and Female Offspring of DES-Treated Mothers," *J. Rep. Med.* **15,** 29–32 (1975).

11. Gill, W. B., G. F. B. Schumacher, and M. Bibbo, "Structural and Functional Abnormalities in the Sex Organs of Male Offspring of Mothers Treated with Diethylstilbestrol (DES)," *J. Rep. Med.* **16,** 147–153 (1976).

12. Bibbo, M., W. B. Gill, F. Azizi, et al., "Follow-Up Study of Male and Female Offspring of DES-Exposed Mothers," *Obstet. Gynecol.* **49,** 1–8 (1977).

13. Gill, W. B., G. F. B. Schumacher, M. Bibbo, "Pathological Semen and Anatomical Abnormalities of the Genital Tract in Human Male Subjects Exposed to Diethylstilbestrol in Utero," *J. Urol.* **117,** 477–480 (1977).

14. Henderson, B. E., B. Benton, M. Cosgrove, et al., "Urogenital Tract Abnormalities in Sons of Women Treated with Diethylstilbestrol," *Pediatrics* **58,** 505–507 (1976).

15. Herbst, A. L., and R. E. Scully, "Adenocarcinoma of the Vagina in Adolescence: A Report of 7 Cases Including 6 Clear Cell Carcinomas (so-called mesonephromas)," *Cancer* **25,** 745–757 (1970).

16. Herbst, A. L., P. Cole, T. Colton, et al., "Age-Incidence and Risk of Diethylstilbestrol-Related Clear Cell Adenocarcinoma of the Vagina and Cervix," *Amer. J. Obstet. Gynecol.* **128**(1), 43–50 (1977).

17. Lanier, A., K. Noller, D. Decker, and L. Kurland, "Cancer and Stilbestrol: A Follow-Up of 1719 Persons Exposed to Estrogens In Utero and Born 1943–1959," *Mayo Clin. Proc.* **48,** 793–799 (1973).

18. Stafl, A., and R. F. Mattingly, "Vaginal Adenosis: A Precancerous Lesion?," *Amer. J. Obstet. Gynecol.* **120,** 666 (1974).

19. DESAD Project, unpublished data.

20. Kaufman, R. H., et al., "Upper Genital Tract Changes Associated with Exposure In Utero to Diethylstilbestrol," *Amer. Obstet. J. Gynecol.* **128,** 51–59 (1977).

21. Barnes, A. B., T. Colton, J. Gunderson, K. L. Noller, B. C. Tilley, I. Strams, D. E. Townsend, P. Hatab, and P. C. O'Brien, "Fertility and Outcome of Women Exposed *in Utero* to Diethylstilbestrol, *"N. Engl. J. Med.* **302,** 609 (1980).

22. Robboy, S. J., R. H. Kaufman, J. Prat, et al., "Pathologic Findings in Young Women Enrolled in National Cooperative Diethylstilbestrol Adenosis (DESAD) Project," *Obstet. Gynecol.* **53,** 309–316 (1979).

23. Antonioli, D. A., L. Burke, and S. Rosen, "Evolution of Diethylstilbestrol-Associated Lower Genital Tract Abnormalities," *Lab. Invest.* (abstract), 1979.
24. O'Brien, P. C., B. C. Tilley, P. Meier, et al., "Effects of Selection Bias Arising in Observational Studies: An Example from the Study of DES and Genital Abnormalities," submitted for publication.
25. Kaufman, R. H., P. M. Gray, G. L. Binder, and A. A. Gerthoff, "Upper Genital Tract Changes and Pregnancy Outcome in Offspring Exposed In Utero to Diethylstilbestrol," *Amer. J. Obstet. Gynecol.* **302**(11), 609–613 (1980).
26. Herbst, A. L., M. M. Hubby, R. R. Blough, and F. Azizi, "A Comparison of Pregnancy Experience in DES-Exposed and Unexposed Daughters," *J. Reprod. Med.* **24**(2), 62–69 (1980).
27. DES Task Force, *DES Task Force Report,* U. S. Department of Health, Education and Welfare, DHEW Publication No. (NIH) 79-1688, 1978.
28. Professional and Public Relations Committee of the DESAD Project and Office of Cancer Communications, *Information for Physicians—DES Exposure In Utero,* U. S. Department of Health, Education and Welfare, DHEW Publication No. (NIH) 78-1119.

THE LEGAL ASPECTS OF THE DES CASE, Fay A. Rozovsky

1. Dieckmann, W. J., et al., Does the Administration of Diethylstilbestrol during Pregnancy Have Therapeutic Value?, *Am. J. Obstet. Gyn.* **66,** 1062 (1953).
2. *Plaintiff's Brief in Opposition to Defendants' Joint Motion for Partial Summary Judgment, Abel v. Eli Lilly & Co.,* No. 74-030-070 NP (Mich. Cir. Ct. 1977), at pp. 12–13, quoting: E. C. Hambler, M.D.; see Editorial, *JAMA* **114,** 1650 (1940), and Henry, J. S., *Can. Med. Assoc. J.* (1945).
3. *T. J. Hooper,* 60 F. 2d 737 (2nd Cir. 1932).
4. *Supra* at p. 740.
5. *Helling* v. *Carey,* 83 Wash. 2d 514 (1974).
6. Herbst, A. L., et al., Adenocarcinoma of the Vagina, *N. Engl. J. Med.* **284,** 878 (1971).
7. See note, DES and A Proposed Theory of Enterprise Liability, *Fordham Law Review* **46,** 963 (1978).
8. *Abel* v. *Eli Lilly & Co., appeal pending,* Supreme Court of Michigan.
9. *Supra* note 2 at Appendix I.
10. *Griffin* v. *U.S.* 351 Supp. 10 (E.D. Pa, 1972), 353 F. Supp. 324 (E.D. Pa, 1973), *aff'd in part, rev'd in part and remanded* 500 F. 2d 1059 (3rd Cir. 1974).
11. *Payras* v. *U.S.,* No. 77-148-Orl—Cir Y (M.D. Fla, 1978) and *Gray* v. *U.S.,* 445 F. Supp. 337 (S.D. Tex, 1978).

12. *Gray* v. *U.S., supra* note 11 at p. 340.
13. Id. at p. 339.
14. New York Laws, 12177, March 30, 1976.

A LOOK AT PRENATAL DIAGNOSIS WITHIN THE CONTEXT OF CHANGING PARENTAL AND REPRODUCTIVE NORMS, Regina H. Kenen

1. *The New York Times,* Clues to Fetus Found in Mother's Blood, April 10, 1979; Prenatal Test Detects Hemophilia, April 26, 1979.
2. Meyerwitz, S., and M. Lipkin, Jr., Psychosocial Aspects, in R. Brent et al. (eds.), *Prevention of Embryonic, Fetal. and Perinatal Disease,* DHEW Publication No. (NIH) 76-8537, Government Printing Office, Washington, D. C., 1976.
3. Emery, A., Changing Patterns in a Genetic Counseling Clinic, in H. Lubs and F. deLa Cruz (eds.), *Genetic Counseling,* Raven Press, New York, (1977).
4. *Current Population Reports* **51,** 16 (1975).
5. National Center for Health Statistics, *Monthly Vital Statistics Report, Annual Summary for the United States, 1976,* U.S. Department of Health, Education and Welfare, 1977, p. 2.
6. Espenshade, T., The Value and Cost of Children, *Population Bull.* **32**(#1) (1977).
7. Berelson, B., The Value of Children: A Taxonomical Essay, in J. Wells (ed.), *Current Issues in Marriage and the Family,* 2nd ed., Macmillan, New York, 1979.
8. Olshansky, S., Chronic Sorrow: A Response to Having a Mentally Defective Child, *Social Casework* 43, 190 (1962).
9. Fletcher, J., Parents in Genetic Counseling: The Moral Shape of Decision-making, in B. Hilton et al. (eds.), *Ethical Issues in Human Genetics: Genetic Counseling and the Use of Genetic Knowledge,* Plenum, New York, 1973.
10. Birenbaum, A., On Managing a Courtesy Stigma, *J. Health Social Behavior* **11,** 196 (1970).
11. *The New York Times,* More Couples Adopting Victims of Genetic Defects, March 8, 1979.
12. Editors of *Ebony* magazine, The Pros and Cons of Parenthood, in J. Wells (ed.), *Current Issues in Marriage and the Family,* 2nd ed., Macmillan, New York, 1979.
13. Mazor, M., Barren Couples, *Psychology Today,* May, 1979.
14. Veevers, J. E., The Moral Careers of Voluntarily Childless Wives: Notes on the Defense of a Variant World View, in P. Stein et al. (eds.), *The Family: Functions, Conflicts, and Symbols,* Addison-Wesley, Reading, Mass., 1977.

15. Rossi, A., Transition to Parenthood, in P. Stein et al. (eds.), *The Family: Functions, Conflicts, and Symbols,* Addison-Wesley, Reading, Mass., 1977.
16. Hollerbach, P. H., Parental Choice and Family Planning: The Acceptability, Use, and Sequelae of Four Methods, in Y. Hsia et al. (eds.), *Counseling in Genetics,* Liss, New York, 1979.
17. Shaw, M., Review of Published Studies of Genetic Counseling: A Critique, in H. Lubs and F. deLa Cruz (eds.), *Genetic Counseling,* Raven Press, New York, 1977.
18. Francoeur, R. T., *Utopian Motherhood,* Doubleday, Garden City, New York, 1970.
19. Consensus Development Conference on Antenatal Diagnosis, Draft, Task Force Report: Predictors of Hereditary Disease or Congenital Defects, Public Health Service, National Institutes of Health, 1979.
20. Cassidy, R., Personal communication, (1979).
21. Fletcher, J. The Brink: The Parent-Child Bond in the Genetic Revolution, *Theological Studies* **33,** 475 (1972).

ANTENATAL DIAGNOSIS, Elaine Locke

1. Milunsky, A., Genetic Counseling in Obstetric Practice, *Contemporary Ob/Gyn* **8,** 107, (1976). Motulsky, A., Brave New World? *Science* **185,** 657 (1974).
2. Task Force on Predictors of Hereditary Disease or Congenital Defects, Draft Report for the Consensus Development Conference on Antenatal Diagnosis, National Institutes of Health, DHEW, Washington, D.C., 1979, pp. 61, 114; Lebel, R., Ethical Issues Arising in the Genetic Counseling Relationship, *Birth Defects:* Original Article Series, XIV, National Foundation/March of Dimes, White Plains, New York, 1978, p. 31.
3. Task Force (NIH), *op. cit.,* pp. 163–164.
4. *Ibid.,* p. 123.
5. Milunsky, *op. cit.,* p. 106; Rosenstock, I., B. Childs, and A. Simopoulos, *Genetic Screening: A Study of the Knowledge and Attitudes of Physicians,* National Academy of Sciences, Washington, D.C., 1975, pp. 77–79.
6. Milunsky, *op. cit.,* p. 110.
7. Lebel, *op. cit.,* pp. 27–28.
8. Task Force (NIH), *op. cit.,* p. 146.
9. *Ibid.,* p. 17.
10. *Ibid.,* p. 61.
11. Powledge, T., and J. Fletcher, Guidelines for the Ethical, Social and Legal Issues in Prenatal Diagnosis, *New England J. Med.* **300,** 171 (1979). Task Force (NIH), *op. cit.,* pp. 17–18, 160, 161.
12. *Ibid.,* p. 109.

13. Lebel, *op. cit.,* pp. 24, 25.
14. *Ibid.,* pp. 19, 20.
15. Childs, B., and A. Simopoulos, *Genetic Screening: Procedural Guidance and Recommendations,* National Academy of Sciences, Washington, D.C., 1979, pp. 40–44.
16. Task Force (NIH), *op. cit.,* pp. 172–175; Fletcher, J., Moral and Ethical Problems of Pre-natal Diagnosis, in: *Problems of Birth Defects from Hippocrates to Thalidomide and After,* University Park Press, Baltimore, 1977, p. 366.

THE POLITICS OF PRENATAL DIAGNOSIS, Susan Rae Peterson

1. Notice that this formulation of the moral question avoids the moral term "rights," and therefore gets down to a more basic level of moral judgment than the rather legal set of judgments such as "Doctors have the right to diagnose" or "Patients have a right to know," etc.
2. In my Medical Ethics courses, usually filled with nurses, fallacy finding meets with student enthusiasm. Nurses go back to their jobs and provide a logical critique of a standard and fallacious argument given to them by a superior, and are gratified to have been able to make their point (although sometimes this endangers a livelihood). One convenient and short paperback about fallacies with amusing examples from politicians is: Kahane, H., *Logic and Contemporary Rhetoric,* Wadsworth, Belmont, California, 1978.
3. A very accessible and accurate discussion of this is given in chapter 8 of Veatch, R., *Case Studies in Medical Ethics,* Harvard, Cambridge, Mass., 1978.
4. Masculinist here is as opposed to feminist; so some women may not be feminist and some men not masculinist. Since feminists support values that guarantee the well-being and rights of women, masculinists support values that maintain the *status quo* of privilege and success among men.
5. A moral agent is a human being who is old enough to be able to predict the consequences of his or her actions, who has thus reached moral maturity, who is not insane, and who is in general capable of being held liable for responsibilities. Historically, the people who have traditionally been held to be nonresponsible are women, children, and the insane.
6. Rationality is the minimum condition under which contracts are valid. Since rationality is defined as maximizing one's own self-interest, and since slavery most absolutely denies that very thing, such a contract would be null and void, however much the would-be slave protested.
7. See especially work done by John Ladd, such as Legalism in Medical Ethics, in *Contemporary Issues in Biomedical Ethics,* Davis, J., et al., eds., Humana, Clifton, NJ, 1978.
8. Lawrence Kohlberg, Stage and Sequence: The Cognitive-Developmental

Approach to Socialization, in *Handbook of Socialization Theory and Research,* Cosan, D., ed., Rand McNally, New York, 1969. Prof. Picciarelli, "Kohlberg and Women's Moral Reasoning: An Ideological Critique" a paper read at the October 1979 New York Society for Women in Philosophy (SWIP) meeting. Requests for more information on this can be sent to Prof. Patricia Picciarelli, Dept. of Social Sciences, 1855 Broadway, New York Institute of Technology, New York, New York.

9. See pp. 5–21 in Jagger, A., Political Philosophies of Women's Liberation, in *Feminism and Philosophy,* Littlefield-Adams, Totowa, New Jersey, 1977.
10. If the means of reproduction are more basic than the means of production, since women produce the producers, then women ought logically to occupy a more powerful or potentially powerful position than do men. There is a real problem here insofar as women produce future laborers for the marketplace. Marx (in *The Economic and Philosophical Manuscripts of 1844*) foresaw this and said that capitalism would find ways either to increase or to decrease the labor market as it saw fit. Of course women are doubly oppressed in such cases.
    See also my "The Ruling Sex: An Argument for the Ownership of the Means of Reproduction," given at the Women and Society Conference, St. Michael's College, Winooski, Vermont, March, 1979.
11. Firestone, S., *The Dialectic of Sex,* Bantam, New York, 1972.
12. Sara Ann Ketchum, Department of Philosophy, SUNY at Oswego, Oswego, New York, presented a paper, "Abortion and the Ownership of Bodies," at the National Project on Philosophy and Engineering Ethics Conference, August, 1978, Rensselaer Polytechnic Institute, Troy, New York.
13. Janet Farrell Smith (Dept. of Philosophy, Smith College) presented a paper, "Violence and Women's Oppression," at the Women and Society Conference, St. Michael's College, Winooski, Vermont, March, 1979, in which she analyzed the differences in forms of power.

NEONATOLOGY, Maureen Edwards

1. Pierre Budin in Paris in the late 19th century was one of the earliest physicians with an interest in the problems of the premature. He is credited with the development of tube feeding, the incubator, and the report of marked improvement in survival of low-birth-weight infants when "normal" body temperatures were maintained. Budin's pupil Martin Couney brought this technology to the United States in 1898 when (perhaps ironically for current specialists) premature infants and their incubators were "exhibited" at a large number of expositions including the New York World's Fair in 1939, and became a permanent concession at the Park in Coney Island. Although this showmanship aura of the beginning of American neonatology seems incongruous by modern standards, Couney provided advanced care for his era and laid a foundation for later

specialists in this field. Julian Hess, acquainted with and influenced by Couney, opened the first premature center in the United States in Chicago in 1922.

Clement Smith, one of the founders of modern neonatology published the first edition of a major scientific text in the field, *The Physiology of the Newborn Infant* in 1945. Schaeffer's clinical text followed in 1960.

2. The American Academy of Pediatrics did not address the issue of Neonatal Intensive Care in its *Standards and Recommendations for Hospital Care of Newborn Infants* until its fifth edition in 1971.
3. Swyer, P. R., in *Neonatology,* Avery, G. B., ed, Lippincott, Philadelphia, 1975, p. 15.
4. Tooley, W. H., and R. H. Phibbs, in *Ethics of Newborn Intensive Care,* Jonsen, A. R., and M. J. Garland, eds., Institute of Governmental Studies, Washington, DC, 1976, p. 11.
5. Stahlman, M. T., in *Problems of Neonatal Intensive Care Units,* Reports of the 59th Conference on Pediatric Research, Lucey, J. F., ed., Columbus, Ross Laboratories, 1966, p. 17.
6. Teberg, A., J. E. Hodgman, P. K. Y. Wu, and R. L. Spears, "Recent Improvement in Outcome for the Small Premature Infant. Follow-Up of Infants with a Birth Weight of Less Than 1,500 Grams," *Clin. Pediatrics* **16**(4) 307–313 (Apr. 1977).
7. Pape, K. E., R. J. Buncic, S. Ashby, and P. M. Fitzhardinge, "The Status at Two Years of Low-Birth Weight Infants Born in 1974 with Birth Weights of Less Than 1,001 gm," *J. Pediatrics* **92**(2) 253–260 (Feb. 1978).

DECISIONS ABOUT HANDICAPPED NEWBORNS, Diana E. Axelsen

1. Darling, R., Parents, Physicians, and Spina Bifida, *Hastings Center Report* 7(4), 10 (1977).
2. Freeman, J., Ethics and the Decision Making Process for Defective Children, in D. J. Roy (ed.), *Medical Wisdom and Ethics in the Treatment of Severely Defective Newborn and Young Children,* Eden Press, Montreal, Canada, 1978.
3. Darling, op. cit., p. 13.
4. Stein, J., *Making Medical Choices: Who Is Responsible,* Houghton Mifflin, Boston, 1978, pp. 120–121.
5. Stein, ibid., p. 104.
6. Rush, A., *Getting Clear: Body Work for Women,* Random House, New York, 1973, pp. 238–239.
7. These arguments might also be used to defend the primacy of maternal choice in the case of abortion, but there would be differences in other aspects of the ethical analysis.
8. Zimmerman, D., Are Test-Tube Babies the Answer for the Childless?, *Woman's Day,* 22 (May 22, 1979).

9. Thomson, J. J., A Defense of Abortion, *Philosophy and Public Affairs* **1,** 47–66 (1971).

10. Much can be learned about the integration of reverence for life into every aspect of human activity, through study of the world views of Native Americans. For example, David Villaseñor offers the following description of attitudes toward hunting:

> The success of the truly sincere hunter is legendary among the American Indians. Guided by the unseen force, he often went directly to his prey, but also he would utter a silent prayer before releasing the fatal arrow, saying: "Forgive me little brother, but I take your life in order to preserve life as I in turn will be taken." But never did he kill more than for his own need, or the need of his people.

To understand such accounts fully, however, it is important to study them within the context of the entire cosmology and ceremonial life of Native Americans. Villaseñor, D., *Tapestries in Sand: The Spirit of Indian Sandpainting,* Naturegraph, Healdsburg, CA, 1963, p. 83.

11. Freeman, op. cit., p. 37.

12. I am indebted to Dr. Mary Harris, former director of the Sickle Cell Foundation of Georgia, for providing information on the composition of NIH advisory boards and on legislation in the area of genetic diseases.

RIGHTS OF A HANDICAPPED NEONATE, Helga M. Bendix

1. *Advocacy and Service Provision to the Developmentally Disabled and Their Families,* John F. Kennedy Institute for Handicapped Children, Maryland, c. 1978, pp. 181–182.
2. Ibid., p. 182.
3. *Federal Register* **42,** No. 86, Wednesday, May 4, 1977.
4. Martin, R., *Workshop Materials, Educational Rights of Handicapped Children,* Research Press Company, Champaign, Illinois, c. 1977, p. 1.

LIVING WITH AN IMPAIRED NEONATE AND CHILD, E. Virginia Sheppard Lapham

1. Friedan, B., *The Feminine Mystique,* Dell, New York, 1974, p. 4.
2. *Ibid.,* p. 57.
3. Bernard, J., *The Future of Motherhood,* Penguin, New York, 1974, p. 275.

4. McBride, A. B., *The Growth and Development of Mothers,* Harper and Row, New York, 1973, pp. 128, 129.
5. Roskies, E., *Abnormality and Normality: The Mothering of Thalidomide Children,* Cornell University Press, Ithaca, 1972. Roskies found that one of the crucial factors in mothering a child deformed by thalidomide was finding some aspect of the child such as bright eyes or normal intelligence that enabled the mother to view her child as "like me."
6. Hall, J., Gains Being Made in Battle Against Birth Defects. *Gannett Westchester Newspapers,* June 14, 1979.
7. Darling, R. B., Parents, Physicians, and Spina Bifida, *The Hastings Center Report* **7** (4), 11 (1977). Ms. Darling, a sociologist who interviewed parents of 25 children with spina bifida said:

> Many [parents] candidly admitted that, if given a choice, they would not have wanted their children to have been born. The typical parental attitude I found might best be described as "realistic acceptance." All the parents would have preferred a normal child but they were still able to love the defective child they had.

8. See for example: Lonsdale, G., Family Life with a Handicapped Child: The Parents Speak, *Child: Care, Health and Development,* **4,** 99 (1978); Lapin, C. L., and A. Donnellan-Walsh, Advocacy and Research: A Parent's Perspective, *Journal of Pediatric Psychology* **2,** 191 (1977); Cunningham, C. C., and T. Sloper, Parents of Down's Syndrome Babies: Their Early Needs, *Child: Care, Health and Development* **3,** 325 (1977); Culbertson, F. M., The Search for Help of Parents of Autistic Children or Beware of Professional "Groupthink," *Journal of Clinical Child Psychology* **1,** 63 (1977); Dembinski, R. J., and J. Mauser, What Parents of the Learning Disabled Really Want from Professionals, *Learning Disabil.* **10,** 578 (1977); Gorham, K. A., A Lost Generation of Parents, *Exceptional Children* **41,** 521 (1975); Gayton, W. F., and L. Walker, Down's Syndrome: Informing the Parents: A Study of Parental Preferences, *Amer. J. Diseases Children* **127,** 510 (1974); Also see the bi-monthly periodical *Exceptional Parents.*
9. The Boston Women's Health Book Collective, *Our Bodies, Ourselves,* 2nd ed., Simon and Schuster, New York, 1976, p. 249.
10. *Ibid.,* p. 250.
11. Jonsen, A. R., and G. Lister, Newborn Intensive Care: The Ethical Problems, *The Hastings Center Report* **8,** 15 (1978).

> Over the past ten to fifteen years a considerable body of data has been developed to guide scientific and technical advances in the medical treatment of seriously ill newborn infants. A neonatal intensive care unit brings together sophisticated equipment and specially trained personnel to provide the optimal environment for assisting the endangered infant through a critical stage in the transition to extrauterine life.

12. See footnote 8 for references on this topic.
13. Retrolental Fibroplasia (RFL) is an abnormal condition of the eyes of premature infants that causes blindness. In the 1950s scientists discovered that excessive oxygen in the incubators caused RFL, so that today few premature infants are now treated in this way unless it is the only way to save the baby's life.
14. Oelsner, L., More Couples Adopting Victims of Genetic Defect, *The New York Times,* March 8, 1 (1979).
15. Jacoby, S., The $73,000 Abandoned Babies, *The New York Times Magazine,* March 6, 55 (1977).
16. Scheflen, A., and A. Ferber, Critique of a Sacred Cow, in A. Ferber et al. (eds.), *The Book of Family Therapy,* Boston, Houghton Mifflin, 1973, p. 674.
17. Anonymous, Life with a Brain-Damaged Child, *The New York Times,* March 28, Op Ed page (1978).
18. This woman, parent of a son, now 22, who was born with multiple handicaps as a result of maternal rubella, is now writing about her experiences with her family. All of her other five children are writing their reactions and feelings and memories too.
19. Barsch, R. H., *The Parent of the Handicapped Child,* Charles C. Thomas, Springfield, Illinois, 1968, p. 352.
20. Jacoby, *op. cit.,* pp. 56, 57.
21. Public Law 94–142, *The Education for All Handicapped Children Act of 1975.*
22. Barsch, *op. cit.,* p. 366.
23. *Ibid.,* p. 362.
24. Darling, *op. cit.,* p. 11.
25. Sharlin, S. A., and N. A. Polansky, The Process of Infantalization, *Amer. J. Orthopsychiatry,* 92–102 (1972).
26. Heisler, V., *A Handicapped Child in the Family,* Grune and Stratton, New York, 1972, p. 7.
27. Debuskey, M., *The Chronically Ill Child and His Family,* Charles C. Thomas, Springfield, Illinois, 1970, p. 82.
28. This review of more than 100 books and articles on research reported in the literature was done in 1974. It included: Barsch, *op. cit.;* Roskies, *op. cit.;* Hewett, S., with J. and E. Newson, *The Family and the Handicapped Child: A Study of Cerebral Palsied Children in Their Homes,* Aldine, Chicago, 1970; McMichael, J. K., *Handicapped: A Study of Physically Handicapped Children and Their Families,* Staples, London, 1971.
29. Schreiber, M., Introduction, *Social Work and Mental Retardation,* John Day, New York, 1970.
30. Heisler, *op. cit.,* p. 7.
31. Resolution on the Handicapped, submitted by The Commission on Social Action of Reform Judaism (November 19, 1977); Pastoral Statement of the U.S. Catholic Bishops on Handicapped People, U.S. Catholic Conference (November 16, 1977); Resolution on the Church and

Persons with Handicaps, National Council of Churches in the USA, adopted by the Governing Board (November 9, 1977).
32. Dillon, D., Opening Doors to the Handicapped, July-August 1979 issue of *New World Outlook,* p. 41.
33. Bernard, *op. cit.,* p. 292.
34. Nagy, K., Rehumanization and the Helping Services, *Rehabilitation Literature* **34**(2), 42 (1975).
35. *Our Bodies, Ourselves: A Book By and For Women,* 2nd edition, The Boston Women's Health Book Collective, New York, Simon and Schuster, 1976, p. 249.
36. Hall, *op. cit.*

INTRODUCTION, Janice G. Raymond

1. Daly, M., *Gyn/Ecology: The Metaethics of Radical Feminism,* Beacon, Boston, 1978, p. 232.

TECHNICAL ASPECTS OF SEX PRESELECTION, M. Ruth Nentwig

1. Gordon, M. J., The Control of Sex, *Scient. Amer.* **236**(6), 87 (1977).
2. O'Ferrall, G. J. M., The Artificial Control of the Sex Ratio in Mammals—A Review, *The Irish Vet. J.* **18,** 81 (1964).
3. Unterberger, F., Use of the Acid-Alkali Method for Sex Control, *Deutsche Med. Wochenschr.* **56,** 304 (1931).
4. Ericsson, R. J., C. N. Langevin, and M. Nishino, Isolation of Fractions Rich in Human Y Sperm, *Nature* **246,** 421 (1973).
5. Campbell, C., The Manchild Pill, *Psychology Today,* p. 86 (August, 1976).
6. Kleegman, S. J., Therapeutic Donor Insemination, *Fertil. Steril.* **5,** 7 (1954).
7. Shettles, L. B., Conception and Birth Sex Ratios: A Review, *Obstet. Gynecol.* **15,** 122 (1961).
8. Department of Obstetrics and Gynecology, Teitung Hospital of Anshan Iron and Steel Company, Fetal Sex Prediction by Sex Chromatin of Chorionic Villi Cells during Early Pregnancy, *Chinese Medical J.* **1,** 117. (1975).
9. Leff, D. N., Boy or Girl: Now Choice Not Chance, *Medical World News* **16,** 45 (1975).
10. Manual, M., I. J. Park, and H. W. Jones, Prenatal Sex Determination by Fluorescent Staining of Cells for the Presence of Y Chromatin, *Amer. J. Obstet. Gynecol.* **119,** 853 (1974).

FUTURISTIC IMPLICATIONS OF SEX PRESELECTION, Roberta Steinbacher

1. Westoff, C. F., and R. R. Rindfuss, Sex Preselection in the United States: Some Implications, *Science* **184,** 633 (1974).

2. Williamson, N. E., Boys or girls? Parental Preferences and Sex Control, *Population Bull.* **33** (1), 1978.

3. Coombs, L. C., Preference for Sex of Children among U.S. Couples, *Family Planning Perspectives* **9,** 259 (1977).

4. Dinitz, S., R. R. Dynes, and A. C. Clarke, Preference for Male or Female Children: Traditional or Affectional?, *Marriage and Family Living* **16,** 128 (1954).

5. Largey, G., Sex Control, Sex Preferences, and the Future of the Family, *Soc. Biol.* **19,** 379 (1972).

6. Markle, G. E., Sex Ratio at Birth: Values, Variance, and Some Determinants, *Demography* **11,** 131 (1974).

7. Markle, G. E., and C. B. Nam, Sex predetermination: Its Impact on Fertility, *Soc. Biol.* **18,** 73 (1971).

8. Rent, C. S., and G. S. Rent, More on Offspring Sex-Preference: A Comment on Nancy E. Williamson's "Sex Preference, Sex Control, and the Status of Women." *Signs: J. of Women in Culture and Society* **3,** 505 (1977).

9. Altus, W. D., Birth Order and Its Sequelae, *Science* **151,** 44 (1966).

10. Campbell, C., What Happens When We Get the Manchild Pill?, *Psychology Today* **10**(3), 86 (1976).

11. Etzioni, A., Sex Control, Science and Society, *Science* **161,** 1107 (1968).

12. Jones, R. J., Sex Predetermination and the Sex Ratio at Birth, *Soc. Biol.* **20,** 203 (1973).

13. Mason, A., and N. G. Bennett, Sex Selection with Biased Technologies and its Effect on the Population Sex Ratio, *Demography* **14,** 285 (1977).

14. Pohlman, E., Some Effects of Being Able to Control Sex of Offspring, *Eugenics Quart.* **14,** 274 (1967).

15. Postgate, J., Bat's Chance in Hell, *New Scientist* (Apr. 5), 13 (1973).

16. Coombs, L. C., Comparative Fertility Analysis: A Project of the International Union for the Scientific Study of Population, paper presented at the annual meetings of the Population Association of America, University of Michigan, Population Studies Center, Ann Arbor, 1973.

17. Freedman, D. S., R. Freedman, and P. K. Whelpton, Size of Family and Preference for Children of Each Sex, *Amer. J. Soc.* **66,** 141 (1960).

18. May, D. A., and D. M. Heer, Son Survivorship Motivation and Family Size in India: A Computer Simulation, *Pop. Studies* **22,** 199 (1968).

19. Williamson, N. E., *Sons or Daughters? A Cross-Cultural Study of Parental Preferences,* Sage Publications, Beverly Hills, (1976).

20. Markle, G. E., paper presented to Population Socialization Conference, Honolulu, (1973).

UNNATURAL SELECTION, Tabitha M. Powledge

1. Dmowski, W. P., L. Gaynor, R. Rao, M. Lawrence, A. Scommegna, Use of Albumin Gradients for X and Y Sperm Separation and Clinical Experience with Male Sex Preselection, *Fertil. Steril.* **31,** 52 (1979).
2. Schelling, T. C., "On Exercising Choice," acceptance paper for the Frank H. Seidman Distinguished Award in Political Economy, 1979.
3. McMillen, M. M., Differential Mortality by Sex in Fetal and Neonatal Deaths, *Science* **204,** 89 (1979).
4. Bouvier, L. F., U.S. Population in 2000—Zero Growth or Not?, *Population Bull.* **30**(5) (1975).
5. Ibid.
6. Ibid.
7. Etzioni, A., Sex Control, Science and Society, *Science* **161,** 1107 (1968).
8. Postgate, J., Bat's Chance in Hell, *New Scientist* **58,** 12 (1973).
9. Department of Obstetrics and Gynecology, Tietung Hospital of Anshan Iron & Steel Co., Fetal Sex Prediction by Sex Chromatin of Chorionic Villi Cells during Early Pregnancy, *Chinese Medical Journal* **1,** 117 (1975).
10. Herzenberg, L. A., D. W. Bianchi, J. Schroeder, H. M. Cann, and G. M. Iverson, Fetal Cells in the Blood of Pregnant Women: Detection and Enrichment by Fluorescence-Activated Cell Sorting, *Proceedings of the National Academy of Sciences* **76,** 1453 (1979).

RESPONSE, Denise Connors

1. Cavin, S., "Lesbian Origins Sex Ratio Theory," *Sinister Wisdom* #9, 14–19 (1979).
2. Daly, M., *Beyond God the Father: Towards a Philosophy of Women's Liberation,* Beacon Press, Boston, 1973, p. 40.
3. Stanley, J., "The Stylistics of Belief," paper presented at the Conference on College Composition and Communication, Anaheim, CA., April 1974. (Paper available by writing to the author c/o English Department, Univ. of Nebraska, Lincoln, Nebraska 68588.)

SEX PRESELECTION: A Response, Janice G. Raymond

1. Rich, A., "Lesbian Existence and Compulsory Heterosexuality," draft of an article to be published in *Signs: A Journal of Women in Culture and Society,* Summer, 1980.
2. Conversation with Pat Hynes, Montague, Massachusetts, August, 1979.
3. Daly, M., *Gyn/Ecology: The Metaethics of Radical Feminism,* Beacon Press, Boston, 1978, p. 28.

4. Postgate, J., "Bat's Chance in Hell," *New Scientist,* 14–15 (April 5, 1973).
5. Luce, C. B., "Fewer Moms Would Slow Pop Clock," *The Seattle Times,* Sunday, August 6, 1978, p. K6.
6. See Illich, I., *Medical Nemesis: The Expropriation of Health,* Pantheon, New York, 1976.
7. Barker-Benfield, G. J., *The Horrors of the Half-Known Life,* Harper & Row, New York, 1976, p. 88.

MANIPULATIVE REPRODUCTIVE TECHNOLOGIES: OVERVIEW, Betty B. Hoskins

1. Gordon, P., *Journal of Irreproducible Results* **24**(3), 29 (1978).

BIOLOGICAL MANIPULATIONS FOR PRODUCING AND NURTURING MAMMALIAN EMBRYOS, Rosalind L. Herlands

1. Huxley, A. L., *Brave New World,* Bantam Books, New York, 1932, p. 3.
2. Kaufman, M. H., The Experimental Production of Mammalian Parthenogenetic Embryos, in *Methods in Mammalian Reproduction,* Daniels, J. C., ed., Academic Press, New York, 1978, pp. 21–49.
3. Gates, A. H., Maximizing Yield and Developmental Uniformity of Eggs, in *Methods in Mammalian Embryology* [*MME*], Daniels, J. C., ed., Freeman, San Francisco, pp. 64–75; Mintz, B., Allophenic Mice of Multi-Embryo Origin, *MME,* pp. 186–214; Whitten, W. K., and A. K. Champlin, Pheromones, Estrus, Ovulation, and Mating, in *Methods in Mammalian Reproduction* [*MMR*], Daniels, J. C., Academic Press, New York, 1978, pp. 403–418.
4. Murray, F. A., Embryo Transfer in Large Domestic Mammals, *MMR,* pp. 288–307.
5. Edwards, E. G., Advances in Reproductive Biology and Their Implications for Studies on Human Congenital Defects, in *Birth Defects,* Motulsky, A. G., and W. Lenz, eds. Excerpta Medica, Amsterdam, 1974, pp. 92–104.
6. Dukelow, W. R., Laparoscopic Research Techniques in Mammalian Embryology, *MMR,* 1978, pp. 438–457.
7. Mintz, op. cit.; Dickmann, A., Egg Transfer, *MME,* 1971, pp. 133–145.
8. McLaren, A., *Mammalian Chimeras,* Cambridge University Press, Cambridge, 1976.
9. McGaughey, R. W., In Vitro Oocyte Maturation, *MMR,* 1978, pp. 1–20; Biggers, J. D., W. K. Whitten, and D. G. Whittingham, The Culture of Mouse Embryos in Vitro, *MME,* 1971, pp. 86–116.

10. McLaren, op. cit.
11. Biggers, et al., op. cit.
12. Lin, T. P., Egg Micromanipulation, *MME,* 1971, pp. 157–171.
13. New, D.A.T., Methods for Culture of Post-Implantation Embryos of Rodents, *MME,* 1971, pp. 305–319; Daniel, J. C., Jr., Culture of the Rabbit Blastocyst Across the Implantation Period, *MME,* 1971, pp. 284–289; Hsu, Y.-C., In Vitro Development of Whole Mouse Embryos beyond the Implantation Stage, *MMR,* 1978, pp. 229–246; Hsu, Y.-C., In Vitro Development of Individually Cultured Whole Mouse Embryos to Early Somite Stage, *Dev. Biol.* **68,** 453–461 (1979).
14. Hsu (1978; 1979), op. cit.
15. New, op. cit.
16. Whittingham, D. G., Survival of Mouse Embryos after Freezing and Thawing, *Nature,* **233,** 125–126 (1971); Whittingham, D. G., S. P. Liebo, and P. Mazur, Survival of Mouse Embryos Frozen to –196° and –269° C, *Science* **178,** 411–414 (1972).
17. Liebo, S. P., and P. Mazur, Methods for Preservation of Mammalian Embryos by Freezing, *MMR,* 1978, pp. 179–202.
18. Ibid.
19. Muller, H. J., Means and Aims in Human Genetic Betterment, in *Control of Heredity and Evolution,* Sonneborn, T. M., ed., Macmillan, New York, 1963.
20. Kolata, G. B., In Vitro Fertilization: Is It Safe and Repeatable? *Science* **201,** 698–699 (1978).
21. Ibid.
22. Chang, M. C., Fertilization of Rabbit Ova in Vitro, *Nature* **184,** 466–467 (1959).
23. Grobstein, C., External Human Fertilization, *Sci. Amer.* **240**(6), 57–67 (1979).
24. Stevens, L. C., and D. S. Varnum, The Development of Teratomas from Parthenogenetically Activated Ovarian Mouse Eggs, *Dev. Biol.* **37,** 369–380 (1974).
25. Cole, C. J., The Value of Virgin Birth, *Natural History,* Jan., 56–63 (1978).
26. Kaufman, M. H., The Experimental Production of Mammalian Parthenogenetic Embryos, *MMR,* 1978, pp. 21–49.
27. Graham, C. F., The Production of Parthenogenetic Mammalian Embryos and Their Use in Biological Research, *Biol. Rev.* **49,** 399–422 (1974).
28. Graham, C. F., Virus Assisted Fusion of Embryonic Cells, *Acta Endocrinologica* (suppl.) **153,** 154–167 (1971).
29. Kaufman, M. H., and L. Sachs, Complete Preimplantation Development in Culture of Parthenogenetic Mouse Embryos. *J. Embryol. Exptl. Morph.* **35,** 179–190, 1976. Kaufman, op. cit.
30. Balakier, H., and A. K. Tarkowski, Diploid Parthenogenetic Mouse Embryos Produced by Heat Shock and Cytochalasin B, *J. Embryol. Exptl. Morph.* **35,** 25–39 (1976).

31. Briggs, R., and T. J. King, Transplantation of Living Nuclei from Blastula Cells into Enucleated Frogs' Eggs, *PNAS* **38,** 455–463 (1952).

32. Gurdon, J. B., The Developmental Capacity of Nuclei Taken from Intestinal Epithelium Cells of Feeding Tadpoles, *J. Embryol. Exptl. Morph.* **10,** 622–640 (1962).

33. Lasky, R. A., and J. B. Gurdon, Genetic Content ofAdult Somatic Cells Tested by Nuclear Transplantation from Cultured Cells, *Nature* **228,** 1332–1334 (1970). Gurdon, J. B., R. A. Laskey, and O. R. Reeves, The Developmental Capacity of Nuclei Transplanted From Keratinized Skin Cells of Adult Frogs, *J. Embryol. Exptl. Morph.* **34,** 93–112, 1975.

34. Bromhall, D., Nuclear Transplantation in the Rabbit Egg, *Nature* **258,** 719–721 (1975).

35. Graham, C. F., The Fusion of Cells with One and Two-Cell Mouse Embryos, in *Heterospecific Genome Interaction,* Defendi, V., ed., Wistar Institute Symposium Monograph 9, Wistar Press, Philadelphia, 1969, pp. 19–35.

36. Modlinski, J. A., Haploid Mouse Embryos Obtained by Microsurgical Removal of One Pronucleus, *J. Embryol. Exptl. Morph.* **33,** 897–905 (1975).

37. Tarkowski, A. K., Development of Single Blastomeres, *MME,* 1971, pp. 172–185.

38. Soupart, P., M. L. Anderson, and J. E. Repp, Initiation of Embryonic Development by Experimental Mammalian Oocyte Fusion, *Theriogenology* **9,** 102 (1978); Graham (1971) op. cit.

39. Mintz, op. cit; McLaren, op. cit.

40. Gardner, R. L., Production of Chimeras by Injecting Cells or Tissue into the Blastocyst, *MMR,* 1978, pp. 137–157.

41. Ibid.

42. Markert, C. L., and R. M. Peters, Manufactured Hexaparental Mice Show That Adults Are Derived from Three Embryonic Cells, *Science* **202,** 56–58 (1978).

43. McLaren, op. cit.

44. Mintz, B., and K. Illmensee, Normal Genetically Mosaic Mice Produced from Malignant Teratocarcinoma Cells, *PNAS* **72,** 3585–3589 (1975); Papaioannou, V. E., M. W. McBurney, and R. L. Gardner, Fate of Teratocarcinoma Cells Injected into Early Mouse Embryos, *Nature* **258,** 70–73 (1975).

45. Glenister, T. W., Methods for Studying Ovoimplantation and Early Embryo-Placental Development In Vitro, *MME,* 1971, pp. 320–333; Sherman, M. I., Implantation of Mouse Blastocysts in Vitro, *MMR,* 1978, pp. 247–258.

46. Kirby, D. R. S., The Transplantation of Mouse Eggs and Trophoblast to Extrauterine Sites, *MME,* 1971, pp. 146–156.

47. Bergstrom, S., Experimentally Delayed Implantation, *MMR,* 1978, pp. 419–437.

48. Zapol, W. M., T. Kolobow, J. E. Pierce, G. G. Varek, and R. L. Bowman, Artificial Placenta: Two Days of Total Extrauterine Support of the Isolated Premature Lamb Fetus, *Science* **166,** 617–618 (1969).

49. Kieffer, G. H., *Bioethics,* Addison-Wesley, Reading, Mass., 1979.
50. Colinet-Lagneaux, D., F. Geubelle, R. Lambotte, and J. Lecomte, Les Echanges Transplacentaires de l'Oxygene chez la Femme, *J. Gyn. Obst. Biol. Repr.* **6,** 611–623 (1977).

Abbreviated Bibliography

Bromhall, D., The Great Cloning Hoax, *New Statesman,* 734 (June 2, 1978).
Daniel, J. C., Jr., ed., *Methods in Mammalian Embryology,* Freeman, San Francisco, 1971.
Daniel, J. C. Jr., ed., *Methods in Mammalian Reproduction,* Academic Press, New York, 1978.
Edwards, R. D., Advances in Reproductive Biology and Their Implications for Studies on Human Congenital Defects, in *Birth Defects,* A. G. Motulsky and W. Lenz, eds., Excerpta Medica, Amsterdam, 1974.
Grobstein, C., External Human Fertilization, *Scientific American* **240,** 57 (1979).
Johnson, H., Can Science Make Carbon Copies of You?, *Ebony* 95–102 (June 1978).
Kolata, G. B., *In Vitro* Fertilization: Is It Safe and Repeatable?, *Science* **201,** 698 (1978).
Markert, C. L., and Peters, R. M., Manufactured Hexaparental Mice Show That Adults Are Derived from Three Embryonic Cells, *Science* **202,** 56–58 (1978).

ETHICS AND REPRODUCTIVE TECHNOLOGY, Susan Anthony Salladay

1. For a more complete understanding of Kohlberg's theory in relation to moral education and decision-making see Bereiter, C., The Morality of Moral Education, *Hastings Center Report* **8**(2), 20 (1978).
2. The concept of the "trap" milieu is insightfully discussed by Frederic Flack in his book *The Secret Strength of Depression,* Lippincott, Philadelphia, 1974; see especially pages 39–52 and 200–219: "Human beings have a strong tendency to reaffirm inner constrictions and deprivations by building external traps, and then to live within them in unhappy equilibrium until something sufficiently dramatic occurs to wake them up to their dilemma."
3. Maguire, D., The Freedom to Die, *Commonweal* (Aug. 11, 1972).
4. Fletcher, J., Ethical Aspects of Genetic Controls, *New England Journal of Medicine* **285,** 776 (1974).
5. *Report: HEW Support of Research Involving Human In Vitro Fertilization and Embryo Transfer, Chapter VI: Conclusions,* Ethics Advisory Board, Department of Health, Education and Welfare, Washington, DC, 1979.

6. Consider that this principle rests on a legal notion that "legitmates" children that are claimed or acknowledged as offspring of a man. Children are illegitimate not because they lack a mother, but because they lack a father. Marriage and the family are the structures that perpetuate this distinction. "The basic social unit is the family, in which the woman is a possession of her husband." Griffin, S., *Rape: The All American Crime,* in *Feminism and Philosophy,* Braggin *et al.* eds, Littlefield, Adams, Totowa, New Jersey, 1977. "He dominates woman both to imprison another consciousness which reflects his own and to provide him with children that are securely his (fear of illegitimacy)." Mitchell, J., *Social Structure and Sexual Oppression.*

7. Rich, A., *On Lies, Secrets, and Silence,* Norton, New York, 1979, p. 16.

8. Griffin, *op. cit.,* p. 320.

9. Phelps, L., Female Sexual Alienation, in *Philosophy for a New Generation,* Bierman and Gould, eds., Macmillan, New York, 1977, p. 487.

RESPONSE, Theresa Mayrand

1. Grobstein, C., External Human Fertilization, *Scientific American* **240,** 57 (June, 1979).

2. Mastroianni, L., Reproductive Technologies: In Vitro Fertilization, *Encyclopedia of Bioethics,* volume 4, 1st ed., Macmillan, New York, 1978, pp. 1448–1451. Walters, L., *Ethical Issues in Human In Vitro Fertilization and Research Involving Early Human Embryos,* Report to the Ethics Advisory Board, Department of Health, Education, and Welfare, September 8, 1978.

THE CASE AGAINST IN VITRO FERTILIZATION AND IMPLANTATION, Ruth Hubbard

1. I want to thank Dr. Michelle Harrison for thinking and talking with me about this.

IN VITRO FERTILIZATION AND EMBRYO TRANSFER Robert F. Murray, Jr.

1. Soupart proposed to harvest human oocytes from donors undergoing gynecological surgery (mostly tubal ligations), to fertilize them with sperm from donors, and to examine the early embryos for an abnormal number or arrangement of chromosomes or for abnormal appearance when studied under the electron microscope. Soupart also proposed to attempt to preserve human embryos resulting from human fertilization by freezing under controlled conditions. This technique was intended to circumvent adverse effects of IVF of possible trauma to the ovary in the process of removing the oocyte. By fertilizing and temporarily freezing a human embryo, then placing it back in the uterus during the next menstrual cycle, the ovary would function normally to release the hormones that support pregnancy.

When the Board considered Dr. Soupart's proposal, there was some difference of opinion among the expert witnesses from his field about its usefulness; the Board came to the conclusion that, in light of current knowledge in the field, his application should be reevaluated by the appropriate peer review committee from the Institute of Child Health and Human Development.

2. A moratorium on research on early embryos had been established in 1975.
3. The members of the Ethics advisory Board (on January 1, 1978) were as follows: James C. Gaither, J.D., Chairman (San Francisco, California); David A. Hamburg, M.D., Vice Chairman (President, Institute of Medicine, Washington, D.C.); Sissela Bok, Ph.D. (Cambridge, Massachusetts); Henry W. Foster, M.D. (Professor and Chairman, Department of Obstetrics and Gynecology, Meharry Medical College, Nashville, Tennessee); Donald A. Henderson, M.D. (Dean, Johns Hopkins School of Health and Hygiene, Baltimore, Maryland); Richard A. McCormick, S.T.D. (Rose Kennedy Professor of Christian Ethics, Kennedy Center for Bioethics, Washington, D.C.); Robert F. Murray, M.D. (Division of Medical Genetics, Howard University College of Medicine, Washington, D.C.); Mitchell W. Spellman, M.D. (Dean for Medical Services, Harvard Medical School, Boston, Massachusetts); Daniel C. Tosteson, M.D. (Dean, Harvard Medical School, Boston, Massachusetts); Agnes N. Williams, LL.B. (Potomac, Maryland); Eugene M. Zweiback, M.D. (Omaha, Nebraska).
4. A complete listing of the issues that were developed as a result of the public testimony received from more than 25 expert witnesses with backgrounds in science, philosophy, law, and public policy appears in the appendix to the report of the board to the Secretary of HEW.

THE BIOLOGY OF UTOPIA, Dennis Livingston

1. Livingston, D., in *Handbook of Futures Research,* Fowles, J., (Ed.), Greenwood Press, Westport, Connecticut, 1978.
2. McKinnell, R. G., *Cloning: A Biologist Reports,* University of Minnesota Press, Minneapolis, 1979. Hamilton, Michael P., (Ed.) *The New Genetics and the Future of Man,* Grand Rapids, Michigan: William B. Eerdmans, 1972. Francoeur, R. T., *Utopian Motherhood: New Trends in Human Reproduction,* A. S. Barnes, Cranbury, New Jersey, 1973.
3. Cowper, R., *Clone,* Pocket Books, New York, 1979.

4. Rorvik, D., *In His Image: The Cloning of a Man,* Pocket Books, New York, 1978.
5. Levin, I., *The Boys From Brazil,* Random House, New York, 1976.
6. LeGuin, U. K., *Introductory Psychology Through Science Fiction,* H. A. Katz, P. Warrick, & M. H. Greenberg, eds., Rand McNally, Chicago, 1974.
7. Wilhelm, K., *Where Late the Sweet Birds Sang,* Harper & Row, New York, 1976.
8. Herbert, F., *The Eyes of Heisenberg,* Berkley, New York, 1976 (1966).
9. Brunner, J., *The Shockwave Rider,* Harper & Row, New York, 1975; *Stand on Zanzibar,* Ballantine, New York, 1976 (1969).
10. Huxley, A., *The Sociology of the Possible,* Ofshe, R. ed., Prentice-Hall, Englewood Cliffs, N.J., 1977.
11. Berger, H. L., *Science Fiction and the New Dark Age,* Bowling Green University Popular Press, Bowling Green, Ohio, 1976. See also, Sibley, Mulford Q., *Technology and Utopian Thought,* Bergess, Minneapolis: 1971.
12. Piercy, M., *Woman on the Edge of Time,* Knopf, New York, 1976.
13. Sargent, P., ed. *More Women of Wonder: Science Fiction Novelettes by Women about Women,* Random House, New York, 1976, p. 42; Rich, A., p. xli.
14. Esfandiary, F. M., *Woman in the Year 2000,* M. Tripp, ed., Dell, New York, 1974, p. 336.
15. Le Guin, U. K., *The Dispossessed,* Harper & Row, New York, 1974.
16. McIntyre, V., *Dreamsnake,* Houghton Mifflin, Boston, 1978.
17. Gilman, C. P., *Herland,* Pantheon, New York, 1979 (1915).
18. Charnas, S. M., *Motherlines,* Berkley Putnam, New York, 1978.
19. Russ, J., *The Female Man,* Ballantine, New York, 1975.

ECTOGENESIS AND IDEOLOGY, Rebecca L. Logan

1. Gardner, S., The Last Woman, in *When Women Rule,* S. Moskowitz, ed., Walker, New York, 1972.
2. Cowper, R., *Clone,* Doubleday, Garden City, 1973.
3. Ehrenreich, B., & D. English, *For Her Own Good: 150 Years of the Experts' Advice to Women,* Doubleday, Garden City, 1978; and Salzman, F., Are Sex Roles Biologically Determined? *Science for the People* 9(4), 27 (1977).
4. Ehrenreich and English, *op. cit.,* p. 106.
5. Reilly, P., *Genetics, Law, and Social Policy,* Harvard, Cambridge, 1977, pp. 125–126.
6. Rorvik, D. M., *In His Image: The Cloning of a Man,* Lippincott, Philadelphia, 1978.

MANIPULATIVE REPRODUCTIVE TECHNOLOGIES DISCUSSION III

1. Barker-Benfield, G. J., *The Horrors of the Half-Known Life,* Harper & Row, New York, 1976, p. 96. See also: Harris, S., *Women's Surgeon,* Macmillan, New York, 1950.

Biographies

The following biographies outline the personal histories of those of our authors with substantial contributions in this volume. Discussants' biographies that do not appear here will be found in the companion volume, *Birth Control and Controlling Birth.*

Fredric Abramson: I have been a feminist and women's rights advocate since the mid-60s when my career involved me in studies of induced and spontaneous abortion. My PhD thesis at Michigan (Human Genetics and Population Planning) dealt with the Epidemiology of Spontaneous Abortion. In addition, I have been a genetic counselor, a medical school faculty member, and a director of a research design biostatistics laboratory, have owned my own consulting firm, have attended MIT's Sloan School of Management as a Sloan Fellow, have worked on Secretary Califano's Alcohol Program and Policy Review, and have developed a career training program for women in management. I enjoy slo-pitch softball, reading, travel, and classic movies.

Mary G. Ampola: I was raised and attended college and medical school in Syracuse, NY. After four years in pediatric training in DC, I moved on to Boston for three years of fellowship in genetics and amino acid diseases. For the past 13 years I have been on the staff of the Boston Floating Hospital with active clinic responsibilities in the areas of birth defects, mental retardation, genetic counseling, and amino acid diseases. Directing a clinical and research lab for amino acid studies and teaching as an Associate Professor of Pediatrics at Tufts University School of Medicine round out my professional activities. Home means my delightful family—husband Vincent, daughter Leanna, age 11, and son David, age 9. My inclinations include commitment to individual liberty, the scientific method, capitalism, technology, and feminism.

Diana E. Axelsen: After growing up on a farm in Idaho, I attended college in Minnesota, Massachusetts, and California, where I received a BA and, later, a PhD in philosophy at Stanford. Since 1969, I have taught at Spelman, a women's college in the historically black Atlanta University Center. Also, I've team-taught a two-year course, "Human Values in Medicine," at the Morehouse College School of Medicine. I'm working on a master's in community counseling at Georgia State. I enjoy yoga, sports, and travel—especially visits with my five nephews, one god-daughter, and several "nieces by friendship."

G. J. (Ben) Barker-Benfield: Member of Evaluation Team. Department of History, State University of New York at Albany.

Susan E. Bell: I am presently completing work on my doctoral dissertation (on DES) in Sociology at Brandeis University. I have taught as a part-time instructor at colleges in the Boston area for the past five years. I have been an active participant in the women's health movement since 1972 when I first began to carry out research into the relationship between the development of birth control technology in the US in the early 20th century and the concurrent social and political environment. My work has continued as a member of a women's health collective, and most recently as a facilitator in a Women-Controlled Birth Control self-help group.

Helga M. Bendix: I have my BA from Barnard College, my MA from Teachers College, Columbia University, and received a Fulbright to Nepal. I am a former teacher of English as a Second Language and German, and the mother of four children, one of whom is handicapped. My current activities include service as a community volunteer and parent advocate for special education services, for group homes for the retarded, and for a range of community services for the handicapped. I help monitor public policy decisions and implementation of recent legislation affecting the handicapped—and am a member of assorted committees at various levels of government (school district, municipal, county and state). I was a member of the New York State delegation to the White House Conference on the Handicapped in May 1977. I am an avid traveler.

Claudia Card: Member of Evaluation Team. Department of Philosophy, University of Wisconsin/Madison.

Wendy Carlton: After graduating from Oberlin (1970), I taught in the experimental high school program in Philadelphia. At the same time I began working on a PhD in Sociology at the University of Pennsylvania. In 1976, I got my PhD and found a tenure-track appointment at the University of Notre Dame. Most of my teaching and research is in medical sociology. My husband, Mark Needleman, and our son, Joshua, and I live in an 1883 Victorian house in South Bend. My hobbies include reading, cooking, and gardening (by the *laissez-faire* method).

Denise D. Connors: In 1966, I graduated from nursing school and then worked for four years in a stroke intensive care unit. While evolving through the "health care system," I obtained a BS and MS in Community Health at Boston College. I have taught nursing at various levels for five years from a progressively more radical perspective. For the past two years I have been teaching at Fitchburg State College with a focus on women as both "professionals" and "patients." In the fall I will begin a doctoral program in Sociology at Brandeis.

Emily Erwin Culpepper: I am a rebellious white woman, originally from Georgia. Before entering the otherworld of academia, I was an adoption social worker. Currently, I am immersed in my doctoral dissertation at Harvard on feminist myth-making as social change. My work has appeared in diverse feminist and academic publications. Menstruation fascinates me, leading me to collect oral, artistic and health information about our periods. I conduct workshops with *Period Piece,* a film I made about menstrual images and folklore. I urge all women to explore our witch-healer wisdom and to bond together past the bondages of patriarchy. Now, I see women reaching new power through breaking silences and inactions concerning race, ethnic, and class realities. I am proud to be a Lesbian and feel blessed to have supportive women friends. I am passionately committed to the cause of female freedom.

Anne J. Davis: In 1976–1977 I was a Kennedy postdoctoral fellow in bioethics at Harvard. Recently I was elected as a fellow at Hastings Institute of Society, Ethics and the Life Sciences. I have lived and worked on four continents. Presently I am a Professor in the School of Nursing, University of California, San Francisco. I have written three books—two in bioethics—and numerous research papers. I am a member of the National Mental Health Advisory Council.

Maureen C. Edwards: I am a native Washingtonian (DC). I attended undergraduate school at Marquette University in Milwaukee, then returned to DC where I graduated from the George Washington University Medical School in 1970. I completed my pediatric and neonatal subspecialty training at the Children's Hospital National Medical Center, after which I joined the staff there working in the Intensive Care Nursery. I moved to the position of Director of Nurseries at the George Washington University Medical Center in 1978. I am the mother of three children, ages 10, 6, and 4, which is a great asset in my particular profession. To keep my life in scale, my current additional interest is making and collecting dollhouse miniatures.

Robin Erhart: I have long been interested in progressive/alternative birth, and in 1976 was selected by a local (Olympia, WA) community group to be trained as a midwife (in response to an offer by the Fremont Women's birth service). I became involved in legislative efforts to update and expand midwifery legislation. I am within a quarter of graduation from The Evergreen State College, where I am also employed as a supervisor of secretarial services for the faculty. When at home, on 5 acres, I enjoy gardening, raising chickens, keeping bees, photography, and spinning.

Maureen A. Flannery: Member of Evaluation Team. Mountain Comprehensive Health, Whitesburg, Kentucky.

Michael Gross: As a graduate student in the history of science (at Princeton) I focused on biomedical thought since the nineteenth century. During some five years of teaching at Hampshire College I have developed concurrent interests in problems of biology and society, especially in theories of biological determinism and the uses of science for social control.

Although gay men are not necessarily sympathetic to feminism, for me that evolving body of political and philosophical thought continues to be of great inspiration. I am also interested in the theories of, and periodically a participant in, various forms of therapy or meditation that strive toward body-mind integration.

Rosalind Herlands: I am almost a native Californian, having arrived in San Francisco from London on my first birthday. After receiving my BA in biology from Stanford University, I pursued studies in developmental and cell biology at the University of California, Irvine. In 1974, I received my PhD and moved on to my first teaching position at Stockton State College in rural southern New Jersey. Since arriving in New Jersey, I have given birth to and am raising two very active boys and have delved into areas outside my specialization, such as bioethics and women's studies. My hobbies are reading, camping, and gardening.

Helen Bequaert Holmes: I was born in Boston, raised in Cambridge, Massachusetts, and received a BA in chemistry from Oberlin College in 1951 and an MS in zoology from Cornell University in 1953. Then I moved to Amherst, Massachusetts, gave birth to and raised three children, was active in Girl Scouting and the Quaker meeting, and taught in high school. Later, at the age of 40, I completed a PhD in zoology (population genetics) at the University of Massachusetts. I have had an assortment of temporary college teaching posts and two year-long sojourns in The Netherlands. My hobbies are reading, canoeing, and hiking. I prefer to be called "Becky."

Joan Hirsch Holtzman: Quite early I had the call of philosophy: "Follow the path of reason; find a life of order and meaning." One PhD and several teaching jobs later a still small voice kept asking: "Where is the reason and sense in public policy? Why are so few philosophers addressing issues of public concern?" The result is that I now direct Programs in Public Philosophy, an organization dedicated to taking remedial action. Naturally, when asked to contribute to this conference and volume, I could only respond with pleasure. The sound of other voices gives me pleasure too, pre-eminently those of my two children, but also those of the muses—I like to sculpt and play the piano. Fortunately I am married to a psychiatrist who helps me deal with all the voices I hear.

Betty B. Hoskins: Constitutionally I'm a generalist with a series of careers. I was trained as a biologist at liberal arts colleges (BA 1956, Goucher; MA 1958, Amherst College; PhD 1973, Texas Women's University—small child rearing in US and Europe in between). At present I'm an Editor of Science Publications at a textbook publishing house. That midlife career change followed six years as a faculty member at an engineering-science college. The diversity of my interests in biology, bioethics, academic advising, and program development led to administrative training and the experience of institutional sexism. I have enjoyed working within professional, women's, and community groups to clarify choices in the applications of our newer biological knowledge, helping people of diverse backgrounds to hear and understand each other. Folkdancing, gardening, friends, and my two teenagers are also enjoyments.

Ruth Hubbard: I am Professor of Biology at Harvard University where I teach courses that deal with the interactions of science and society. My laboratory research has been concerned with how visual pigment molecules in the eyes change when they absorb light and how their changes initiate the signals that travel to the brain where they make us able to see. In recent years I have thought, taught, and written about how scientists work and about how their work is affected by the society in which it is done—what about nature scientists find interesting, why it interests them, what explanations they accept as true or reject, and why. I am particularly interested in the way gender—the fact of one's having grown up female or male—affects such questions. I am also interested in the ways health care and technology affect women, and have written articles and given popular and academic talks about these subjects.

Kathy Karpeles: Observer. Counselor, Hampshire College, Amherst, Massachusetts.

Regina (Reggie) H. Kenen: My middle name is "role conflict," from many years of juggling commitments to teaching, research, husband, four children, and three cats. After receiving a BA (Psychology, Barnard) and an MEd (Tufts) in the mid-1950s, I taught in reading clinics. From 1966 to 1974, interrupted by the birth of my fourth child and semesters spent in Europe and California, I worked toward a PhD in Sociology from Columbia. I am now an Assistant Professor of Sociology at Trenton State College. I publish on the social implications of medical advances, and I have received two grants from the NJ Committee of the Humanities, an affiliate of the NEH to run workshops in this area.

Elizabeth Kutter: Representative of the EVIST Program of the National Science Foundation. Molecular biologist at Evergreen State College, Olympia, Washington.

E. Virginia Sheppard Lapham: I prefer being called Ginny. My current position of Coordinator of Research, Planning, and Development grew out of my social work with families of children with multiple handicaps, which grew out of my earlier career in speech therapy where I was more interested in working with families than teaching children. In between, I lived for ten years in developing countries with my husband of 24 years, alternately initiating projects such as well-baby clinics, feeding centers, and an international kindergarten, with bearing and parenting five children. My hobbies include reading, writing, travel, social and political action, genealogy, and square dancing.

Adele Laslie: Observer. Department of Philosophy, Lehigh University, Bethlehem, Pennsylvania.

Dennis Livingston: I am a father, musician (flute), and political scientist. Also a science fiction freak, walker in the woods, star watcher, and rambler. Way stations include jobs at California/Davis, Case Western Reserve, Scripps Institute of Oceanography, and Rensselaer Polytechnic Institute. My interests include alternative futures, decentralization, utopias, technology and society, soft energy paths, world order, new lifestyles, and feeling good. I am currently a policy analyst with the Massachusetts Executive Office of Communities and Development (Boston), working on anti-poverty strategies.

Elaine Locke: In 1970, I came to The American College of Obstetricians and Gynecologists to develop a government relations program. ACOG (located in Chicago) is the major professional organization for the specialty in America. I received a Masters in Public Administration, Roosevelt University, 1974; my major paper was on the role of schools in programs related to adolescent pregnancy. (My BA was in English Literature, University of Chicago, 1961.) ACOG sent me (1976) to open a Washington, DC, office. Now in Chicago I serve as liaison between the two offices, and specialist in policy analysis and development. I staff various College practice committees, currently including the Task Force on Adolescent Pregnancy (producing a professional guidebook under a HEW grant) and the Committee on Bioethics.

Rebecca Logan: After graduation from Michigan State in 1967, with a BA in Social Science, I spent two years in the Peace Corps in Colombia. I moved to Ithaca to study social policy planning at Cornell, but left to direct a community information/advocacy/organizing center for six years. Now I work for Cornell's Program on Science, Technology, and Society researching attitudes of various groups (workers, Native Americans, Blacks, feminists) towards nuclear power. My interest in this conference comes from my interest in social policy and my feminism. I am the mother of two children. I like to learn/talk about women's spirituality, magic, politics, and utopian dreams.

Gerene Major: After completing a BS degree in public health nursing from Marquette University, I practiced professional nursing in the areas of pediatrics, neonatology, obstetrics-gynecology, public health, and burn nursing. In addition to clinical practice, I taught clinical nursing and designed and implemented the first nurse internship program in Wisconsin. Because of my interest in analysis of clinical practice and related ethical problems I pursued a Master's degree in Philosophy of Science—Philosophy of Law at the University of Wisconsin-Milwaukee. The focus of my study was on the investigation of clinical medicine as science, the nature of clinical decision-making, and compensation for harm in malpractice. Then I began study at the University of Wisconsin-Madison on the doctoral level in that same area. I have three daughters, ages 15, 14, and 12.

Martha Mathis: After graduating from high school in 1969, I spent 5½ years at Northern Illinois University working on my BA and MA, both in Education. After returning to Rockford, I began teaching at a community college (which I do presently), working at an abortion clinic (presently doing), emergency counseling at the Mental Health Center, and involving myself in many other community activities. In 1977, I took time out to get married to a man also interested in understanding and encouraging better women's health care. As of summer 1979, I have enrolled once again at NIU to pursue the big one: PhD in Education, part-time. No children of the human species, but two of the canine family.

Theresa Mayrand: I received my BS from Siena Heights College in 1965, and began a career in secondary science education. A grant in field biology took me to California's Sonoma State College in the summer of 1970. I obtained my MS in biology from Michigan State University in 1973. Interest in bioethics led me to become a Hastings associate and incorporate bioethics units in my courses. Among other biology courses, I teach several sections each year of "Physiology of Woman." I truly enjoy teaching, designing new courses, and working with high school people in a variety of ways, such as taking small groups on Appalachian experiences. My hobbies are hiking and nature photography.

Barbara Eck Menning: I founded and direct a small, national, nonprofit organization called RESOLVE that offers counseling and referral to infertile couples. My interest in this area is twofold: first I am a nurse, with an advanced degree in Maternal-Child Health. Second, I was personally acquainted with the pain of infertility in my marriage. I am now single again and mother of three young multiracial adopted children. Two of the best years of my life were devoted to teaching and practicing midwifery with the Peace Corps in Afghanistan. I attained fluency in Farsi—a skill I've never needed since! In my few spare moments I enjoy jogging, gardening, keeping a journal of personal experiences, and meeting new people. I am very eager to exchange viewpoints with the participants of this Workshop.

Robert F. Murray, Jr.: I am a medical geneticist; I received my MD from the University of Rochester in 1958. I was trained in internal medicine at the University of Colorado Medical Center. I was a staff investigator from 1962–65 at the NIH; I was a fellow in medical genetics and from 1965–1967 worked on a Masters Degree in Genetics at the University of Washington, which was awarded in 1968. Currently I am a professor of Pediatrics, Medicine and Oncology and Chief of the Division of Medical Genetics. I am married, have four children, and special interests in genetic counseling, biochemical genetics, inherited susceptibility to disease, and bioethics. I am a Fellow of the Hastings Center and a member of their board of directors, and was a member of the Ethics Advisory Board to the Secretary of HEW.

Catherine A. Musemeche: I graduated from the University of Texas at Austin in 1978, with a BA in Biology, and I have just completed my first two years of medical school at the University of Texas Medical School at Houston. I have recently been involved in initiating myself into an awareness of women's concerns relating to the medical profession. This has led me to spend most of my free time working with a new Women in Medicine organization at my school as well as learning about other women's groups in Houston and women's issues in general.

M. Ruth Nentwig: I received my PhD in anatomy from Upstate Medical Center—State University of New York in 1972. Since that time I have been involved in teaching and research in anatomy, developmental biology, and neuroendocrinology. My interest in the Workshop stemmed from my concerns as a feminist/biologist and a desire to learn and share with others. I enjoy golf, tennis, nature, animals, music, reading, painting, crafts, and sea shell collecting.

Susan Rae Peterson: I teach philosophy and interdisciplinary studies at SUNY at Old Westbury, and at Long Island University. Originally from Milwaukee, I studied at the University of Wisconsin, Madison, received a Bachelor's Degree in Humanities from the New School in Manhattan, and an MA in Philosophy from San Francisco State University. During graduate studies in philosophy and criminology at the University of Toronto, I was cofounder of the Toronto Rape Crisis Center in 1974, and published and lectured on both the cause of rape and the treatment of victims. Recently I was director of the Nassau Rape Crisis Center (Nassau County, Long Island). I am currently completing a PhD in philosophy at the City University of New York Graduate Center, but still find time to swim, run, dance, and watch basketball.

Tabitha M. Powledge: A burden, that name, but people remember (and mispronounce) it. Call me Tammy. BA in English lit (University of Michigan), MS in human genetics (Sarah Lawrence), "on leave" from a doctorate in physical anthropology (CUNY), but I don't expect to finish. I've written used car commercials, worked on Wall St., and now commute daily from a

Brooklyn brownstone to the Hastings Center, where I took a temporary job 6½ years ago. Since genetics is all-important in my life, you should know that my ancestry is Irish, Scots, and Norwegian, that my parents worked for the Hearst newspaper in Chicago during *The Front Page* days, and that my sister and daughter are both aspiring novelists. Despite these biological determinants, I try hard to write only facts.

Janice G. Raymond: This year, Beacon Press published my first book, *The Transsexual Empire: The Making of the She-Male,* which is a feminist ethical analysis of sex conversion surgery and the social context in which it arises. My academic background is in religion and ethics. I am interested in the theological basis of biomedicine and how it functions as a secular religion. I have been active in lesbian-feminist and feminist writers' groups. At present, I am working on a book about genetic technology and the future of women, and one on philosophies of female friendship.

Fay A. Rozovsky: I am an attorney licensed to practice law in Florida and Massachusetts. I have an AB from Providence College (1973, *summa cum laude*), a JD from Boston College Law School (1976), and an MPH from the Harvard School of Public Health (1977). I am a specialist in health law. Formerly on the faculty of the Wright State University School of Medicine in Dayton, Ohio I have written and lectured extensively on various aspects of health and hospital law. A particular area of interest to me is women's health law issues. I now reside in Halifax, Nova Scotia where my husband Lorne Elkin Rozovsky (also a Health Lawyer, and a member of the Nova Scotia bar) and I, work together writing, lecturing and consulting in health and hospital law.

Susan Anthony Salladay: I am natively rooted in Spokane, WA, and the great Northwest, a graduate of Whitman College (Walla Walla), an immigrant to Boston shores for my doctorate (in philosophy at Boston College), and currently a midwesterner teaching biomedical ethics in a psychiatric hospital (at the University of Nebraska College of Medicine). Through this odyssey I discover myself as feminist (the "Anthony" is my mother's and her family; the "Susan" is tribute to my *great* aunt!), as artist (aspiring poet), and as explorer (charting the ineffable of reality for new languages of faith and freedom).

Janet Farrell Smith: Observer. Department of Philosophy, University of Massachusetts at Boston.

Roberta Steinbacher: I am currently Chairperson, Department of Urban Studies, Cleveland State University. After receiving a PhD in Psychology from St. Louis University in 1967, I codirected a Ford Foundation Project in Cleveland, Ohio, on ethnic attitudes. One of my areas of research has been in sex differences in persuasibility. My special interest for the last several years has been sex preselection and its implications for women. In 1975, I co-founded a coalition of women's groups in Cleveland (now numbering 60 groups), am active in the Women's Political Caucus, President of Ohio Women, Inc., a statewide organization to implement the Houston resolutions in Ohio, and am a faculty member of the Institute for Women Today.

Barbara C. Tilley: I am a biostatistician, feminist and jogger. For 3½ years I coordinated the DESAD Project, a study of women exposed *in utero* to DES. I recently finished my PhD in Biometry at the University of Texas School of Public Health. I am now Assistant Professor of Preventive Oncology and Biomathematics at M.D. Anderson Hospital and Tumor Institute. I am the mother of two sons, 18 and 20 years old (I started college when they started school.)

Caroline Whitbeck: I did my doctoral work in the philosophy of physics at MIT during which time I became actively involved in peace work. My first full time teaching job was in the Philosophy Department at Yale in 1968, the year before Yale began coeducation. That experience made me a feminist activist; it was during this period that I became deeply involved in the women's movement. I survived in that situation for three years and then did two years of research in the Psychiatry Department at Yale. During this time I bore my daughter, Evelyn, who is a great joy in my life. Since then I have taught at SUNY/Albany, had a post-doc at the Hastings Center and am now associate professor at the Institute for the Medical Humanities at the University of Texas Medical Branch, Galveston. Being a feminist and being a Friend (Quaker) are the key (highly compatible) sources of my understanding of my life. I am happy.

Index†

†Topics marked with an asterisk * are treated at much greater depth in our companion volume, *Birth Control and Controlling Birth.* Page numbers in **boldface** indicate the major contribution of an author or the major treatment of a topic.